Test	Normal adult values
Serum calcium (ionized)	4.75-5.2 mg/dl
Folic acid (serum folate)	2.0-10.0 mg/ml
Prothrombin time	10-13 sec
Partial thromboplastin time	25-39 sec (usually stated to be within 10 sec of control)
Blood platelets	150,000-400,000/mm^3
Bleeding time	Ivy: 2-7 min
	Duke: 5 min
Coagulation factors concentration	
V	60%-140%
VII	70%-130%
VIII	50%-200%
IX	60%-140%
Fibrin degradation products	<10 μg/ml

URINE VALUES (FROM URINALYSIS)

Laboratory test	Normal adult values
Urinalysis/microscopic analysis	
Bilirubin	Negative
Color	Clear, golden yellow
Bacteria	Negative
Casts	0-4 hyaline casts per low-power field
Red blood cells	0-5 per high-power field
White blood cells	0-5 per high-power field

BLOOD DISORDERS

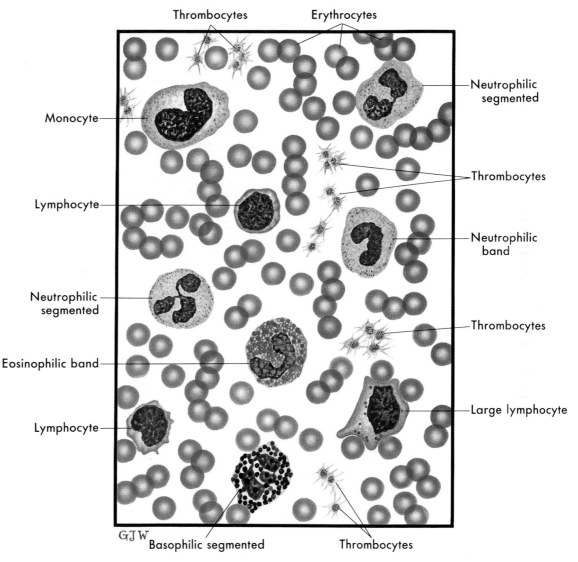

Thrombocytes Erythrocytes

Monocyte

Lymphocyte

Neutrophilic
segmented

Eosinophilic band

Lymphocyte

Neutrophilic
segmented

Thrombocytes

Neutrophilic
band

Thrombocytes

Large lymphocyte

GJW
Basophilic segmented   Thrombocytes

Components of normal blood cells

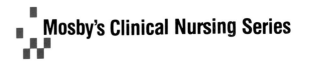

Mosby's Clinical Nursing Series

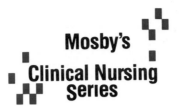

Mosby's Clinical Nursing Series

Cardiovascular Disorders
by Mary Canobbio

Respiratory Disorders
by Susan Wilson and June Thompson

Infectious Diseases
by Deanna Grimes

Orthopedic Disorders
by Leona Mourad

Renal Disorders
by Dorothy Brundage

Neurologic Disorders
by Esther Chipps, Norma Clanin, and Victor Campbell

Cancer Nursing
by Anne Belcher

Genitourinary Disorders
by Mikel Gray

Immunologic Disorders
by Christine Mudge-Grout

Gastrointestinal Disorders
by Dorothy Doughty and Debra Broadwell Jackson

Blood Disorders
by Anne Belcher

Ear, Nose, and Throat Disorders
by Barbara Sigler and Linda Schuring

AIDS and HIV Infection
by Deanna Grimes and Richard Grimes

Skin Disorders
by Marcia Hill

Women's Health Care
by Valerie Edge and Mindi Miller

BLOOD DISORDERS

ANNE E. BELCHER, PhD, RN

Professor of Oncology Nursing,
American Cancer Society;
Associate Professor,
University of Maryland School of Nursing,
University of Maryland at Baltimore,
Baltimore, Maryland

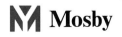 **Mosby**

St. Louis Baltimore Boston Chicago London Philadelphia Sydney Toronto

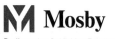
Mosby
Dedicated to Publishing Excellence

Publisher: Alison Miller
Editor: Sally Schrefer
Developmental Editor: Penny Rudolph
Project Manager: Mark Spann
Production Editors: Julie Zipfel, Christine O'Neil
Layout: Doris Hallas

Acknowledgment
The author wishes to acknowledge the contributions of the University of Maryland School of Nursing, the University of Maryland Cancer Center, and the Shock Trauma Center STAT Laboratory and Blood Bank of the University of Maryland Hospital.

Printed in the United States of America

Mosby–Year Book, Inc.
11830 Westline Industrial Drive
St. Louis, Missouri 63146

Library of Congress Cataloging-in-Publication Data

Belcher, Anne E.
    Blood disorders / Anne E. Belcher.
        p.   cm. — (Mosby's clinical nursing series)
    Includes bibliographical references and index.
    ISBN 0-8016-7801-3
    1. Blood—Diseases—Nursing.   I. Title   II. Series.
    [DNLM: 1. Blood—nurses' instruction.   2. Hematologic Diseases—
    —nursing.   WY 152.5 B427b 1993]
    RC636.B37   1993
    616.1′5—dc20
    DNLM/DLC   93-7369
    for Library of Congress   CIP

93 94 95 96 97 CL/CD/VH 9 8 7 6 5 4 3 2 1

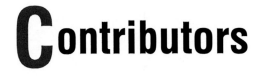Contributors

CHRISTINE L. MUDGE-GROUT, RN, MS, CNN

Clinical Nurse Specialist,
Assistant Clinical Professor,
University of California at San Francisco,
San Francisco, California
(Lymph Node Assessment)

KATHERINE STEFOS

The University of Texas
M.D. Anderson Center,
Division of Pharmacy,
Houston, Texas
(Pharmacologic Agents)

ROBERTA STROHL, RN, MN

Clinical Nurse Specialist,
Department of Radiation Oncology,
University of Maryland at Baltimore,
Baltimore, Maryland
(Radiation Therapy)

CAROL S. VIELE, RN, MS

Clinical Nurse Specialist, Department of Nursing,
Oncology/Hematology, Bone Marrow Transplant;
Assistant Clinical Professor,
University of California at San Francisco,
San Francisco, California
(Bone Marrow Transplantation)

Original illustrations by

GEORGE J. WASSILCHENKO
Tulsa, Oklahoma
and

DONALD P. O'CONNOR
St. Peters, Missouri

Original photography by

PATRICK WATSON
Poughkeepsie, New York

Preface

Blood Disorders is the eleventh volume in *Mosby's Clinical Nursing Series*, a new kind of resource for practicing nurses.

The *Series* is the result of the most elaborate market research ever undertaken by Mosby. We first surveyed hundreds of working nurses to determine what kinds of resources practicing nurses want to meet their advanced information needs. We then approached clinical specialists, proven authors and experts, and asked them to develop a format that would meet the needs of nurses in practice. This format was presented to nine focus groups composed of working nurses and refined between each group. In the later stages we published a 32-page, full-color sample so that detailed changes could be made to improve physical layout and appearance, section by section and page by page. The result is a new genre of professional books for nursing professionals.

Blood Disorders begins with a clear and concise discussion of the anatomy and physiology of the blood and blood-forming organs. The first chapter includes a variety of illustrations that depict sometimes difficult-to-visualize aspects of normal and abnormal cellular generation and function.

Chapter 2 is a pictorial guide to the nurse's assessment of the body systems affected by blood disorders. Clear, full-color photographs show proper position and technique in sharp detail, augmented by concise instructions, rationales, and tips.

Chapter 3 presents the latest in diagnostic tests, using full-color photographs of equipment, techniques, monitors, and output. A consistent format for each procedure provides information about the purpose of the test, indications and contraindications, and nursing care associated with each test, including patient teaching. Inside the front cover of the book are tables of normal laboratory values.

Chapters 4 through 9 present the nursing care of patients experiencing specific blood disorders and the major surgical and therapeutic interventions. Chapter 4 focuses on erythrocytic disorders; Chapter 5 on leukocytic disorders; Chapter 6 on thrombocytic disorders; Chapter 7 on myelodysplastic syndromes; Chapter 8 on multiple myeloma; and Chapter 9 on lymphomas. Information on pathophysiology answers questions nurses often have. Definitive diagnostic tests and the physician's treatment plan are briefly reviewed to promote collaborative care among members of the health team.

The heart of the book is the nursing care, presented according to the nursing process. These pages are bordered in blue to make them easy to find and use on the unit. The nursing care is structured to integrate the five steps of the nursing process, centered around appropriate nursing diagnoses accepted by the North American Nursing Diagnosis Association (NANDA). The material can be used to develop individualized care plans quickly and accurately, and it meets the standards of nursing care required by the Joint Commission on the Accreditation of Healthcare Organizations (JCAHO). By facilitating the development of individualized and authoritative care plans, this book can actually save you time to spend on direct patient care.

Chapter 10 describes therapies, including surgery, radiation, chemotherapy, and bone marrow transplantation. Supportive therapies such as blood and blood-component therapy, nutritional support, and pain management are also described.

In response to requests from scores of nurses participating in our research, a distinctive feature of this book is its use in patient teaching. Background information on diseases and medical interventions enables nurses to answer with authority questions patients often ask. The illustrations in the book, particularly those in the color atlas (Chapter 1) and the chapter on diagnostic procedures (Chapter 3), are specifically designed to support patient teaching. Chapter 11 consists of 15 patient teaching guides written to be copied, distributed to patients and their families, and used for self-care after discharge. In addition, patient teaching sections in each care plan provide nurses with checklists of concepts to teach, promoting this increasingly vital aspect of care.

The book concludes with a concise guide to drugs used for the treatment of blood disorders, and, inside the back cover, a resource section directs you to organizations and other resources for nurses and patients.

We hope this book contributes to the advancement of professional nursing by serving as a first step toward a body of professional literature for nurses to call their own.

Contents

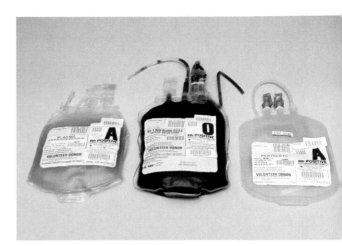

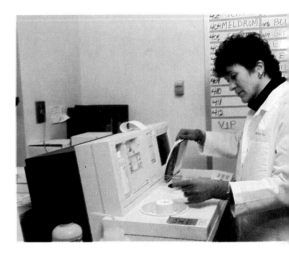

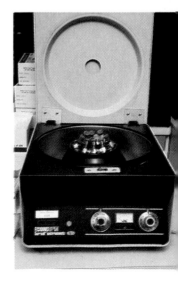

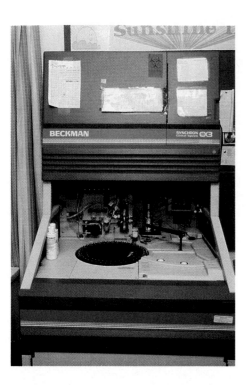

4 Erythrocytic disorders, 51

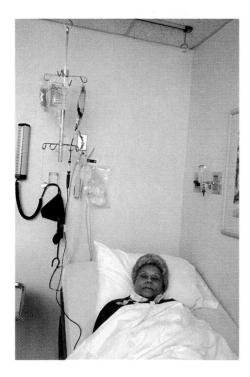

5 Leukocytic disorders, 93

6 Thrombocytic disorders, 112

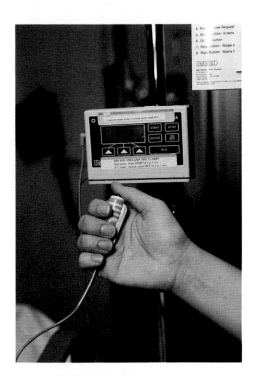

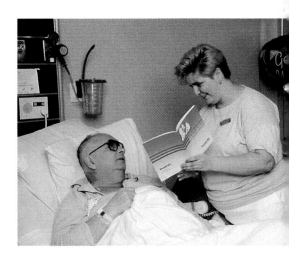

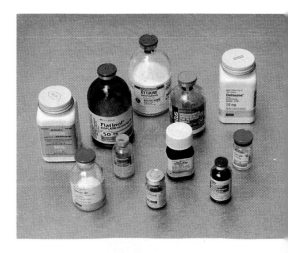

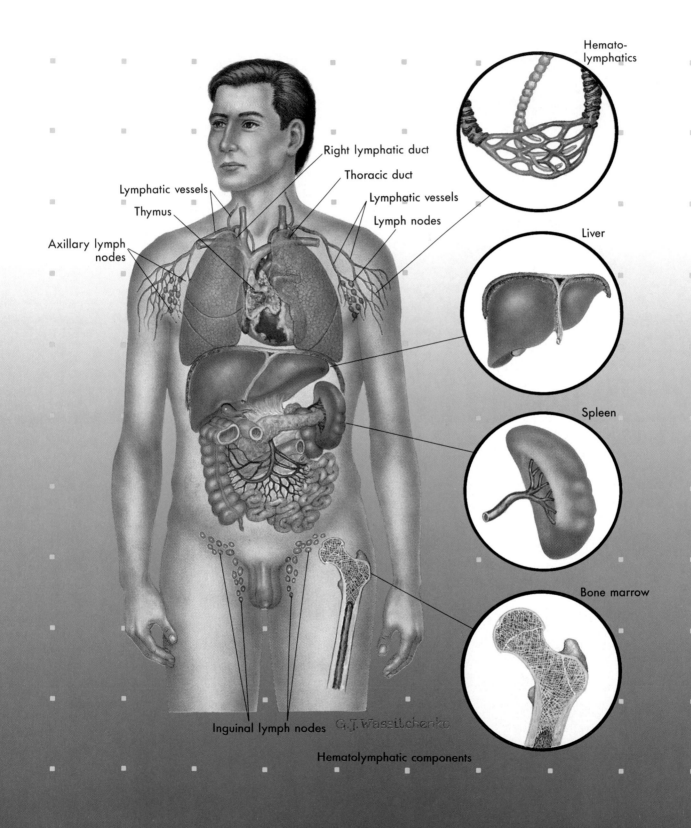

Right lymphatic duct

Thoracic duct

Lymphatic vessels

Lymphatic vessels

Thymus

Lymph nodes

Axillary lymph
nodes

Inguinal lymph nodes

Hemato-
lymphatics

Liver

Spleen

Bone marrow

G.J.Wassilchenko

Hematolymphatic components

CHAPTER 1

Color Atlas of the Blood and Blood-Forming Organs

HEMATOLYMPHATIC SYSTEM

The hematolymphatic system is composed of blood and blood-forming organs, the bone marrow, spleen, liver, and lymphatics.

BLOOD AND ITS COMPONENTS

Blood, which circulates continuously through the heart and vascular system, performs numerous vital functions (see box).

The major characteristics of blood include color (arterial blood is bright red; venous blood is dark red); viscosity (blood is three to four times thicker than water); reaction (the pH is 7.35 to 7.4); and volume (adults have approximately 70 to 75 ml/kg of body weight, or 5 to 6 L).

Blood is a suspension of particulate matter in an aqueous solution of colloid and electrolytes that serves as a medium of exchange between body cells and the exterior. It also has protective properties that benefit the body and the blood itself. The liquid portion of blood, **plasma,** is a suspension of colloid, electrolytes, proteins, and numerous other substances (Table 1-1). The concentration of these substances varies on the basis of diet, metabolic demand, hormones, and vitamins. **Serum** is plasma that has had fibrinogen (a clotting factor) or some other unwanted or unneeded substance removed from the sample in the laboratory.

Plasma is about 90% water and 10% dissolved substances (solutes). The dominant substances in weight are the plasma proteins, which are classified as albumins; globulins (immunoglobulins and gamma-globulins); and clotting factors, primarily fibrinogen.

The plasma proteins are synthesized in the liver, except for the **immunoglobulins,** which are synthesized by lymphocytes in the lymph nodes and other lym-

---

FUNCTIONS OF BLOOD

Transport of oxygen and absorbed nutrients to cells

Transport of waste products to kidneys, skin, and lungs

Transport of hormones from endocrine glands to other tissues

Protection of the body from life-threatening microorganisms

Regulation of body temperature by heat transfer

Table 1-1

ORGANIC AND INORGANIC COMPONENTS OF ARTERIAL PLASMA

Constituent	Amount/concentration	Major functions
Water	93% of plasma weight	Medium for carrying all other constituents
Electrolytes	Total <1% of plasma weight	Maintain water in extracellular compartment; act as buffers; function in membrane excitability
Sodium (Na^+)	142 mEq/L (142 mM)	
Potassium (K^+)	4 mEq/L (4 mM)	
Calcium (CA^{++})	5 mEq/L (2.5 mM)	
Magnesium (Mg^{++})	3 mEq/L (1.5 mM)	
Chloride (CL^-)	103 mEq/L (103 mM)	
Bicarbonate (HCO_3^-)	27 mEq/L (27 mM)	
Phosphate (mostly HPO_4^{2-})	2 mEq/L (1 mM)	
Sulfate (SO_4^{2-})	1 mEq/L (0.5 mM)	
Proteins	7.3 g/dl (2.5 mM)	Provide colloid osmotic pressure of plasma; act as buffers; bind other plasma constituents (e.g., lipids, hormones, vitamins, metals); clotting factors; enzymes; enzyme precursors; antibodies (immune globulins); hormones
Albumins	4.5 g/dl	
Globulins	2.5 g/dl	
Fibrinogen	0.3 g/dl	
Gases		
Carbon dioxide (CO_2) content	22-20 mmol/L plasma	By-product of oxygenation, most carbon dioxide content is from bicarbonate and acts as a buffer
Oxygen (O_2)	Pao_2 80 torr or greater (arterial); Pvo_2 30-40 torr (venous)	Oxygenation
Nitrogen (N_2)	0.9 ml/dl	By-product of protein catabolism
Nutrients		Provide nutrition and substances for tissue repair
Glucose and other carbohydrates	100 mg/dl (5.6 mM)	
Total amino acids	40 mg/dl (2 mM)	
Total lipids	500 mg/dl (7.5 mM)	
Cholesterol	150-250 mg/dl (4-7 mM)	
Individual vitamins	0.0001-2.5 mg/dl	
Individual trace elements	0.001-0.3 mg/dl	
Waste products		
Urea (BUN)	7-18 mg/dl (5.7 mM)	End product of protein catabolism
Creatinine (from creatinine)	1 mg/dl (0.09 mM)	End product from energy metabolism
Uric acid (from nucleic acids)	5 mg/dl (0.3 mM)	End product of protein metabolism
Bilirubin (from heme)	0.2-1.2 mg/dl (0.003-0.018 mM)	End product of red blood cell destruction
Individual hormones	0.000001-0.05 mg/dl	Functions specific to target tissue

(From Vander, Sherman, and Luciano.)[61a]

phoid tissues. **Albumin** is essential for regulating the passage of water and solutes through the capillaries. Because these molecules are large and do not diffuse freely through the vascular endothelium, they provide the critical colloid osmotic pressure that regulates the passage of water and solutes through the microcirculation. Albumin also serves as a carrier molecule for normal blood components and exogenous agents such as drugs. The immunoglobulins (antibodies) are synthesized by plasma cells in the lymphoid organs. The antibodies are IgA, IgG, IgM, IgD, and IgE, and they are critical for defense against infectious microorganisms.

The **clotting factors** (Table 1-2) stop bleeding from damaged blood vessels. **Fibrinogen,** the most plentiful of the clotting factors, is the precursor of the fibrin clot. **Hemostasis,** which means arrest of bleeding, involves a complex sequence of events, including vasoconstriction, formation of a platelet plug, activation of the coagulation cascade, and formation of a blood clot (Figures 1-1 and 1-2 and box on p. 3).

Other plasma proteins include complement proteins involved in the immune response, a variety of enzymes and their inhibitors, and specific carriers of such elements as iron and copper.

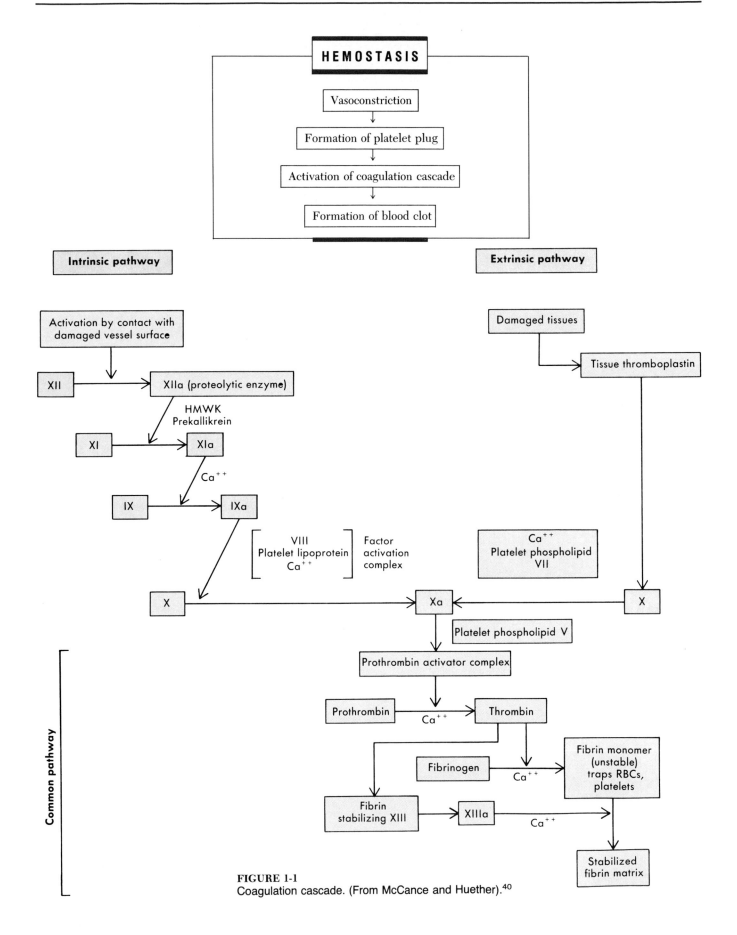

FIGURE 1-1
Coagulation cascade. (From McCance and Huether).[40]

Table 1-2

CLOTTING FACTORS

International nomenclature	Synonym	Substance	Source	Enzymatic function	Pathway of activation
I	Fibrinogen	Plasma protein	Liver	Precursor of fibrin	Final common pathway
II	Prothrombin	Plasma protein	Liver	Precursor of thrombin	Final common pathway
III	Tissue thromboplastin Tissue factor Thrombokinase	Lipoprotein and phospholipid	Released from damaged tissues	Activates prothrombin	Extrinsic pathway
IV	Calcium ion	Ion in plasma	Diet and bones	Activates prothrombin and fibrin formation	All
V	Labile factor Proaccelerin accelerator globulin (AcG) Thrombogen	Plasma protein	Liver	Accelerates conversion of prothrombin to thrombin	Final common pathway
VI	Obsolete; same as V				
VII	Serum prothrombin conversion factor Proconvertin Stable factor	Plasma protein	Liver	Accelerates conversion of prothrombin to thrombin; part of enzyme complex	Extrinsic pathway
VIII	Antihemophilic globulin (AGH) Antihemophilic factor (AHF) Thromboplastinogen Platelet cofactor 1	Plasma protein (three subunits)	Large molecular weight Subunit by endothelium	Associated with platelet factor 3 and Christmas factor (IX), activates prothrombin (II)	Intrinsic pathway
IX	Plasma thromboplastin component (PTC) Christmas factor Antihemophilic factor B Autoprothrombin II (protein C) Platelet cofactor 2	Plasma protein	Liver	Associated with platelet factors 3 and 6; activates prothrombin	Intrinsic pathway
X	Stuart-Prower factor Stuart factor Autoprothrombin III	Plasma protein	Liver and plasma	Activated by Hageman factor	Extrinsic and intrinsic pathway
XI	Plasma thromboplastin antecedent (PTA) Antihemophilic factor C	Plasma protein	Possibly liver	Activated by Hageman factor; accelerates thrombin formation; substrate for activator enzymatic complex	Intrinsic pathway
XII	Hageman factor Contact factor Glass factor Antihemophilic factor D	Plasma protein	Liver and (plasma?)	Involved in first step of activation of intrinsic pathway; activates XI	Intrinsic pathway

Table 1-2

CLOTTING FACTORS—cont'd

International nomenclature	Synonym	Substance	Source	Enzymatic function	Pathway of activation
XIII	Fibrin-stabilizing factor (FSF) Fibrinase Fibrinoligase Laki-Lorand factor (LLF) Plasma transglutaminase	Plasma protein	Present in plasma and platelets Liver	Produces stronger fibrin clot; stabilizes clot formation	Common
High-molecular-weight kininogen	HMWK Fitzgerald factor Williams factor Fluajeac factor Reid factor Washington factor	Alpha-globulin	Tissues	Activates contraction of clot	Intrinsic kinin cascade
Prekallikrein	Fletcher factor	Gamma-globulin	Tissues	Activates contraction of clot	Intrinsic kinin cascade

The factors are numbered in the order of their discovery. Numerals do not denote their sequence of activation in the coagulation cascade. (From McCance and Huether.)[40]

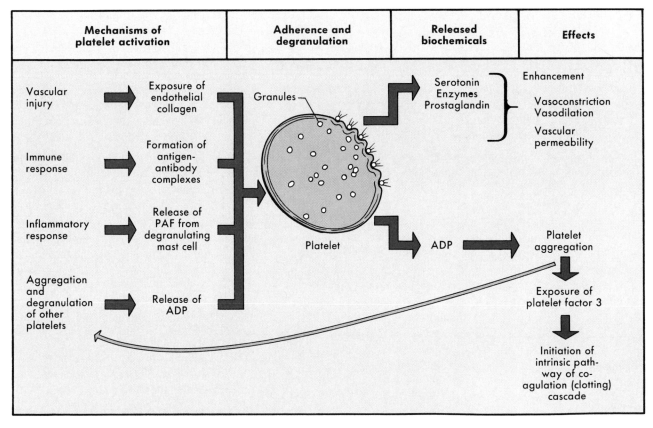

FIGURE 1-2
Platelet degranulation. PAF, Platelet-activating factor. (From McCance and Huether).[40]

Table 1-3

CELLULAR COMPONENTS OF THE BLOOD

Cell	Structural characteristics	Normal amounts in circulating blood	Function	Life span
Erythrocyte (red blood cell)	Nonnucleated cytoplasmic disk containing hemoglobin	4.2-6.2 million/mm^3	Gas transport to and from tissue cells and lungs	80-120 days
Leukocyte (white blood cell)	Nucleated cell	5,000-10,000/mm^3	Bodily defense mechanisms	See below
Lymphocyte	Mononuclear immunocyte	25%-33% of leukocyte count (leukocyte differential)	Humoral and cell-mediated immunity	Days or years, depending on type
Monocyte and macrophage	Large mononuclear phagocyte	3%-7% of leukocyte differential	Phagocytosis; mononuclear phagocyte system	Months or years
Eosinophil	Segmented polymorphonuclear granulocyte	1%-4% of leukocyte differential	Phagocytosis; antibody-mediated defense against parasites, allergic reactions; associated with Hodgkin disease, recovery phase of infection	Unknown
Neutrophil	Segmented polymorphonuclear granulocyte	57%-67% of leukocyte differential	Phagocytosis, particularly during early phase of inflammation	4 days
Basophil	Segmented polymorphonuclear granulocyte	0-0.75% of leukocyte differential	Unknown, but associated with allergic reactions and mechanical irritation	Unknown
Thrombocyte (platelet)	Irregularly shaped cytoplasmic fragment (not a cell)	140,000-340,000/mm^3	Hemostasis following vascular injury; normal coagulation and clot formation/retraction	8 to 11 days

(From McCance and Huether.)[40]

Lipoproteins are carried through the blood as complexes with **plasma proteins.** The lipoproteins include the plasma lipids, triglycerides, phospholipids, cholesterol, and fatty acids.

The **electrolytes** (sodium, potassium, calcium, magnesium, chloride, bicarbonate, phosphate, and sulfate) maintain the osmolarity and pH of the blood within a physiologic range.

The cellular elements of the blood include red blood cells (erythrocytes), white blood cells of several types (leukocytes), and platelets (thrombocytes) (Table 1-3). All of these cells are believed to be derived from a single stem cell, which divides and matures to produce three distinct types of cells with different functions, properties, and characteristics (Figure 1-3). Blood cell production (**hematopoiesis**) occurs in the bone marrow; it is a two-stage process involving mitotic division (**proliferation**) and maturation (**differentiation**). Each type of blood cell has parent cells (**stem cells**), which undergo mitosis when they receive specific biochemical signals that populations of circulating blood cells have decreased to a certain point. Proliferation continues until the required number of mature daughter cells has entered the circulation. Hematopoiesis continues throughout life. Blood cell production in tissues other than bone marrow usually is a sign of disease.

Erythrocytes

Erythrocytes have several principal functions:

- Transport of oxygen to the tissues
- Transport of carbon dioxide to the lungs
- Maintenance of normal blood pH through a series of intracellular buffers

There are approximately 5 million erythrocytes per cubic millimeter of blood; normal hemoglobin is 15 g/dl of blood. Erythrocytes are produced in the red

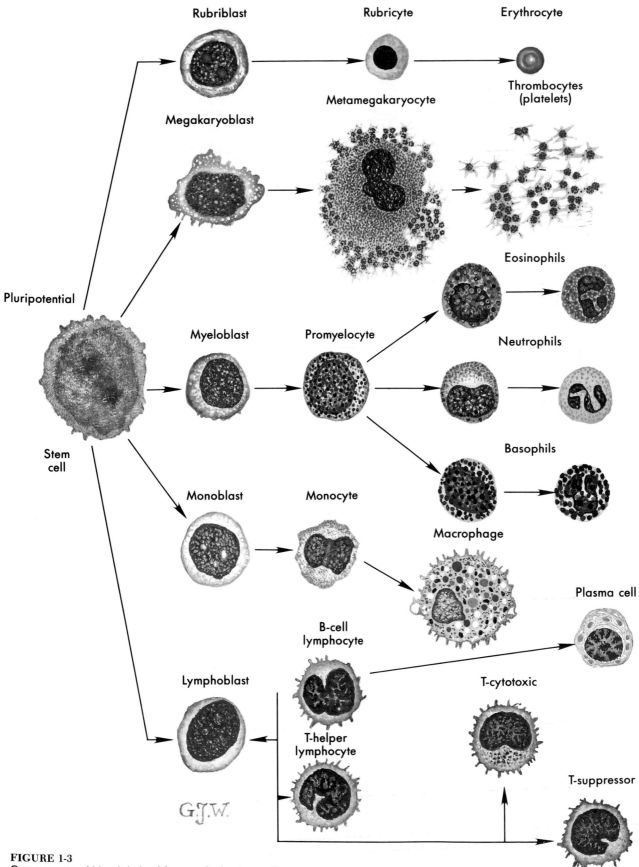

FIGURE 1-3
Components of blood derived from a single stem cell.

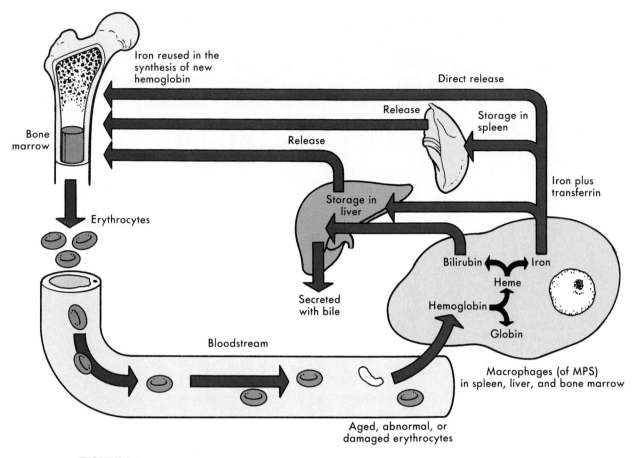

FIGURE 1-4

Iron cycle. Iron (Fe) released from gastrointestinal epithelial cells circulates in the bloodstream associated with its plasma carrier, transferrin. It is delivered to erythroblasts in the bone marrow, where most of it is incorporated into hemoglobin. Mature erythrocytes circulate for approximately 120 days, after which they become senescent and are removed by the mononuclear phagocyte system (MPS). Macrophages of the MPS (mostly in the spleen) break down ingested erythrocytes and return iron to the bloodstream directly or after storing it as ferritin or hemosiderin. (From McCance and Huether.)[40]

bone marrow and found in the ribs, sternum, skull, vertebrae, and bones of the hands, feet, and pelvis. Numerous nutrients are needed for normal cell formation, including iron, vitamin B_{12}, folic acid, and pyridoxine. The young reticulocytes released from the bone marrow circulate for 4 days while maturing into adult erythrocytes. The average life span of an erythrocyte is 115 to 130 days; dead cells are eliminated by phagocytosis in the mononuclear phagocyte system, particularly in the spleen and liver.

The size and shape of the erythrocyte are ideal for its function as a gas carrier. It is a small disk with the unique characteristics of biconcavity and reversible deformability. The flattened, biconcave shape provides a surface area to volume ratio that is optimal for the diffusion of gases into and out of the cell. Reversible deformity enables the cell to alter its shape to squeeze

through the microcirculation and then return to normal.

Hemoglobin, the iron-containing substance of the red blood cell, is composed of a simple protein called globin and a red compound called heme, which contains iron and porphyrin. Each erythrocyte contains 200 million to 300 million molecules of hemoglobin, which combine chemically with oxygen to form oxyhemoglobin. Hemoglobin also combines with carbon dioxide. These two capacities enable the blood to carry oxygen to the tissues and carbon dioxide to the alveoli and thus to the atmosphere.

Total iron in the body ranges from 2 to 6 g, two thirds of which is contained in hemoglobin (Figure 1-4 illustrates the iron cycle). The rest is stored in the bone marrow, spleen, and liver. Iron is obtained from such rich dietary sources as liver; oysters; lean meat;

kidney beans; green, leafy vegetables; apricots; and raisins.

When hemoglobin is phagocytosed in the liver or spleen, it breaks down into its heme and globin factors. The iron is reused by the liver to produce fresh hemoglobin, and the porphyrin is converted into bilirubin, which is excreted by the body in feces and urine.

Leukocytes

Leukocytes are white blood cells that defend the body against infective microorganisms and remove debris, including dead or injured host cells. There are about 5,000 to 10,000 leukocytes per cubic millimeter of blood. Leukocytes act primarily in the body tissues but are transported in the circulation. They are divided into three major categories: granulocytes, lymphocytes, and monocytes.

Granulocytes, which make up 70% of all white blood cells, are produced by the bone marrow and function according to the type of granule. Polymorphonuclear leukocytes (PMNs or neutrophils), which constitute about 55% of the total leukocyte count in adults, fight bacterial infections through a process of phagocytosis; foreign particulate matter, or breakdown products from cells, is also digested. These cells are present during the early, acute phase of an inflammatory reaction. Soon after bacterial invasion or tissue injury, the neutrophils migrate from the capillaries into the inflamed area, where they ingest and destroy microorganisms and debris. When they die, in a day or two, digestive enzymes are released from their cytoplasmic granules. These enzymes dissolve cellular debris and prepare the site for healing.

Eosinophils have a similar phagocytic function and are particularly important in digesting bacteria. They ingest antigen-antibody complexes and are induced by IgE-mediated hypersensitivity reactions to attack parasites. They also appear to play a role in combating allergic reactions.

Basophils have cytoplasmic granules that contain vasoactive amines (histamine, bradykinin, and serotonin) believed to play a role in combating acute systemic allergic reactions. They also contain heparin, an anticoagulant.

Agranulocytes (monocytes, macrophages, and lymphocytes) do not contain lysosomal granules in their cytoplasm. **Lymphocytes,** which are produced mainly in the lymph nodes, make up about 25% of the leukocytes. They are primarily involved in producing antibodies and maintaining tissue immunity. The most important lymphocytes are T cells, B cells, and mature B cells (plasma cells).

Monocytes and macrophages make up the mononuclear phagocyte system (formerly called the reticuloendothelial system) and are responsible for the phagocytosis of dead erythrocytes and leukocytes in the blood. They are also important in the processing of antigenic information. Monocytes are immature macrophages. After being formed in and released by the bone marrow, they enter the bloodstream and circulate for about 36 hours while maturing. Some of the circulating macrophages migrate out of the blood vessels in response to infection or inflammation in the body, whereas others migrate to fixed sites in lymphoid tissues of the liver, spleen, lymph nodes, peritoneum, or gastrointestinal tract, where they remain active for months or years.

Thrombocytes

Thrombocytes, also called **platelets,** are disk-shaped cytoplasmic fragments formed in the bone marrow. They maintain capillary integrity, initiate coagulation, and retract clots. Because platelets lack a nucleus, they have no DNA and are incapable of mitotic division. There are 250,000 to 500,000 platelets per cubic millimeter of blood. One third of the body's available platelets are in a reserve pool in the spleen. Platelets live approximately 10 days, after which time they die and are removed by macrophages, mostly in the spleen.

THE LYMPHATIC SYSTEM

The lymphatic system's primary organs are the thymus and bone marrow. Its secondary organs are the spleen, lymph nodes, tonsils, and Peyer's patches of the small intestine (Figure 1-5). The lymphatic system has numerous functions, including:

- Transport of lymph
- Production of lymphocytes and antibodies
- Phagocytosis
- Absorption of fats and fat-soluble matter from the intestine.

The lymphatic system has three major characteristics: (1) the formation of lymph is regulated by the exchange of fluid between capillaries and tissue spaces; (2) the muscle pump is responsible for the movement of lymph; and (3) the amount of lymphoid tissue and the distribution of lymph nodes are related to age.

Spleen

The spleen is a mass of lymphoid and mononuclear phagocyte cells found under the ribs in the upper left quadrant of the abdomen. It is a concave, encapsulated organ that weighs about 150 g and is about the size of a fist. Its structure allows close interaction among lymphocytes, macrophages, and materials carried in the bloodstream. Blood that circulates through

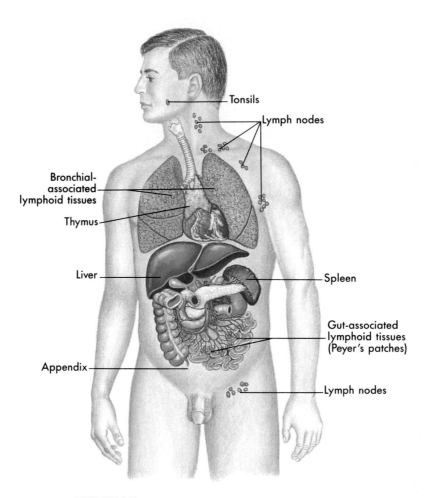

Tonsils

Lymph nodes

Bronchial-associated lymphoid tissues

Thymus

Liver

Spleen

Gut-associated lymphoid tissues (Peyer's patches)

Appendix

Lymph nodes

FIGURE 1-5
Components of the lymphatic system. (From Seidel.)[50]

the spleen comes from the splenic artery, which branches from the descending aorta and reenters the circulatory system via the splenic vein. The arterial blood that enters the spleen encounters the white splenic pulp first. This pulp consists of masses of lymphoid tissue containing lymphocytes and macrophages. This is the chief site of immune and phagocytic function in the spleen. Some of the blood continues through the microcirculation of the spleen and enters storage areas, called **venous sinuses.** However, most of the blood oozes through the permeable capillary walls into the red pulp. Here the resident macrophages phagocytose old, damaged, or dead blood cells, micro-

organisms, and debris. Hemoglobin from phagocytosed erythrocytes is catabolized, and heme is stored in the cytoplasm of the macrophages or released back into the plasma. The macrophages can also remove particulate inclusions from the red blood cells without harming them. Blood that filters through the red pulp finds its way into the venous sinuses and the portal circulation.

The venous sinuses and the red pulp can store more than 300 ml of blood. A sudden drop in blood pressure causes the sympathetic nervous system to stimulate constriction of the sinuses, which can expel as much as 200 ml of blood into the venous circulation, helping to restore blood volume or pressure in

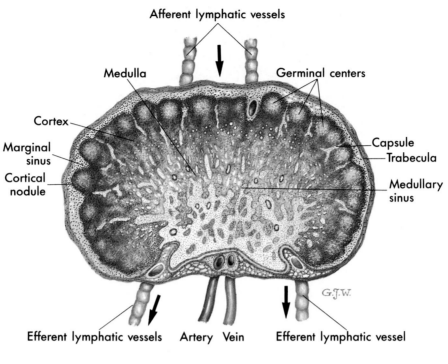

Afferent lymphatic vessels

Medulla

Germinal centers

Cortex

Marginal sinus

Cortical nodule

Capsule

Trabecula

Medullary sinus

Efferent lymphatic vessels   Artery   Vein   Efferent lymphatic vessel

FIGURE 1-6
Structures of a lymph node.

the circulation. This mechanism can also increase the hematocrit by as much as 4%.

Although the spleen is not necessary to sustain life, its absence is marked by leukocytosis (a high level of circulating leukocytes), which indicates that the spleen exerts some control over the rate of proliferation of stem cells in the bone marrow or their release into the bloodstream. The absence of the spleen is also associated with a decrease in the amount of iron in the circulation, a decrease in immune function, diminished antibody production in response to soluble antigen, and an increase in the number of morphologically defective blood cells.

Lymph Nodes

Lymph nodes, the most numerous components of the lymphatic system, are present in virtually every area of the body. They are clustered around the lymphatic veins, which collect interstitial fluid from the tissues and transport it back into the circulatory system near the heart. The most familiar nodes are those palpable in the neck and groin. They serve as filters along the course of lymphatic channels and have a rich blood supply, which is important in transporting lymphocytes (Figure 1-6). During an infection macrophages

proliferate rapidly in the lymph nodes, causing the nodes to enlarge and become tender. Lymph flows slowly through the nodes, which facilitates phagocytosis of foreign substances in the nodes and prevents these substances from reentering the blood.

Thymus

The thymus is located in the thorax anterior to the upper part of the heart and great vessels. It contains lymphatic follicles and lymphocytes, and it is here that the T cells of the immune system are produced.

Bone Marrow

The bone marrow is considered an important part of the lymphoid system, because millions of lymphocytes are scattered throughout it. In an adult active marrow is found in the pelvic bones, vertebrae, cranium and mandible, sternum and ribs, and extreme proximal portions of the humerus and femur. Stem cells in the hematopoietic marrow receive the necessary oxygen and nutrients from the primary, or nutrient, arteries of the bone.

The **mononuclear phagocyte system (MPS)** consists of a line of cells originating in the bone marrow; these include monoblasts, promonoblasts, and monocytes in

Table 1-4

MONONUCLEAR PHAGOCYTE SYSTEM (MPS) (FORMERLY RETICULOENDOTHELIAL SYSTEM)

Name of cell	Location
Committed stem cells	Bone marrow
Monoblasts	Bone marrow
Promonoblasts	Bone marrow
Monocytes	Bone marrow and peripheral blood
Macrophages	Tissue
Kupffer cells (inflammatory macrophages)	Liver
Alveolar macrophages	Lung
Histiocytes	Connective tissue
Macrophages	Bone marrow
Fixed and free macrophages	Spleen and lymph nodes
Pleural and peritoneal macrophages	Serous cavities
Microglial cells	Nervous system
Mesangial cells	Kidney
Osteoclasts	Bone
Langerhans cells	Skin
Dendritic cells	Lymphoid tissue

(From Robbins, Cotran, and Kumar[46a] and from Halma, Daha, and Van Es.)[29a]

bone marrow; monocytes in peripheral blood; and macrophages in tissue (Table 1-4). The cells of the MPS ingest and phagocytose unwanted materials in the blood and in organs. During the inflammatory process, they engulf and digest foreign protein particles, microorganisms, debris from injured or dead cells, injured or defective erythrocytes, and dead neutrophils. The MPS is also the main line of defense against bacteria in the bloodstream; it cleanses the blood by removing a variety of cells, coagulation products, antigen-antibody complexes, and macromolecules such as lipids and carbohydrates.

Monocytes and macrophages secrete **colony-stimulating factor (CSF)**, which is necessary for the formation and growth of colonies of macrophages and granulocytes in the bone marrow. The macrophages also secrete prostaglandin E, which inhibits colony-forming cells. They may also indirectly regulate erythrocyte differentiation by producing erythropoietin, which stimulates erythrocyte production in the bone marrow.

CHAPTER 2

Assessment

Hematologic assessment naturally involves more than just the hematologic system itself, since the circulatory system interacts with every other body system. Assessment should involve careful, systematic evaluation of a person's medical, family, social, cultural, psychologic, and occupational history, and a systematic physical examination. The extent to which other body systems are affected by hematologic, or blood, disorders will be noted as the assessment process is described.

HISTORY AND INTERVIEWING

An effective assessment depends on the nurse's ability to put the patient at ease, such as by using everyday language appropriate for the patient's age, ethnicity, and life experiences. Because it is essential that the patient approach this process as a team member, working with medical staff to assess his or her own needs, the purposes of the assessment should be shared with the patient from the beginning. These purposes are to evaluate current signs and symptoms, health status, mental and emotional status, life-style and occupational influences, and family health history, and to examine all these aspects in light of their effect on the current disorder or suspected dysfunction. Sharing these purposes often enables the patient to relax and to recognize the value of his input. The interview format of this process provides an opportunity for nurse and patient to establish a rapport; by showing interest and concern, the nurse can elicit valuable information for evaluating risks and symptoms.

Perhaps the best way to determine a patient's chief complaint is to begin by asking, "What has brought you here today?" By contrast, asking the tired, cliched,

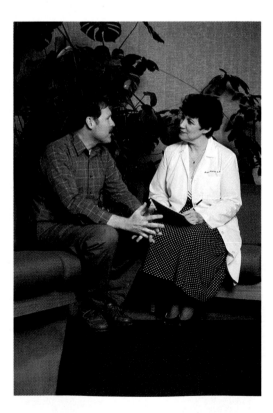

HEALTH HISTORY

General information

Name
Age
Gender
Ethnicity
Date and place of birth
Marital status

Presenting complaint

Severity: Location, quality, and quantity
Temporality: Onset, duration, frequency, precipitators
Alleviating or aggravating factors
What the patient thinks may be happening

Concurrent disorders

Cardiac disease
Pulmonary disease
Diabetes
Obesity
Renal disease

Previous state of health

Infancy and childhood
Previous disorders
Injuries
Hospitalizations and surgeries
Allergies

Present state of health and life-style

Prescription and over-the-counter medication pattern
Diet and fluid intake
Oral hygiene and dental status
Sleep patterns
Elimination patterns
Educational level
Occupation, including exposure to chemicals
Cultural and religious or spiritual values
Economic resources, including health insurance
Life-style, including exercise, consumption of caffeine, alcohol ingestion, use of tobacco products, sexual practices, exposure to sun, self-examination practices, safety measures

Family medical history

Age and state of health of family members, including grandparents, parents, siblings, children; if any one of these is deceased, specify cause of death; if any one of these has been diagnosed as having a blood disorder, specify type and outcome

General review of systems

Weight—present weight, usual weight
Performance status—present level of activity, usual level of activity, fatigue, weakness
Skin and mucous membranes—color, integrity, turgor, color of nail beds, presence of edema, petechiae or ecchymoses, pruritus, flushing, sweating, enlarged lymph nodes, clubbing of fingers, fever
Head and neck—dysphagia, swelling, hoarseness, nasal discharge, asymmetry
Respiratory tract—hemoptysis, dyspnea with or without exertion
Cardiovascular function—hypertension, tachycardia
Gastrointestinal function—anorexia, abdominal pain or bloating, nausea, vomiting, hematemesis, change in bowel pattern, melena, date and result of Hemoccult or guaiac stool test
Urinary tract and bladder—hematuria, pelvic or flank pain, cloudy urine, frequency, urgency, dysuria
Gynecologic system—abnormal vaginal bleeding, pelvic pain, pattern of menses, sparse hair, underdeveloped vulva
Breasts—underdeveloped
Musculoskeletal system—swelling, pain, stiffness, redness, limitation of movement
Neurologic function—headache, convulsions, visual disturbances, altered pupillary reflex, syncope, vertigo, sensory deficit, altered reflexes

"How are you?" usually elicits the equally noncommunicative, "Fine." After encouraging a description of what is really bothering the patient, the nurse's line of questioning is guided by the conversation itself and is aimed at determining (1) when the symptoms began; (2) precipitating or aggravating factors; (3) location, radiation, quality, and quantity of the symptoms; (4) relieving factors; (5) associated findings; and (6) treatments sought.

During this interview the nurse watches for nonverbal cues (e.g., facial expression, body position, and tone of voice) while recording the patient's responses in his own words. Although coping methods and responses to stress are difficult to assess in this initial interview, direct questions about specific, recent stressful events and life changes often can elicit pertinent information. However, the nurse must keep in mind that just how stressful an event is can be truly determined only by the person experiencing it.

After this initial interview, physical assessment is the next step. Because the circulatory system is involved in numerous far-ranging interactions, the functions of a variety of body systems must be evaluated.

PSYCHOSOCIAL/DEVELOPMENTAL ASSESSMENT

A complete psychosocial/developmental assessment involves taking into account the individual's life developmental processes and the phases of growth and maturing through which he has progressed. Naturally, the tool for accomplishing this phase of assessment is the interview and a review of the patient's history (see the box on the next page). Discussing developmental phases, stages, or crises can provide both the nurse and the patient with a broader insight into the patient's life situation and its bearing on health or illness. It can also be useful for patients to review their past and compare it with the present. This demonstrates to the patient two basic premises: that growth and development are continuous throughout the life cycle and that human beings have a remarkable ability to change over time while maintaining a unique core of individuality. An awareness of these two principles can be a valuable resource to the patient in learning to cope with disease, since some blood disorders can be long-term conditions and can affect the person's life-style.

PHYSICAL EXAMINATION

The physical examination of a person in whom a blood disorder is suspected should include all body systems, with an emphasis on identifying deviations from normal structure and function. These areas should be further assessed with specific diagnostic procedures. A family history of a genetic disorder may guide the examiner in assessing such aspects of structure as delayed secondary sexual characteristics, as is seen in sickle cell anemia.

SKIN, HAIR, AND NAILS

Examination of the skin and its appendages begins with a general inspection, using the two major techniques of inspection and palpation. The skin is inspected for color and vascularity and for evidence of perspiration, edema, injuries, or skin lesions (Figure 2-1). During the examination the examiner should think about the underlying structures and the particular kind of exposure of a body part. It is also helpful to note changes in the skin that indicate past injuries and habits (e.g., calluses, stains, scars, needle marks, and insect bites) and the grooming of the hair and nails.

Skin color varies from person to person and from one part of the body to another, ranging from a whitish

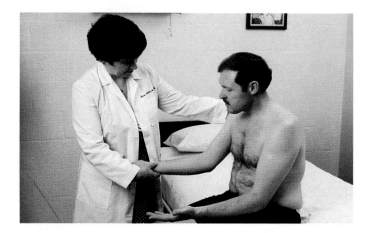

FIGURE 2-1
Inspection of skin.

pink to a dark brown, depending on race. Exposed areas are noticeably different. The vascular flush areas are the cheeks, the bridge of the nose, the neck, the upper chest, the flexor surfaces of the extremities, and the genital area. These areas may be involved in a vascular disturbance or may demonstrate increased color caused by blushing or temperature elevation. They should be compared with areas of less vascularity. The pigment labile areas are the face, the backs of the hands, the flexors of the wrists, the axillae, the mammary areolae, the midline of the abdomen, and the genital area. These areas may demonstrate normal systemic pigmentary changes.

> Alterations in platelet count and clotting mechanisms may result in petechiae, ecchymosis, or hematoma formation.

Other changes in skin color should be noted as evidence of systemic disease. These signs can be particularly helpful in diagnosing blood disorders or related conditions. For example, cyanosis, a dusky blue color, may be observed in the nail beds, lips, and oral mucosa (Figure 2-2). It results from decreased oxyhemoglobin binding or decreased oxygenation of the blood. The yellow or green hue of jaundice, which develops when tissue bilirubin increases, may be noted first in the sclerae and then in the mucous membranes and skin. Pallor, or decreased color in the skin, results from decreased blood flow to the superficial vessels or from a decrease in the amount of hemoglobin in the blood; it is most evident in the face, palpebral conjunctivae, mouth, and nails. Generalized redness of the skin may be caused by fever, whereas defined areas of redness may be caused by a localized infection or sunburn.

Skin palpation is used to amplify the findings ob-

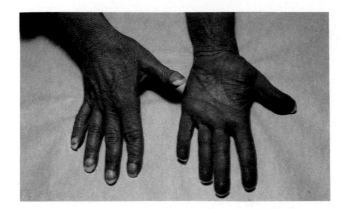

FIGURE 2-2
Cyanosis of hand and fingers. (Also note severe clubbing.)
(From Cannobio.)[10]

served through inspection and usually is carried out as each body part is examined. Changes in temperature, moisture, texture, and turgor are detected by palpation.

The *hair* over the entire body is examined to determine the distribution and pattern, quantity, and quality (texture and color). Persons receiving cancer chemotherapeutic agents may experience partial or complete alopecia as well as loss of body hair.

The assessment of the *nails*, for overall condition and possible evidence of systemic disease, includes examination for shape, normal dorsal curvature, adhesion to the nail bed, regularity of the nail surface, color, and thickness. The skinfolds around the nails are examined for color changes, swelling, increased temperature, and tenderness. Certain anemias may cause alterations in nail shape or size; for example, iron deficiency anemia results in thin, brittle, and "spoon-shaped" or concave nails.

LYMPHATIC ASSESSMENT
Superficial Lymph Nodes

Lymph nodes are located along the lymphatic vessels; they can be identified as superficial nodes in the subcutaneous connective tissue or as deep nodes under the muscular fascia.* They rarely are found isolated, but rather are grouped in chains or clusters. The exact number of lymph nodes varies from one individual to another, but smaller lymph nodes appear to be more proliferative.

Physical assessment of the superficial lymph nodes enables the nurse to detect enlarged, tender, or mobile lymph nodes, providing functional information about the immune system.

*The entire discussion on lymphatic assessment is from Mudge-Grout CL: *Immunologic disorders*, St. Louis, 1992, Mosby–Year Book.

Lymph node assessment includes inspection and palpation. Using a centimeter ruler may be helpful in measuring the exact size of the lymph node being examined. When a node has been identified, it must be evaluated according to location, size, surface characteristics, consistency, symmetry, fixation and mobility, tenderness and pain, erythema, heat, and increased vascularity (see box on the next page). *Assessment of the lymph nodes begins with the neck nodes and proceeds to other nodal areas as each related area of the body is examined.*

Inspect the body for prominent lymph nodes, erythema, and red streaks that follow lymphatic drainage patterns. Palpate the lymph nodes using the pads of the second, third, and fourth fingers. Start by pressing very lightly, using a rotary motion; gradually increase the pressure. Heavier pressure can move the node before it can be felt. Concern is warranted when the node is firm and fixed. When enlarged nodes are identified, evaluate the adjacent areas and those regions drained by the involved nodes for infection or malignancy (Figure 2-3).

Generally lymph nodes are not palpable in a healthy, well-developed adult. In a child, thin adult, or someone who has had a viral infection, they will be easier to feel. When lymph nodes are palpable, they should be smooth, symmetric, slightly soft, and mobile and have clearly defined edges. The node should have no pain, tenderness, erythema, or warmth to touch.

Normal lymph nodes vary considerably in size, from next to unidentifiable to the size of a coffee bean or even as large as an olive. They usually are round or oval in shape. However, they have also been observed as flat and elongated or cylindric. Generally lymph nodes closer to the middle of the body are smaller than

- Inflamed, tender, fixed, or matted nodes indicate a problem and require further evaluation.
- Hard, firm, immobile, irregularly shaped, and nontender nodes often involve a malignancy.
- Generalized lymphadenopathy involving three or more nodal regions may indicate an inflammation, infection, autoimmune disorder, or neoplastic process.

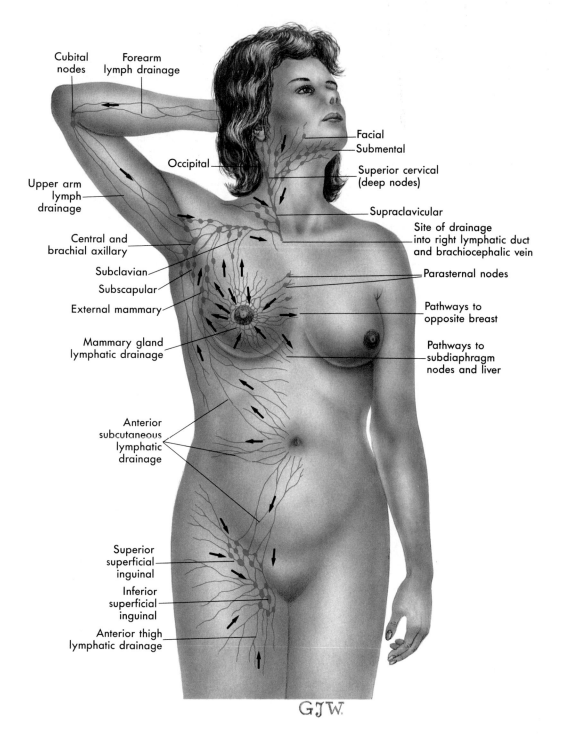

FIGURE 2-3
Lymphatic drainage. (From Mudge-Grout.)[42a]

ASSESSMENT CHARACTERISTICS OF LYMPH NODES OR MASSES

Location: Be specific in describing the site; use imaginary body lines or bony prominences to relate findings; draw pictures when appropriate.

Size: Define the volume in centimeters, using a tape measure, from the three dimensions of length, width, and thickness; state the total volume; accurately describe the shape (round, cylindric); if irregular, draw pictures.

Surface characteristics: Describe accurately as smooth, nodular, or irregular.

Consistency: Describe as hard, firm, soft, resilient, spongy, cystic (cysts usually are transluminal; nodes are not).

Symmetry: Describe symmetry, and compare with other structures; clearly define the edges.

Fixation and mobility: Describe the exact mobile parameters in centimeters; if the mass is fixed in position, identify whether fixation is to underlying or overlying tissue by trying to move it with your fingers; matted nodes are enlarged nodes that feel like a mass.

Tenderness and pain: Describe whether present without stimulation or elicited by palpation or movement; indicate whether direct, referred, or rebound; malignant nodes generally are nontender; inflamed and infected nodes generally are painful.

Erythema: Describe the extent of color change, if present, and the area of distribution.

Heat: Describe the extent if present.

Increased vascularity: Describe the prominence of overlying veins or cyanosis of the area.

---

those that are more superficial. For example, the axillary and inguinal lymph nodes typically are larger than the supraclavicular or iliac lymph nodes. Small, movable nodes less than 1 cm in size are of minimal concern. For example, an occasional small, firm node found in the cervical or inguinal regions is called a "shotty" node; these shotty nodes usually are clinically insignificant.

Infants and children under 2 years of age often have widespread lymph node enlargement, which usually decreases with age. Fibrosis and fatty degeneration typically are found on pathologic examination of nodes in the elderly.

Head and Neck Lymph Nodes

A systematic approach to assessing the lymph nodes of the head and neck is mandatory. If a meticulous method is not used during the assessment, portions of the lymph node chain probably will be overlooked.

Inspect the regions where the lymph nodes are located. Have the patient slightly rotate his head to either side and tilt it backward. Look for any obvious swollen or reddened lymph nodes, asymmetry, masses, or lesions. Ask the patient if he has any tenderness in his head or neck.

Most of the nodes in the body that are palpable are located in the head and neck. Identifying the anterior and posterior triangles at the lateral side of the neck can assist the examiner in palpating the lymph nodes of the head and neck.

The lymph nodes of the head and neck are palpated with the patient in a sitting position. The patient's neck should be flexed slightly forward and toward the side being examined. Face the patient, and place the fingertips of your right hand at the location of the preauricular nodes, just anterior to the ear (Figure 2-4). Use your left hand to support the patient's head. By using the pads of the index finger and middle fingers of both hands, the skin is rolled in a gentle but firm circular motion (not pushed) over the underlying tissue. Gentle, firm, and consistent pressure should be applied (pushing too hard on the nodes will obliterate them in the deeper soft tissue). Next, sequentially palpate the postauricular nodes located behind the ear, the occipital nodes at the base of the skull, and the tonsillar nodes. Then, move your fingertips to the underside of the mandible on the side you are examining. Pull the skin and subcutaneous tissue laterally over the ramus of the mandible at the location of the submandibular nodes, between the chin and the angle of the mandible (Figure 2-5). Sequentially palpate the submandibular, sublingual, and submental nodes. Examine the other side.

The posterior **cervical nodes** (spinal nerve chain and posterior superficial cervical chain) are examined next (Figure 2-6). The patient should be in a sitting position. Inspection of the neck begins with having the patient raise his chin and tilt his head slightly backward. Look for asymmetry, swelling, obvious lymph nodes, or masses, and palpate these areas.

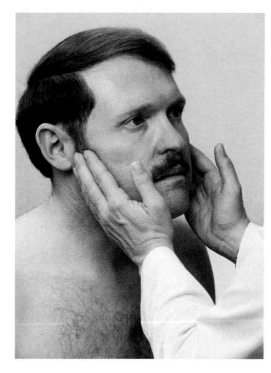

FIGURE 2-4
Palpation of the preauricular lymph nodes.

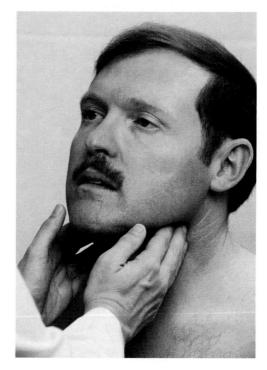

FIGURE 2-5
Palpation of the submandibular lymph nodes.

Table 2-1

REGIONAL LYMPH NODE ASSESSMENT

Lymph node region	Normal findings	Abnormal findings
Head and neck nodes	Small (<1 cm), smooth, nontender, possibly firm (as in a "shotty node"), and with well-defined edges	Tender or enlarged nodes
Cervical nodes	Palpable in children and adolescents; gradually diminish with age, and by fifth decade are reduced by 50%	Nodes with a diameter of ≥1 cm indicate a malignancy; enlarged nodes in children usually are due to an infection
Supraclavicular nodes	Should not be palpable	Enlarged, firm, fixed nodes in patients >35 yr indicate malignancy; tender nodes suggest infection or inflammation
Axillary nodes	Most are not palpable; of the central axillary nodes, one or two nontender, small nodes may be palpable	Enlarged or tender nodes may indicate a malignancy; this mandates reexamination of the supraclavicular and infraclavicular nodes
Upper extremity nodes: epitrochlear node	Not palpable or very small (<1 cm)	Enlargement may suggest secondary syphilis or inflammation
Lower extremity nodes: popliteal and inguinal nodes	Popliteal nodes generally are not palpable; inguinal nodes are larger than other nodes in the body (approximately 1 cm) and may be palpable; if so, they should be small, soft, and mobile	Enlarged inguinal nodes (>1 cm) indicate a lesion or inflammation in the vulva, lower aspect of the vagina, penis, or scrotal surface

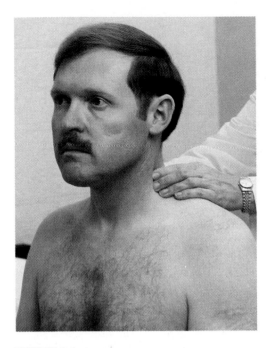

FIGURE 2-6
Palpation of the postcervical lymph nodes.

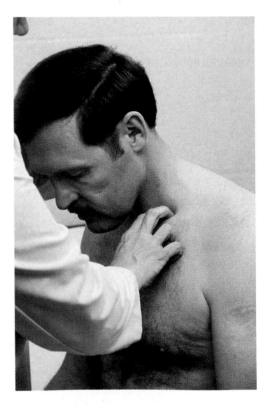

FIGURE 2-7
Palpation of the supraclavicular lymph nodes.

PALPATING LYMPH NODES AND NECK

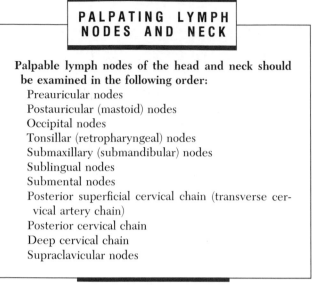

Palpable lymph nodes of the head and neck should be examined in the following order:
Preauricular nodes
Postauricular (mastoid) nodes
Occipital nodes
Tonsillar (retropharyngeal) nodes
Submaxillary (submandibular) nodes
Sublingual nodes
Submental nodes
Posterior superficial cervical chain (transverse cervical artery chain)
Posterior cervical chain
Deep cervical chain
Supraclavicular nodes

Palpation may be initiated from either in front or in back of the patient. To examine the posterior cervical nodes, support the patient's head with one hand and with the fingertips of the other hand palpate along the anterior surface of the trapezius muscle. Use a circular motion, moving toward the posterior surface of the sternocleidomastoid muscle. Examine the other side.

The anterior triangle, which harbors the deep cervical chain, is largely obstructed by the overlying sternomastoid muscle. However, it is possible to palpate the nodes at either end of this chain, the tonsillar and supraclavicular nodes, respectively. To examine the anterior triangle, hold the patient's chin in your left hand and gently palpate the nodes of this chain. Start with the tonsillar node and move the fingertips down the neck to the terminal node of this chain, the supraclavicular node. Then examine the other side.

For examination of the **supraclavicular nodes** (Virchow's nodes), the patient should be in a sitting position. Encourage the patient to relax the muscles of the upper body and allow the clavicles to drop. Bend the patient's head forward with your left hand (this promotes relaxation of the sternocleidomastoid muscle and the anterior neck, promoting exposure of the scalene triangle) (Figure 2-7). Inspect the area for nodal enlargement or erythema. To palpate these nodes, hook your right index finger over the clavicle lateral to the tendinous portion of the sternocleidomastoid muscle. The index finger should probe deeply in a rotary motion into the scalene triangle to allow the supraclavicular nodes to be palpated. At the completion of the examination, the entire neck is lightly palpated for nodes.

Axillary Nodes

Examination of the axillary nodes is approached by visualizing the area as a four-sided pyramid with its apex being the most superior point. The apex is located at the level between the first rib and clavicle in the axilla (the apex is the uppermost part of the armpit).

The axillary nodes are **inspected** with the patient in a sitting position. Observe for any obvious swollen or reddened lymph nodes. Inspect the skin of each axilla, and observe for evidence of a rash, erythema, or changes in pigmentation.

To palpate the axillary nodes, stand in front of the patient and ask him to relax his left arm down (Figure 2-8). Assist him by supporting his left forearm with your right hand. To palpate the patient's left axilla, cup the fingers of your right hand and reach high into the apex of the patient's axilla. Slowly bring your fingers down in a rotary motion over the surface of his ribs, milking the axillary contents downward. Feel for the central nodes by compressing them against the chest wall and muscles of the axilla. Continue to palpate in a rotary motion deep inside the anterior and posterior axillary folds and along the upper humerus to feel for the pectoral (anterior), subcapsular (posterior), and lateral axillary nodes. If these last nodes are difficult to palpate, they may be more easily palpated by standing behind the patient. Then examine the other side.

Lymph Nodes of the Extremities

The **epitrochlear node** is the only peripheral lymph center in the upper extremities. It is located on the medial surface of the arm above the elbow in the depression above and posterior to the medial condyle of the humerus.

The epitrochlear nodes are **inspected** with the patient in a sitting position. Observe for any obvious swollen or reddened lymph nodes. Inspect the skin, and check for evidence of nodules, rash, erythema, or changes in pigmentation. To palpate the epitrochlear nodes, support the patient's elbow with one hand and assess the nodes with the other. Use the same rotary motion with the pads of the first three fingers. Examine the other side.

The lower extremities are made up of an extensive network of deep and superficial lymphatic ducts. Only the superficial ducts are palpable. They drain lymph from the legs primarily into the **popliteal** and **superficial inguinal lymph centers.** The popliteal lymph center comprises two or three nodes. It is located posterior to the knee close to the terminal end of the saphenous vein. There are two groups of superficial inguinal lymph centers, the horizontal (superior) group and the vertical (inferior) group (Figure 2-9).

The horizontal group comprises five or six nodes lo-

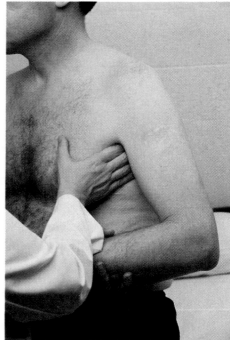

FIGURE 2-8
Palpation of the axillary lymph nodes.

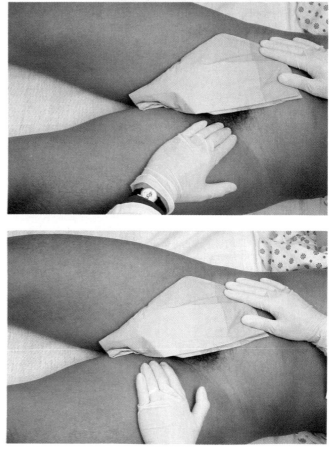

A

B

FIGURE 2-9
Palpation of the inguinal lymph nodes. **A,** Superior (horizontal). **B,** Inferior (vertical). (From Mudge-Grout.)[42a]

cated just inferior and parallel to the inguinal ligament. The vertical group comprises four or five large lymph nodes located just inferior to the junction of the saphenous and femoral veins. Only the horizontal and vertical superficial inguinal lymph nodes are palpable. The nodes are examined with the patient in the supine position, legs slightly apart, with the examiner to one side. Maintain the patient's modesty by covering the genitalia during the examination.

Inspect the nodal area for edema, redness, and changes in the skin. Observe for enlarged nodes. Palpate the vertical inguinal lymph nodes by placing your right thumb on top of the upper aspect of the patient's right thigh. Then use the pads of the first three fingers, which should cup right over to the medial aspect of the leg, to palpate these inguinal nodes. Continue to use a rotary motion when palpating for these nodes. To palpate for the horizontal nodes, move the fingers of the right hand to the area just below the inguinal ligament, using the same rotary motion. Examine the other side.

CARDIOVASCULAR FUNCTION

Assessment of cardiovascular function often is divided into three parts: inspection, palpation, and auscultation. Inspection and palpation should be done before applying the stethoscope for auscultation.

The precordium is best examined with the examiner standing on the patient's right side. Inspection and palpation are performed primarily with the patient in the supine position; auscultation, however, should be done with the patient in the forward sitting, supine, and left lateral recumbent positions because each position brings various parts of the heart closer to the chest wall (Figure 2-10).

A thorough examination includes the peripheral pulses (i.e., the radial, brachial, femoral, popliteal, dorsalis pedis, and posterior tibial pulses). Also included are assessment of the abdominal aorta and assessment of the blood pressure in the upper and lower extremities in the sitting, standing, and lying positions. These components may be assessed during this portion of the physical examination or may be integrated into other portions.

The purpose of both inspection and palpation is to determine the presence and extent of normal and abnormal pulsations over the precordium. Together the two techniques provide valuable information on left, right, and combined ventricular hypertrophy. Inspection includes inspecting the chest wall and epigastrium for size and symmetry and then for any pulsations, retractions, heaves, or lifts. The location and timing of all impulses should be noted. Palpation builds on and expands the findings gleaned from inspection. The entire precordium is palpated methodically, beginning

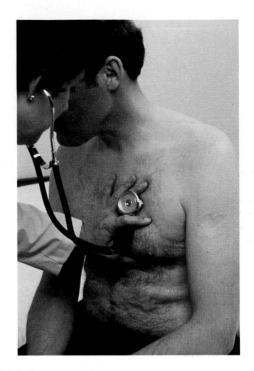

FIGURE 2-10
Auscultation of heart sounds.

at the apex, moving to the left sternal border, and then to the base of the heart. Other areas may be included as need is indicated. During palpation the examiner is searching for the apical impulse at or near the apex and for any abnormal heaves, thrills, or retractions elsewhere on the precordium.

In auscultation, the stethoscope gathers and slightly amplifies sound before it is transmitted to the ears. The stethoscope's chestpiece should be equipped with both a bell and a diaphragm, each of which selectively transmits different frequencies of sound. Throughout auscultation the patient should be asked to change from sitting to supine to left lateral recumbent positions, since auscultation in only one position is inadequate. A systematic method may begin at the apex and move toward the left sternal border and up to both right and left intercostal spaces.

> Persons with anemias are particularly vulnerable to cardiac dysfunction as a result of increased blood pressure and increased cardiac output as compensatory mechanisms in the presence of blood loss, or inadequate hemoglobin, whether acute or chronic. Platelet and clotting disorders also stress cardiovascular function due to blood loss into the tissues as well as from the body.

In each area examined the nurse listens selectively to each component of the cardiac cycle. First she notes rate and rhythm; then, at each auscultatory area, she concentrates initially on S_1, then S_2, then systole, then diastole.

RESPIRATORY FUNCTION

The equipment needed includes a stethoscope with a bell and diaphragm, a marking pencil, and a centimeter rule. Inspection is performed to measure and assess the pattern of respirations; to assess the skin and the overall symmetry and integrity of the thorax; and to assess thoracic configuration.

For adequate inspection of the thorax, the patient should be sitting upright without support and uncovered to the waist. The examiner first observes the general shape of the thorax and its symmetry. Although no individual is absolutely symmetric in both body hemispheres, most individuals are reasonably similar side to side. The examination is regional and integrated, and examination of systems is combined in body regions when appropriate. Since the patient is uncovered to the waist, a large portion of skin and tissue is accessible to inspection. Thoracic configuration, ribs and interspaces, pattern of respiration, and lips and nails are all assessed.

Palpation is performed to further assess abnormalities suggested by the history or observation (e.g., tenderness, pulsations, masses, or skin lesions) and to assess the skin and subcutaneous structures; thoracic expansion; vocal (tactile) fremitus; and tracheal position.

Percussion is the tapping of an object to set underlying structures in motion and consequently to produce a sound, called a percussion note, and palpable vibration. Percussion is used in the thoracic examination to determine the relative amounts of air, liquid, or solid material in the underlying lung and to determine the positions and boundaries of organs.

The two techniques of percussion are *direct*, or *immediate*, percussion and *indirect*, or *mediate*, percussion. In direct percussion the examiner strikes the area to be percussed directly with the palmar aspect of two, three, or four fingers held together or with the palmar aspect of the tip of the middle finger. The strikes are rapid and downward from the wrist. This type of percussion is not normally used in thoracic examination but is useful in the thorax of an infant or the sinuses of an adult.

In indirect percussion, the examiner strikes an object held against the area to be examined. The middle finger of the examiner's left hand (if the examiner is right-handed) is the pleximeter. The distal phalanx and joint and the middle phalanx are placed firmly on the surface to be percussed. The point to be struck by the plexor should be pressed as tightly as possible against the patient, with all other areas of that hand held off the patient's skin. The plexor is the index finger of the examiner's right hand or the index and middle fingers held together.

With the forearm and shoulder stationary and all movement at the wrist, the pleximeter is struck sharply

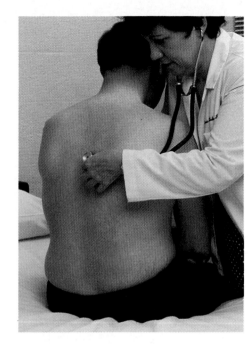

FIGURE 2-11
Auscultation of lungs.

with the plexor. The blow is aimed at the part of the pleximeter that is exerting maximum pressure on the thoracic surface, usually the base of the terminal phalanx, the distal interphalangeal joint, or the middle phalanx. The blow is executed rapidly, and the plexor is immediately withdrawn. The plexor strikes with the tip of the finger at right angles to the pleximeter. One or two rapid blows are struck in each area.

With experience and study, the nurse will be able to differentiate among the five percussion tones—resonant, flat, dull, tympanic, hyperresonant—commonly elicited on the human body and will be able to evaluate them for intensity, pitch, duration, and quality.

> Respiratory function may be altered as a result of blood volume depletion in general or inadequate hemoglobin concentration in particular. The presence of infection also increases respiratory rate and audible congestion, particularly in patients with leukemia.

Before *auscultation* the patient should be directed to breathe through the mouth more deeply and slowly than usual (Figure 2-11). The examiner systematically auscultates the apices and the posterior, lateral, and anterior chest. At each application of the stethoscope, the examiner listens to at least one complete respiration. The examiner should observe the patient for signs of hyperventilation and should stop the procedure if the patient becomes light-headed or faint. The process of auscultation involves (1) analyzing breath sounds, (2) detecting abnormal sounds, and (3) examining the sounds produced by the spoken voice. As with percussion the examiner should use a zigzag procedure, comparing the finding at each point with the corresponding point on the opposite hemithorax.

NEUROMUSCULAR/MUSCULOSKELETAL FUNCTION

Cephalocaudal (head to toe) organization is used in examining the bones, joints, and muscles, because this sequence provides order and helps prevent omissions. Side-to-side comparison is the basic criterion for assessment. A general inspection includes visual scanning for symmetry, contour, size, involuntary movement of the two sides of the body, gross deformities, areas of swelling or edema, and ecchymoses or other discoloration.

The *posture,* or stance, and body alignment are viewed from both in front of and behind the patient. The structural relationships of the feet to the legs and the hips to the pelvis are noted, as are those of the upper extremities, shoulder girdle, and upper trunk. Examination frequently includes *measurement of the extremities* for length and circumference, again, to verify symmetry and any deviation from the norm. These measurements are taken with the patient lying relaxed on a hard surface with the pelvis level and the hips equally adducted. Along these same lines, muscles are examined for gross hypertrophy or atrophy. Although muscle size is largely a function of the use or disuse of the muscle fibers, changes in size may indicate disease. The limbs should be in the same position and the muscles in the same state of tension each time measurements are taken.

Gait is evaluated in both the stance phase and the swing phase to evaluate rhythm and smoothness. Stance consists of three processes: (1) heel strike (the heel contacts the floor or the ground), (2) midstance (body weight is transferred from the heel to the ball of the foot), and (3) push-off (the heel leaves the ground). The swing phase also consists of three processes: (1) acceleration (weight shifts from second foot as first foot swings forward), (2) swing through (the lifted foot travels ahead of the weight-bearing foot), and (3) deceleration (the foot slows in preparation for the heel strike). The description of the patient's gait should include phase, cadence, stride length, trunk posture, pelvic posture, and arm swing.

Bones and joints are examined for deformity or tumors and for integrity by testing resistance to a deforming force. Bones are palpated to check for pain or tenderness, and range of motion is measured by the degree of deviation from a defined neutral zero point for each joint (Figure 2-12). The position of neutral zero is that of the extended extremity or anatomic position. Seven types of joint motion can be measured in this

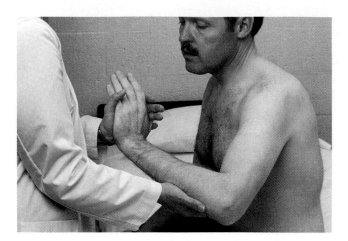

FIGURE 2-12
Examination of joints.

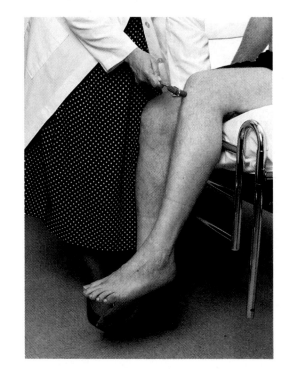

FIGURE 2-13
Eliciting the knee-jerk reflex.

way: flexion, extension, abduction, adduction, internal rotation, external rotation, and circumduction.

The examination of the joints, described above, may be incorporated into *examination of functional muscle groups.* The assessment sequence used in examining muscles is inspection, palpation, and testing of muscle strength. As with the bones, muscles are examined in symmetric pairs; that is, first one and then the other for equivalence in size, contour, tone, and strength. The contralateral, matching muscle pairs should be uniformly positioned while they are examined both at rest

---

MENTAL STATUS

In evaluating mental status, the aim is to determine the patient's problems in living and the psychodynamics underlying them, since these factors can affect treatment planning. It is important to use the patient's own words in describing any symptoms. This information, coupled with certain visible cues, can reveal a lot about the patient's awareness and response to signs and symptoms and orientation for person, place, and time. Orientation usually is lost initially in the sphere of time, followed by place, and finally by person. Deviation from this order should be reported.

Besides obtaining a verbal description of the patient's problems, the nurse should watch for body language, facial expressions, and behaviors that indicate not only level of awareness and education but also speed of response to motor activity instructions, length of attention span, cooperativeness, aggressiveness, and mood.

Patients with anemias may experience irritability or confusion caused by cerebral tissue hypoxia. Those experiencing blood loss as a result of platelet or clotting disorders often become confused and lethargic, and advance to coma if interventions are not initiated in a timely manner.

---

and in a state of contraction. The muscles are palpated to detect swelling, localized temperature changes, and marked changes in shape, consistency, or tone. *Muscle strength* may be assessed throughout the full range of motion for each muscle or group of muscles. A simple screening test can be performed in less than 5 minutes and allows the examiner to find nearly any muscle or reflex abnormality (Figure 2-13). Although muscle weakness in adults generally is mild and transitory, it may be the result of musculoskeletal, neurologic, metabolic, or infectious problems.

> Patients with such clotting disorders as hemophilia are particularly susceptible to bleeding into the joints. Those with anemias often experience fatigue and muscular weakness due to tissue hypoxia.

A concept of clinical importance in the examination of the musculoskeletal system is the distinction between upper and lower *motor neuron involvement*. Lesions of the upper motor neuron produce a spasticity or hypertonicity of the affected muscles, but muscle strength is not diminished. Tendon stretch reflexes are brisk, and Babinski's sign is present if the lesion is in the corticospinal tract. Atrophy occurs only with disuse. By contrast, lesions of the lower motor neurons produce flaccidity or loss of muscle tone. The hypotonus leads to atrophy, fasciculations are seen, and tendon reflexes are depressed or absent. The distinction between the two types of nerve involvement often can be made during palpation of the muscle and tests for muscle strength.

SENSORY FUNCTION

The equipment needed for sensory testing includes a cotton wisp or soft brush, a safety pin, test tubes for cold and warm water, a tuning fork, and calipers or a compass with dull points. Although it is not necessary to evaluate sensation over the entire skin surface, stimuli should be applied strategically to test dermatomes and major peripheral nerves. Test sites should include the forehead, cheek, hand, lower arm, abdomen, foot, and lower leg.

Usually the more distal area of the limb is checked first; the nerve may be assumed to be intact if sensation is normal at its most peripheral extent. If evidence of dysfunction is found, the specific boundaries of the site of dysfunction (the area experiencing loss of sensation) must be localized and mapped in a sketch of the region, and a written description of the sensory change must be included.

Just as the more distal area is checked first, the intensity of the stimulus is also kept to a minimum on initial application. The intensity may be increased gradually until the patient is aware of the stimulus. Of course, skin areas normally vary in sensitivity, with a stronger stimulus required over areas such as the back and buttocks and where the skin is heavily cornified. Symmetry of sensation is established by checking first one spot and then its mirror image area.

Perception of light and deep touch are mediated by different nerve endings. Light touch is tested by touching the skin with a wisp of cotton or a soft brush without perceptibly depressing the skin and without stimu-

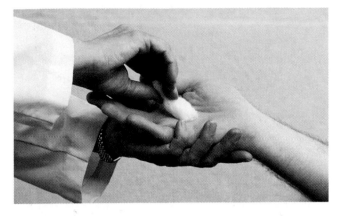

FIGURE 2-14
Examination of sensory function.

lating the sensory fibers of hair follicles (Figure 2-14). The patient is instructed to indicate verbally when he feels the stimulus and to point to the site where the sensation is felt.

Superficial pain and *pressure* tests can be conducted by using the sharp and hub ends of a sterile safety pin or hypodermic needle. The patient is asked to identify sensations as sharp, dull, or "can't tell." At least 2 seconds should be allowed between successive tests to avoid summation effects (several stimuli perceived as one). Deep pressure is tested over the Achilles tendons, forearms, and calf muscles by squeezing the muscle. The patient should experience discomfort.

Temperature sensation need not be evaluated if pain sensation is normal. If temperature sensation must be tested, tubes filled with warm and cold water are rolled against the patient's skin (the examiner first tests the stimuli on her own skin). The patient is asked to identify each sensation as hot, cold, or "can't tell."

Vibration sensation involves testing with a tuning fork. Normally a patient can distinguish vibration when the base of a vibrating tuning fork is applied to a bony prominence such as the sternum, elbow, or ankle. This sensation typically is perceived as a buzzing or tingling. The greatest sensitivity to vibration is seen when the fork is vibrating between 200 and 400 c/s, with vibration lasting longer in proportion to the size of the tuning fork. As a rule, the sites tested include the clavicles, spinous processes, elbows, finger joints, knees, ankles, and toes. The patient is asked to close his eyes and then indicate when he first detects the vibrations and when they stop.

Tactile discrimination is evaluated clinically by testing for three types: (1) stereognosis, (2) two-point discrimination, and (3) extinction. Stereognosis is the recognition of objects through touch and manipulation. Objects used to test stereognosis should be universally familiar items such as a key or a coin. Two-

point discrimination is the ability to sense whether one or two areas of the skin are being stimulated by pressure. This may be done with pins, calipers, or a compass with dull points. One pin is held in each hand, and they are applied to the skin simultaneously. The patient is asked whether he feels one or two pinpricks. Again, perception varies considerably over different areas of the body. For example, on the tongue the minimum distance between two points at which normal adults can sense simultaneous stimulation is 1 mm, on the forearms the minimum distance is 40 mm, and on the thighs it is 75 mm. The extinction phenomenon is tested by simultaneously touching the same body parts bilaterally with a sterile needle point. The patient should be able to detect both stimuli and identify their locations.

Kinesthetic sensation is the ability to identify position, orientation, and motion of limbs and body parts. With his eyes closed, the patient is asked to describe changes in position of a finger on his hand (the finger is always moved to a neutral position before it is moved again). This procedure may be followed for any joint.

Graphesthesia measures the patient's ability to discern the identity of letters or numbers inscribed on the palm of the hand, back, or other areas with a blunt object.

PAIN ASSESSMENT

Pain and temperature nerve fibers both travel in the dorsolateral fasciculus for a short distance, after which they cross and continue to the thalamus in the lateral spinothalamic tract.

Superficial pain evaluation has already been discussed in the section on sensory function. The evaluation can be conducted using the sharp and dull ends of a safety pin, but because recent studies have indicated a risk of infection with safety pins, some examiners use the hub (dull) and point (sharp) of a hypodermic needle.

THE ABDOMEN

Physical assessment of the abdomen includes all four methods of examination (inspection, auscultation, percussion, and palpation). Inspection is done first, followed by auscultation, because the movement or stimulation by pressure on the bowel caused by palpation and percussion is known to alter the motility of the bowel and generally to heighten the sounds. Palpation

> Numerous blood disorders can alter sensory function, particularly the anemias. For example, pernicious anemia with the abnormally low hemoglobin experienced by the patient results in paresthesias of the fingers and feet, as well as difficulty in walking.

is the technique most useful in detecting pathologic conditions in the abdomen.

It is important to note the position that the patient assumes voluntarily. An individual with abdominal pain frequently draws up the knees to reduce tension on the abdominal muscles and to reduce intraabdominal pressure. A patient with generalized peritonitis lies almost motionless with the knees flexed. Marked restlessness has been associated with biliary and intestinal colic and intraperitoneal hemorrhage. Patients with hepatosplenomegaly will be more comfortable sitting up because of abdominal distention.

The best position for the patient during an abdominal examination is supine with the abdominal muscles as relaxed as possible. To prevent tension in the abdominal wall muscles, the patient's arms should be placed comfortably at his sides and a small pillow should be put beneath his knees to help keep the legs in slight flexion.

After positioning the patient, the nurse first does a careful visual inspection of the abdomen to identify the presence or absence of symmetry, distention, masses, visible peristaltic waves, and respiratory movements (Figure 2-15). If the presence of peristalsis is in question, the examiner should carefully study the abdomen for several minutes, first from a sitting position on the right side of the patient with the examiner's head only slightly higher than the patient's abdomen. Then the examiner should inspect the abdomen from a standing position at the foot of the bed or examining table (asymmetry of the abdominal contour may be more readily detected from this position).

Either of two methods of subdividing the abdomen —into four quadrants or nine sections—can help determine the normal position of organs. Certain anatomic structures have been used as landmarks to facilitate the description of abdominal signs and symptoms. These landmarks are the ensiform (xiphoid) process of the sternum, the costal margin, the midline, the umbilicus, the anterosuperior iliac spine, Poupart's (inguinal) ligament, and the superior margin of the os pubis. The abdominal structures protected by the rib cage (the liver, stomach, and spleen) are evaluated by palpation and percussion.

Skin, abdominal contour, respiratory movement, visible peristalsis, and pulsation are all visually assessed; auscultation comes next, preceding percussion to prevent increased stimulation of bowel sounds. The diaphragm of the stethoscope is used to listen to the sounds of air and fluid as they move through the gastrointestinal tract (Figure 2-16). This helps in evaluating bowel motility through the detection of either increased or decreased bowel sounds, arterial sounds, and venous hums.

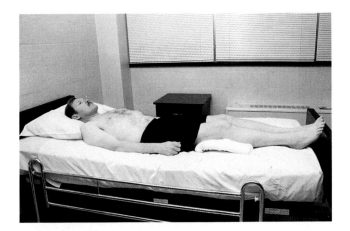

FIGURE 2-15
Patient positioned for inspection of the abdomen.

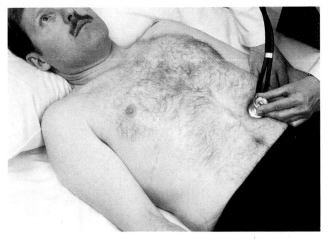

FIGURE 2-16
Auscultation of the abdomen.

The scratch test makes use of the difference in sound over solid as opposed to hollow organs. Actually a percussion technique, it occasionally is used to assess the size of the liver. The peritoneal friction rub provides a rough, grating sound that resembles two pieces of leather being rubbed together. Common causes of friction rubs include splenic infection, abscesses, or tumors.

Percussion of the abdomen is used to detect fluid, gaseous distention, and masses and to assess solid structures in the abdomen. This technique helps delineate the position and size of the liver and spleen (Figure 2-17). The entire abdomen should be percussed lightly for a general picture of the areas of tympany and dullness and for free fluid. Solid masses percuss as dull, as does a distended bladder. Fist percussion is used to vibrate the tissue rather than to produce sound. The palm of the left hand is placed over the region of liver dullness, and the hand is struck a light blow by the fisted right hand.

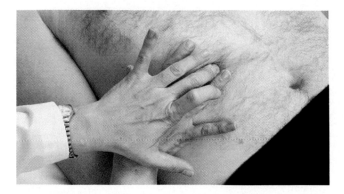

FIGURE 2-17
Percussion of the abdomen, focusing on the liver.

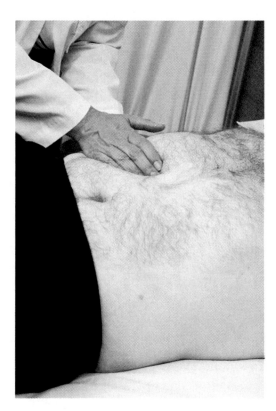

FIGURE 2-18
Palpation of the abdomen.

After careful visual scrutiny, auscultation, and percussion, palpation is used to substantiate findings and to explore the abdomen further. Palpation is used to evaluate the major organs of the abdomen, which are examined for shape, position and mobility, size, consistency, and tension (Figure 2-18). Thorough and systematic screening is performed to detect areas of tenderness, muscular spasm, masses, or fluid. Light palpation is used to assess hypersensitivity and muscle spasticity;

moderate palpation is used to assess organs that move with respiration, such as the liver and spleen; deep palpation is used to assess deeper structures such as retroperitoneal organs (e.g., the kidneys) and may be used to obtain more specific information about a lesion or mass detected by lighter palpation. Bimanual palpation may be used when additional pressure is needed to overcome resistance or to examine a deep abdominal structure, to determine the size of a mass, or to detect a pulsatile mass. Ballottement is a palpation technique used to assess a floating object.

The above techniques are used to examine the liver, gallbladder, spleen, pancreas, kidneys, urinary bladder, and umbilicus.

RENAL FUNCTION

Palpation of the kidneys is best accomplished with the patient in the supine position and with the examiner standing on the patient's right side. For the left kidney, the examiner reaches across the patient with the left arm, placing the hand behind the left flank. Elevating the left flank displaces the kidney anteriorly. The examiner uses the palm of the right hand to palpate deeply through the abdominal wall (Figure 2-19).

The kidneys usually are not palpable in an adult, and only the lower pole of the right kidney can be felt in very thin people. The kidneys may be more readily palpated in the elderly because of the loss of muscle tone and elastic fibers that accompanies aging. The left kidney generally is not palpable.

The examiner remains on the patient's right side to examine the right kidney. The right flank is similarly elevated with the left hand, and the right hand is used to palpate deeply for the right kidney. The lower pole of the right kidney may be felt as a smooth, rounded mass that descends on inspiration.

Splenic and kidney enlargement may be differentiated by percussion. The percussion note over the spleen is dull, since the bowel is displaced downward, whereas resonance is heard over the kidney because of the intervening bowel. Also, the free edge of the spleen is sharper in contour and tends to enlarge caudally and to the right.

> Patients with sickle cell anemia experience difficulty with urination as a result of occlusion of the microcirculation by sickling cells, particularly during sickle cell crisis.

The urinary bladder normally is not palpable unless it is distended with urine. When it is distended with urine, it may be felt as a smooth, round, rather tense mass. Percussion may be used to define the outline of the distended bladder, which may extend up as far as the umbilicus.

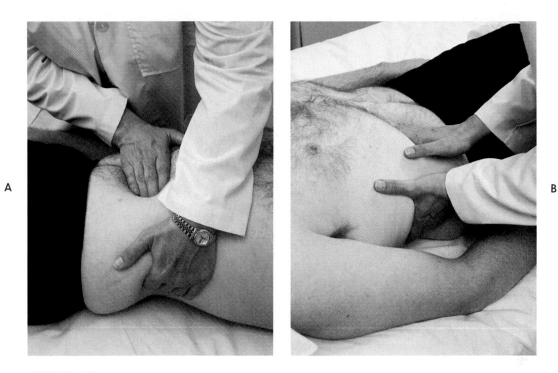

FIGURE 2-19
Technique for kidney palpation. **A,** Left kidney. **B,** Right kidney.

GENITAL/SEXUAL FUNCTION
Male Genitalia

Inspection and palpation are performed consecutively for each portion of the genitalia. After the inguinal and genital areas are exposed, the skin, hair, and gross appearance of the penis and scrotum are inspected. The size of the penis and the secondary sex characteristics are assessed in relationship to the patient's age and general development. If inflammation or lesions are observed or suspected, gloves are used for the examination. Pubic hair and enlarged testes appear by 16 years of age, and penile enlargement and seminal emission generally occur by age 17.

The penis is assessed for color, lesions, nodules, swelling, inflammation, and discharge. If the patient is uncircumcised, he is asked to retract the prepuce from the glans, and the glans and foreskin are examined carefully. The prepuce should retract easily from the glans and return easily to its original position.

The scrotum normally appears asymmetric because the left testis generally is lower than the right testis. Scrotal skin is more darkly pigmented than that of the rest of the body. The examiner should remember to inspect the posterior and posterolateral and anterior and anterolateral skin areas, the contents of each half of the scrotal sac, and each epididymis. The testes are palpated simultaneously between the thumb and the first two fingers and assessed for consistency, size, shape,

and tenderness. All scrotal masses should be described by their placement, size, shape, consistency, and tenderness and by whether they transilluminate.

In an ambulatory patient the prostate gland is most easily examined with the patient standing, hips flexed, toes pointed toward each other, and upper body resting on the examining table. This allows the gland and seminal vesicles to be palpated with the pad of the index finger.

> Persons with sickle cell anemia experience delayed sexual maturity, which may be manifested by small breasts or penis and sparse body hair.

Female Genitalia

Regional examination of the female genital system consists of seven steps: (1) the abdominal examination, (2) inspection of the external genitalia, (3) palpation of the external genitalia, (4) the speculum examination, (5) obtaining specimens, (6) the bimanual vaginal examination, and (7) the rectovaginal examination.

For the abdominal examination, the patient lies supine on the examination table with the examiner facing her right side (see the section on the Abdomen, above). For the inspection and palpation of the external genitalia and the speculum examination, the patient is in the lithotomy position and the examiner is seated on a stool, facing the patient's genitalia. The total skin area is inspected for lesions and parasites. The gloved fingers of one hand are used to spread the hair and labia so that all skin surfaces can be adequately visualized and palpated. The clitoris is examined for size. The labia majora and labia minora should feel soft, and the texture should be homogenous.

Next, the index and middle fingers are inserted into the vagina. First the urethra and the area of Skene's duct openings are gently milked from about 4 cm in on the anterior vaginal wall down to the orifice. This procedure normally should not cause pain or discharge. The examiner next observes the area of Bartholin's glands and their ducts for swelling, erythema, duct enlargement, or discharge; any of these conditions is abnormal. The perineum is inspected for evidence of a healed episiotomy, and the perineal area is palpated between the fingers inside the vagina and the thumb of the same hand.

Finally, in a third intravaginal maneuver, the index and middle fingers are spread laterally, and the patient is asked to push down against them. Urinary stress in-continence, cystocele, rectocele, enterocele, or uterine prolapse can be detected with this technique. The cervical Papanicolaou (Pap) smear is obtained during the vaginal examination.

The speculum examination allows the cervix to be inspected for color, position, size, projection into the vaginal vault, shape, general symmetry, surface characteristics, shape and patency of the os, and discharge.

For the bimanual and rectovaginal examinations, the patient remains in the lithotomy position, and the examiner stands. The bimanual examination involves palpation of the pelvic contents between the examiner's two hands. One hand is used to press the abdominal and pelvic contents toward the intravaginal hand. In addition to examination of the cervix, the size, shape, surface characteristics, consistency, position, mobility, and tenderness of the uterine body and fundus are assessed. In the rectovaginal examination the uterine position is confirmed, and the area of the rectovaginal septum and cul-de-sac is palpated. The uterosacral ligaments may be palpable. Skin and hair distribution are examined, and the anus is inspected.

CHAPTER 3

Diagnostic Procedures

COMPLETE BLOOD COUNT AND DIFFERENTIAL

The complete blood count (CBC) and differential count are a series of seven tests of the peripheral blood that provide information about the hematologic system and, because of its wide range of systemic effects, many other organ systems as well. These tests are performed as a quick, easy, and inexpensive screening test on almost every patient who enters the hospital (Figure 3-1).

Approximately 7 to 10 ml of peripheral venous blood is collected in a red-top tube and sent to the hematology laboratory for analysis.

See the box on page 33.

CONTRAINDICATIONS

None

PATIENT TEACHING

Explain the procedure. Advise the patient that although few complications are associated with this procedure, bleeding from the venipuncture site sometimes is seen in patients with thrombocytopenia.

A discussion of the seven tests included in the CBC series follows.

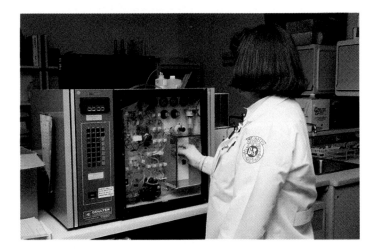

FIGURE 3-1
Medical technologist running a complete blood count.

RED BLOOD CELL (ERYTHROCYTE) COUNT

The red blood cell (RBC) count is a count of the number of circulating RBCs in a cubic milliliter of peripheral venous blood. Normal values vary according to sex and age. When the value is decreased by more than 10% of the expected normal value, the patient is said to be anemic.

RBC counts above normal can be physiologically induced if the body requires greater oxygen-carrying capacity (such as at high altitudes). Diseases that produce chronic anoxia (e.g., congenital heart disease) also provoke this physiologic increase in RBCs.

COLLECTING A BLOOD SPECIMEN

Instruct the patient in the procedure, and assemble the equipment: appropriate tubes for the tests being performed, 10- to 30-ml syringes (depending on the amount of blood needed for the test; often less blood is required for children), 21-gauge needle (butterfly), gloves, alcohol swabs, tourniquet, one 2 × 2 sterile gauze pad, plastic bandage strip (e.g., Band-Aid), and appropriate labels and forms. Wash your hands, and then clean the area with an alcohol swab in a circular motion from the inside out to remove superficial dirt and body oil. Allow the area to dry. Apply the tourniquet, and put on the gloves. Identify the vein, and perform the venipuncture, drawing up the appropriate amount of blood for the test.

Remove the tourniquet and then the needle, applying pressure to the site with the sterile gauze. Insert the needle with the syringe of blood into the appropriate tubes, and apply the plastic bandage strip to the venipuncture site.

Label the tubes, and complete the appropriate forms. The following information should be on all forms and tubes: patient's name, date, time the blood was drawn, and whether the blood was obtained peripherally or from a central line. Finally, send the specimen to the appropriate laboratory for testing. Many institutions have more than one laboratory for testing.

Note: Procedures for drawing blood from central or hemodialysis lines vary between institutions. Be sure you are familiar with the procedure in your facility before obtaining a blood sample from such a line.

(From Mudge-Grout).

HEMOGLOBIN CONCENTRATION

The hemoglobin (Hb) concentration test is a measure of the total amount of hemoglobin in the peripheral blood. Hemoglobin serves as a vehicle for oxygen and carbon dioxide transport. As with RBC counts, normal values vary according to sex and age. The clinical implications of this test closely parallel the RBC count. In addition, however, changes in plasma volume are more accurately reflected by hemoglobin concentrations.

HEMATOCRIT, OR PACKED RED CELL VOLUME

Hematocrit (Hct) is a measure of the percentage of RBCs in the total blood volume; thus it closely reflects the hemoglobin and RBC values. The hematocrit in percentage points usually is about three times the hemoglobin concentration in grams per deciliter when the RBCs are of normal size and contain normal amounts of hemoglobin.

MEAN CORPUSCULAR VOLUME

Mean corpuscular volume (MCV) is a measure of the average volume, or size, of a single red blood cell and is therefore useful in classifying anemias. It is derived by dividing the hematocrit by the total RBC. Normal values vary according to sex and age. When the MCV value is increased, the RBC is said to be abnormally large, or *macrocytic*. When the MCV value is decreased, the RBC is said to be abnormally small, or *microcytic*.

MEAN CORPUSCULAR HEMOGLOBIN

Mean corpuscular hemoglobin (MCH) is a measure of the average amount of hemoglobin in an RBC. This value is derived by dividing the total hemoglobin concentration by the number of RBCs. Because macrocytic cells generally have more hemoglobin and microcytic cells generally have less, the causes for these values closely resemble those for the MCV value.

MEAN CORPUSCULAR HEMOGLOBIN CONCENTRATION

The mean corpuscular hemoglobin concentration (MCHC) is a measure of the average concentration or the percentage of hemoglobin in a single RBC. This value is derived by dividing the total hemoglobin concentration by the hematocrit. When values are decreased, the cell has a deficiency of hemoglobin and is said to be *hypochromic*.

INDICATIONS FOR COMPLETE BLOOD COUNT (CBC)

Red blood cell count

To detect:
Anemia
Hemorrhage
Dietary deficiencies
Drug ingestion
Chronic illness (tumor, sepsis)
Chronic anoxia (congenital heart disease)
Hemolysis
Genetic aberrations
Marrow failure
Other organ failure (renal disease)

Hemoglobin concentration

To detect:
Hemorrhage
Dietary deficiency
Drug ingestion
Chronic illness (tumor or sepsis)
Overhydration
Dehydration
Hemolysis
Genetic aberrations
Marrow failure
Other organ failure (renal disease)
Expanded blood volume in pregnancy

Hematocrit or packed red cell volume

To detect:
Hemorrhage
Dietary deficiency
Drug ingestion
Chronic illness (tumor, sepsis)
Hemolysis
Genetic aberrations
Marrow failure
Other organ failure (renal disease)

Mean corpuscular volume (MCV); mean corpuscular hemoglobin (MCH); mean corpuscular hemoglobin concentration (MCHC)

To classify types and causes of anemia

White blood cell (leukocyte) count

To detect a wide range of disorders, including:

Altered neutrophil count

Respiratory disorders
Myelocytic leukemia
Metabolic disorders
Addison's disease
Neutropenia
Various infections
Cushing's syndrome
Aplastic anemia

Altered lymphocyte count

Lymphocytosis
Various infections
Lymphocytic leukemia
Multiple myeloma
Infectious mononucleosis
Lymphocytopenia
Leukemia
Sepsis
Immune deficiency
  diseases/AIDS
Infectious hepatitis

Altered monocyte count

Monocytosis
Chronic ulcerative colitis
Chronic inflammations
Monocytopenia
Viral infections
Tuberculosis

Altered eosinophil count

Eosinophilia
Parasitic infections
Eczema
Autoimmune diseases
Eosinopenia
Allergic reactions
Leukemia
Increased adrenal steroid production

Altered basophil count

Basophilia
Hyperthyroidism
Leukemia
Basopenia
Myeloproliferative disease
Stress/allergic reactions

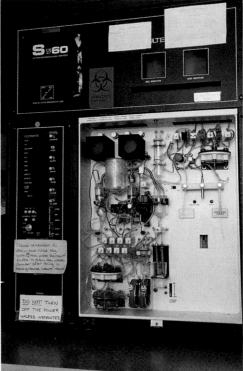

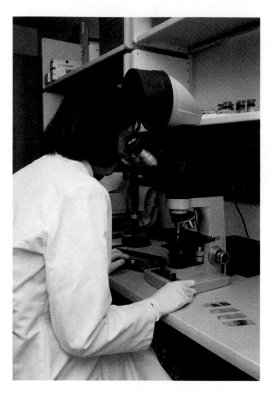

FIGURE 3-2
Medical technologist conducting microscopic examination of white blood cells.

WHITE BLOOD CELL (LEUKOCYTE) COUNT

The white blood cell (WBC) count has two components. One is a count of the total number of WBCs in a cubic milliliter of peripheral venous blood. The other component, the differential count, measures the percentage of each type of leukocyte present in the same specimen (Figure 3-2). An increase in the percentage of one type means a decrease in the percentage of another type. Neutrophils and lymphocytes make up 75% to 90% of the leukocytes. These leukocyte types can be identified easily by the morphology on a peripheral blood smear. Although the total leukocyte count has a wide range of normal values, many diseases can induce abnormal values.

HEMOGLOBIN ELECTROPHORESIS

Hemoglobin electrophoresis allows abnormal forms of hemoglobin to be detected. Each major hemoglobin type is charged to varying degrees. When placed in an electromagnetic field, the hemoglobin variants migrate at different rates and therefore spread apart from each other. Each band can be quantitated as a percentage of the total hemoglobin.

A lavender-top tube, or any tube containing edetate (EDTA), is filled with 7 ml of peripheral venous blood and sent to the hematology laboratory as soon as possible. A small amount of blood is placed on a starch gel or cellulose acetate medium. Electrophoresis ensues within an electromagnetic field, and the hemoglobin variants are separated and quantified by spectrophotometry.

Hb A$_1$ is the major component (98%) of hemoglobin in the normal RBC. *Hb A$_2$* is only a minor component (2% to 3%) of the normal hemoglobin total. *Hb F* is the major hemoglobin in the fetus, yet exists in only minimal quantities in a normal adult. An Hb F value higher than 2% in patients over 3 years of age is considered abnormal. Hb F can transport oxygen when only small amounts of oxygen are available (as in fetal life). In patients requiring compensation for prolonged chronic hypoxia (as in congenital cardiac abnormalities), Hb F may be increased to help transport the available oxygen.

Hb S is an abnormal form of hemoglobin associated with sickle cell anemia, which occurs predominantly in American blacks. Hb S is a relatively insoluble variant. When little oxygen is available, it assumes a crescent (sickle) shape that greatly distorts the RBC morphology. Vascular sludging is a consequence of the localized sickling and may lead to organ infarction.

Hb C is another hemoglobin variant seen in American blacks. RBCs containing Hb C have a decreased life span and are more readily lysed than normal RBCs. Mild hemolytic anemia may result.

INDICATIONS

To detect hemoglobinopathies

CONTRAINDICATIONS

Patients who have received a blood transfusion within the previous 12 weeks should not have hemoglobin electrophoresis. The donor's blood, if normal, can mask and dilute abnormal hemoglobin variation that may exist in the recipient.

PATIENT TEACHING

Explain the procedure to the patient. Ensure that the patient has not had a blood transfusion within the previous 12 weeks, and explain this precaution.

ERYTHROCYTE SEDIMENTATION RATE

The erythrocyte sedimentation rate (ESR) is a test used to detect inflammatory, neoplastic, infectious, and necrotic processes. However, since this test is nonspecific, it is not diagnostic for any specific organ disease or injury. The test is performed by measuring the distance (in millimeters) that RBCs descend (or settle) in anticoagulated blood in 1 hour. Because the disorders mentioned previously increase the protein content of plasma, RBCs have a tendency to stack up on one another, increasing their weight and causing them to descend faster.

The ESR test can be used to detect disease that otherwise is not suspected; it also is a fairly reliable indicator of the course of the disease and can therefore be used to monitor treatment.

Peripheral venous blood is obtained and placed in an oxalate or edetate (EDTA) anticoagulated tube. The blood is immediately taken to the hematology laboratory where the sedimentation rate is measured. The study must be performed within 3 hours of obtaining the specimen.

INDICATIONS

To detect inflammatory, neoplastic, infectious, and necrotic processes; can be used to detect disease that otherwise is not suspected; to differentiate disease entities or complaints
To indicate the course of a disease
To monitor treatment

CONTRAINDICATIONS

None

PATIENT TEACHING

Explain the procedure and that the only discomfort associated with this test is the venipuncture.

PERIPHERAL BLOOD SMEAR

A peripheral blood smear is the most informative of all hematologic tests. All three hematologic cell lines (red cells, white cells, and platelets) can be examined.

A peripheral blood smear is obtained by performing a finger stick. A drop of blood is spread on a slide using a second slide to smear it across the first. The slide is colored with a polychromatic stain (usually Wright's or Giemsa), and the stained slide is examined under a microscope.

Microscopic examination of the RBCs can reveal variation in red cell size, shape, color, or intracellular content. For example, target cells (codocytes) appear as targets with central color and ring of pallor associated with thalassemia, sickle cell anemia, hemoglobin C, iron deficiency, and/or obstructive jaundice. Classification of RBCs is most helpful in identifying the causes of anemia.

The WBCs are examined for total quantity, differential count, and degree of maturity. An increased number of immature WBCs may indicate leukemia. A decreased WBC count indicates marrow failure. Also, the number of platelets can be estimated.

INDICATIONS

To detect one of the following variables in identifying the causes of anemia:
Iron deficiency; thalassemia; reticulosis secondary to increased erythropoiesis; hereditary spherocytosis; hereditary elliptocytosis; hemoglobinopathies; bleeding ulcer; dehydration; hypoxemia; lead poisoning; vitamin B_{12} or folic acid deficiency; liver disorders; postsplenectomy anemia; acquired immunohemolytic anemia; sickle cell anemia; uremia; cardiac disease; RBC deficiency; marrow-occupying neoplasm; reticulocytosis

CONTRAINDICATIONS

None

PATIENT TEACHING

Explain the procedure for obtaining a peripheral blood smear.

RETICULOCYTE COUNT

The reticulocyte count is a test for determining bone marrow function. A reticulocyte is an immature RBC that can be readily identified under the microscope by staining a peripheral blood smear with a supravital stain. The reticulocyte count is a direct measurement of RBC production by the bone marrow. An increased erythrocyte count is expected as physiologic compensation in a patient who is anemic. A normal or low reticulocyte count in an anemic patient indicates that marrow production of RBCs is inadequate, which may be the cause of the anemia. An elevated reticulocyte count in a patient with a normal hemogram indicates increased RBC production (compensated hemolysis or hemorrhage).

INDICATIONS

To determine:
Bone marrow function
Adequate erythropoiesis in anemia

CONTRAINDICATIONS

None

PATIENT TEACHING

Explain the procedure. Advise the patient that although few complications are associated with this procedure, bleeding from the venipuncture site sometimes is seen in patients with thrombocytopenia.

IRON LEVEL AND TOTAL IRON-BINDING CAPACITY

Abnormal levels of iron and total iron-binding capacity (TIBC) are characteristics of many diseases, including iron-deficiency anemia. Most of the iron in the body is found in the hemoglobin of the RBCs. Iron, supplied by the diet, is absorbed in the small intestine and transported to the plasma. There the iron is bound to a globulin protein called transferrin and carried to the bone marrow for incorporation into hemoglobin. The serum iron determination is a measurement of the amount of iron bound to transferrin. Iron deficiency results in decreased production of hemoglobin, which in turn results in a small, pale RBC.

Because serum iron levels may vary significantly during the day, the specimen for them should be drawn in the morning, especially when the results are used to monitor iron replacement therapy.

TIBC, on the other hand, varies minimally according to intake. The TIBC is more a reflection of liver function and nutrition than of iron metabolism. Often TIBC values are used to monitor the course of patients receiving hyperalimentation.

Approximately 7 ml of peripheral venous blood is obtained in a red-top tube (some laboratories require that iron-free needles and iron-free plastic containers be used for collecting the blood). With hemolysis the iron usually contained in the RBC pours out into the serum and causes an artificially high iron level. The serum is transported to the chemistry laboratory for analysis.

INDICATIONS

To detect abnormal levels of iron and total iron-binding capacity, which aids in detecting a number of diseases

CONTRAINDICATIONS

Recent transfusions
Recent ingestion of a meal high in iron
Hemolytic diseases that may be associated with an artificially high iron content

PATIENT TEACHING

Explain the procedure to the patient. Instruct the patient to fast, except for water, for 12 hours before the blood test.

SERUM FERRITIN

The serum ferritin study is a good indicator of available iron stores. Ferritin, the major iron-storage protein, normally is present in the serum in concentrations directly related to iron storage. Decreases are associated with iron-deficiency anemia and are also seen in severe protein depletion. An increased amount is a sign of iron excess and associated disorders. However, a limitation of this study is that ferritin can also be elevated in conditions that do not reflect iron stores (e.g., acute inflammatory diseases, infections, metastatic cancer, lymphomas).

A peripheral venous blood sample is collected in a red-top tube and sent to the hematology laboratory for analysis.

INDICATIONS

To determine:
Iron-deficiency anemia
Iron excess and associated disorders (hemochromatosis, hemosiderosis, megaloblastic anemia, hemolytic anemia, certain liver disorders)

CONTRAINDICATIONS

Recent transfusion
Recent ingestion of a meal high in iron
Hemolytic diseases that may be associated with an artificially high iron content

PATIENT TEACHING

Explain the procedure.

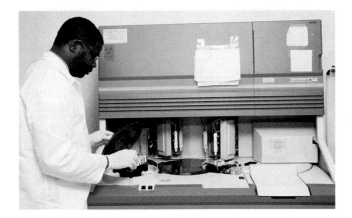

FIGURE 3-3
Medical technologist performing a test to measure serum bilirubin level.

SERUM BILIRUBIN

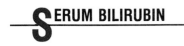

The total serum bilirubin determination measures both direct (conjugated) and indirect (unconjugated) bilirubin (Figure 3-3). The total serum bilirubin is the sum of the direct and indirect bilirubin levels. Many drugs (e.g., antibiotics, sulfonamides, allopurinol, diuretics, barbiturates, steroids, and oral contraceptives) can influence test results to show an elevated serum bilirubin. Serum bilirubin may be decreased in patients with iron-deficiency anemia and in those taking penicillin or large amounts of salicylates.

Peripheral venipuncture is performed, and one red-top tube of blood is collected. A heel puncture is used to collect blood in infants, and two blood microtubes are filled. Patient preparation for this test varies among laboratories; some require the patient to be NPO after midnight except for water.

INDICATIONS
To detect the presence and causes of:
Conjugated hyperbilirubinemia
Unconjugated hyperbilirubinemia

CONTRAINDICATIONS
None

PATIENT TEACHING
Explain the procedure.

SICKLE CELL

Both sickle cell disease and sickle cell trait can be detected by the sickle cell test. Sickle cell anemia is caused by Hb S, an abnormal form of hemoglobin. Hb S is found in 8% to 10% of American blacks.

In the sickle cell test, a deoxygenating agent is added to the patient's blood. If 25% or more of the patient's hemoglobin is of the S variation, the cells assume the crescent (sickle) shape, and the test result is positive. If no sickling occurs, the test result is negative. A negative test result indicates that the patient has no or very little Hb S. Other, less common hemoglobin variants can also cause sickling.

The sickle cell test is only a screening test, and its sensitivity varies according to the method used by the laboratory. Definitive diagnosis is made by hemoglobin electrophoresis.

Approximately 7 ml of peripheral venous blood is drawn, placed in a lavender-top vacutainer, and transported to the hematology laboratory. A small quantity of blood is then mixed with a bisulfite solution and examined on a peripheral blood smear for crescent-shaped RBCs. Tell the patient that the only discomfort associated with this study is the venipuncture.

INDICATIONS
To screen for sickle cell disease and sickle cell trait

CONTRAINDICATIONS
None

PATIENT TEACHING
Explain the procedure.

IMMUNOHEMATOLOGIC TESTS

Immunohematologic tests are used to assess antigens on RBC surfaces. These tests are clinically indicated to monitor potential blood transfusion reactions, hemolytic anemia, blood type (ABO) compatibility and Rh typing, antibody screening (indirect Coombs' test), and antiglobulin testing (direct Coombs' test).

ABO blood typing is performed to decrease the risk of a blood transfusion reaction. Isohemagglutinins are naturally occurring antibodies to RBCs. They are present in all immunocompetent individuals by 2 years of age except for individuals with AB blood type. For example, individuals with type A blood have anti-B isoantibodies, those with type B have anti-A isoantibodies, and persons with type O have both anti-A and anti-B isoantibodies; individuals with type AB have neither. This allows individuals with type O blood to be universal donors and those with type AB to be universal recipients. To determine an individual's specific blood type, separate aliquots of the patient's RBCs are mixed with anti-A serum and anti-B serum. The results depend on the presence or absence of agglutination. For example, patients whose RBCs agglutinate in the presence of anti-A serum will have either A or AB blood type. Patients whose RBCs agglutinate with both anti-A and anti-B serum are AB blood type.

The **antiglobulin test** (**Coombs' test**) is used to detect any immunoglobulin that is bound to antigen by using antiimmunoglobulin.

The **indirect Coombs' test** is a type of *antibody screening* that detects specific serum antibodies to RBC antigens that are not attached to the cell. It is performed by adding antiimmunoglobulins to particles, usually RBCs, that are suspected of having antibodies bound to the antigens on their cell surface. This results in agglutination of the red blood cells, confirming the presence of antibody. This type of testing is performed before RBC transfusions and to detect Rh-positive antibody in maternal blood.

The **direct Coombs' test** is an *antiglobulin test* that detects serum antibodies that coat RBCs but do not result in agglutination. This test is performed by adding antiimmunoglobulin (anti-IgG or anticomplement) to saline-washed RBCs. If immunoglobulin or complement is present, agglutination will occur, indicating a positive reaction. A positive reaction may be useful in the diagnosis of newborn hemolytic disease or autoimmune disorders.

INDICATIONS FOR COOMBS' TESTING

To determine:
Rh factor
To evaluate:
Suspected blood transfusion reaction; SLE; drug reactions; hemolytic anemia

GLUCOSE-6-PHOSPHATE DEHYDROGENASE

The glucose-6-phosphate dehydrogenase (G6PD) test is used to determine if hemolytic anemia is caused by a lack of G6PD (an enzyme normally present in the RBC). The presence of a decreased amount of this enzyme is a sex-linked, recessive trait carried on the X chromosome. Hemolytic episodes in these individuals may be triggered by drugs, infections, or acidotic states. Because there are two common types of G6PD deficiencies (Mediterranean and type A), some drugs cause hemolysis in only one or the other type. The Mediterranean type is found in whites and Orientals; type A is found in blacks.

INDICATIONS

To determine whether a G6PD deficiency is the cause of hemolytic anemia

CONTRAINDICATIONS

None

PATIENT TEACHING

Explain the procedure for venipuncture. Tell the patient that no food or fluid restrictions are associated with this test.

VITAMIN B₁₂ ASSAY (SCHILLING TEST)

The Schilling test is performed to detect vitamin B_{12} absorption. Ingested vitamin B_{12} combines with intrinsic factor produced by the gastric mucosa and is absorbed in the distal part of the ileum. Pernicious anemia results when the body is unable to absorb vitamin B_{12} because of a lack of intrinsic factor.

The Schilling test can determine whether there is a defect in vitamin B_{12} absorption or a deficiency in the intrinsic factor.

The test can be performed in one or two stages. Patients who excrete a normal amount of radioactive vitamin B_{12} in the first stage require no further testing. The second stage is needed to confirm the diagnosis of pernicious anemia.

First stage (without intrinsic factor). After the patient has been kept NPO for 8 to 12 hours, she voids before receiving an oral dose of radioactive vitamin B_{12} and begins a 24- to 48-hour urine collection. After 1 or 2 hours, the patient receives an IM injection of nonradioactive vitamin B_{12} to saturate tissue-binding sites and to permit some excretion of radioactive vitamin B_{12} in the urine. The patient may resume eating after the injection.

Second stage (with intrinsic factor). After being kept NPO for 8 to 12 hours before the test, the patient voids and discards the urine specimen. She then receives an oral dose of radioactive vitamin B_{12} and human intrinsic factor, and a 24-hour urine collection is begun. After 2 hours the patient receives an IM dose of nonradioactive vitamin B_{12}. She may resume eating after the injection. After administration of intrinsic factor and vitamin B_{12} in the second stage, most patients excrete normal amounts of radioactive B_{12}. The second stage usually is performed within 1 week after the first.

A combined assay can also be performed to incorporate stages one and two into one procedure. In this method the fasting patient receives a capsule of cobalt-57–labeled vitamin B_{12} plus intrinsic factor and a second capsule of cobalt-58. One hour later, an IM injection of nonradioactive vitamin B_{12} is given. All urine is then collected for 24 hours, and the percentages of cobalt-57 and cobalt-58 are calculated.

INDICATIONS

To detect vitamin B_{12} absorption
To confirm diagnosis of pernicious anemia

CONTRAINDICATIONS

Within 10 days after a radionuclide scan
Pregnancy and/or lactation

PATIENT TEACHING

Explain the purpose and procedure; provide written instructions.

Advise the patient not to use laxatives the night before the test, because they could decrease the rate of vitamin B_{12} absorption.

Explain the procedure for collecting the 24-hour urine specimen.

Reassure the patient that the tracer dose of radioactive vitamin B_{12} is small and will not harm her or others.

If the patient showed decreased excretion of vitamin B_{12} in the first stage of the test, explain that the second stage usually is performed within 1 week.

SERUM PROTEIN ELECTROPHORESIS

Total serum protein is a combination of albumin and globulins. Albumin is the smaller molecule, which is most important in maintaining the oncotic pressure of plasma (the pressure that keeps water in the bloodstream). The larger molecules are globulins, which are subclassified into alpha, beta, and gamma. Alpha$_1$ globulins include alpha antitrypsin and thyroid-binding globulins. Alpha$_2$ globulins include serum haptoglobins (bind hemoglobin during hemolysis), ceruloplasmin (carrier for copper), prothrombin and cholinesterase (an enzyme used in the catabolism of acetylcholine). Beta$_1$

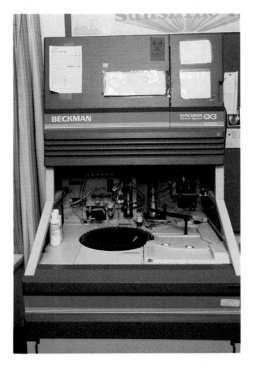

FIGURE 3-4
Equipment used to perform serum protein electrophoresis.

globulins include lipoproteins, transferrin, plasminogen, and complement proteins. Beta$_2$ globulins include fibrinogen. Gamma globulins are the immune globulins (antibodies).

Serum electrophoresis separates and quantifies these components of total protein according to their electrical charge. Many diseases can be associated with an increase or decrease in one or more components.

Seven milliliters of peripheral venous blood is drawn into a red-top tube and taken to the laboratory. The serum is placed on a pH-adjusted gel strip to which an electrical current is applied. Each protein component migrates to a certain point, depending on its electrical charge. The final migration pattern is then identified as either normal or associated with a specific disease (Figure 3-4).

INDICATIONS

To detect possible associated disorders such as:
Malnutrition; nephrotic syndrome; multiple myeloma; gammopathies; specific drug ingestions; chronic liver disease; acute or chronic inflammation; rheumatoid-connective tissue diseases; immune deficiencies

CONTRAINDICATIONS

None

PATIENT TEACHING

Explain the procedure. Advise the patient that although few complications are associated with this procedure, bleeding from the venipuncture site sometimes is seen in patients with thrombocytopenia.

URIC ACID

Uric acid is a nitrogenous compound that is a product of purine (DNA building block) catabolism. It is mostly excreted by the intestinal tract. Determination of the uric acid level usually is included in any multiphasic automated systems analysis of the blood. Some hospitals require that the patient be fasting. Usually for these studies, two red-top tubes of blood are obtained from a peripheral vein.

INDICATIONS

Increased serum levels may be clinically associated with:
Gout
Tophi
Arthritis
Uric acid kidney stones
Cancer chemotherapy
Decreased serum levels may be clinically associated with:
Poor liver function

CONTRAINDICATIONS

None

PATIENT TEACHING

Explain the procedure for obtaining blood. Advise the patient that although few complications are associated with this procedure, bleeding from the venipuncture site sometimes is seen in patients with thrombocytopenia.

If the patient's uric acid level is high, instruct him to avoid foods high in purine (e.g., liver, kidney, heart, brain, sweetbreads, sardines, anchovies, and mince meat). Foods that contain a moderate amount of purine nitrogens include poultry, fish, asparagus, mushrooms, peas, and spinach.

Instruct a patient with an elevated uric acid level to decrease his alcoholic intake, because alcohol causes renal retention of urate.

LACTIC DEHYDROGENASE (LDH)

Lactic dehydrogenase is found in many body tissues, especially the heart, liver, kidneys, skeletal muscle, brain, red blood cells, and lungs. While particularly useful in the diagnosis of myocardial infarction, an increase in LDH levels may also indicate hemolysis. The procedure involves the collection of 7 to 10 ml of venous blood in a red-top tube. It is important to record on the laboratory slip the date and time when blood was drawn for an accurate evaluation of the temporal pattern of enzyme elevations.

INDICATIONS

To detect increased values in:
Myocardial infarction; pulmonary infarction; congestive heart failure; heart disease; red blood cell disease such as hemolytic anemia; neoplastic states; shock; hypotension; renal parenchymal diseases; intestinal ischemia and infarction; cerebrovascular accident (CVA); infectious mononucleosis; heat stroke; pancreatitis; collagen diseases; fractures

CONTRAINDICATIONS

None

PATIENT TEACHING

Explain the procedure. Tell the patient that no fasting is required.

SERUM CALCIUM

The serum calcium test is used to evaluate parathyroid function and calcium metabolism by directly measuring the total amount of calcium in the blood. Total calcium exists in the blood in its free (ionized) form and in its protein-bound form (with albumin). The serum calcium level is a measure of both. As a rule of thumb, the total serum calcium level decreases by approximately 0.8 mg for every 1 g decrease in the serum albumin level.

The ionized form of calcium can also be measured; some physicians consider this measurement more sensitive and reliable than total calcium in detecting primary hyperparathyroidism. However, there is not total agreement on this, and most laboratories do not have the equipment to perform the ionized calcium assay.

Approximately 7 ml of peripheral venous blood is obtained from a nonfasting patient and placed in a red-top tube. The blood is then transported to the clinical chemistry laboratory. The serum calcium determinations usually are done as part of a multiple chemical analysis done automatically by a machine. The patient may be kept fasting for multichemical examinations.

INDICATIONS

Hypercalcemia may indicate:
Metastatic tumor of the bone
Nonparathyroid PTH-inducing tumor
Excessive ingestion of calcium products
Hyperparathyroidism
Vitamin D intoxication
Sarcoidosis
Hypocalcemia may indicate:
Hypoparathyroidism
Hyperphosphatemia in renal failure
Renal failure
Rickets

CONTRAINDICATIONS

None

PATIENT TEACHING

Explain the procedure. Tell the patient that the only discomfort associated with this test is the venipuncture.

FOLIC ACID

The folic acid test evaluates hemolytic disorders and detects folic acid anemia, in which the RBCs are abnormally large due to a deficiency of folic acid (a B vitamin). These RBCs have a shortened life span and impaired oxygen-carrying capacity. The main causes of this deficiency are dietary deficiency, malabsorption syndrome, pregnancy, and certain anticonvulsive drugs. Elevated folic acid levels may be seen in patients with pernicious anemia.

Approximately 7 to 10 ml of peripheral venous blood is collected in a red-top tube and sent to the hematology laboratory for analysis.

INDICATIONS

To detect folic acid anemia
In conjunction with the Schilling test, to detect pernicious anemia
To evaluate hemolytic disorders

CONTRAINDICATIONS

None

PATIENT TEACHING

Explain the procedure. Advise the patient not to drink alcoholic beverages before the test. Also tell him that although few complications are associated with this procedure, bleeding from the venipuncture site sometimes is seen in patients with thrombocytopenia.

BLOOD CULTURE

Blood cultures are used to detect bacteremia (bacteria in the blood). Except in endocarditis or suppurative thrombophlebitis, bacteremia usually is intermittent and transient; thus the blood should be drawn at the time the patient develops chills and fever. At least two culture specimens should be obtained from different sites, in case one produces bacteria and the other does not; it can then be assumed that the bacteria in the first culture are a contaminant and not the infecting agent. When both cultures produce the infecting agent, bacteremia exists. If the patient is receiving antibiotics, the laboratory should be notified, and the blood culture specimen should be taken shortly before the next dose.

To take the blood specimens, two different peripheral venous sites are carefully prepared with povidone-iodine (Betadine). The tops of the vacutainer tubes or culture bottles are cleaned with iodine and allowed to dry. The venipuncture is performed aseptically, and enough blood is aspirated (approximately 8 ml) to allow a dilution ratio of blood to culture broth of about 1:10. The culture bottles should be transported to the laboratory immediately. Culture specimens drawn through an intravenous catheter frequently are contaminated, and tests using them should not be performed unless catheter sepsis is suspected. In these situations, blood culture specimens drawn through the catheter indicate the causative agent more accurately than a culture specimen from the catheter tip.

INDICATIONS

To detect bacteremia

CONTRAINDICATIONS

None

PATIENT TEACHING

Explain the procedure for obtaining a blood culture, as described above. Tell the patient that no fasting is required.

PROTHROMBIN TIME

The prothrombin time (PT) test is used to evaluate the adequacy of the extrinsic system and the common pathway in the clotting mechanism. When the amounts of the clotting factors involved (especially factors V and VII) are deficient, PT is prolonged. Many diseases and drugs are associated with a decrease in the amounts of these factors.

Peripheral venipuncture is performed, and one or two blue-top tubes are filled to capacity with blood (each tube must be filled to capacity, or the PT may be artificially prolonged by the extra citrate in the tube). The blood samples should be transported on ice to the laboratory as soon as possible. There tissue thromboplastin is added, circumventing the intrinsic system of clotting, and the time required for clotting is noted.

INDICATIONS

To detect diseases and drugs associated with decreased levels of clotting factors. These include:
Hepatocellular liver disease
Parenchymal liver disease
Obstructive biliary disease
Coumarin ingestion

CONTRAINDICATIONS

None

PATIENT TEACHING

Explain the procedure. Tell the patient that blood is being drawn to assess how quickly the blood clots. Because of the danger of drug interactions, instruct the patient not to take any medication unless it is specifically ordered by the physician.

PARTIAL THROMBOPLASTIN TIME (ACTIVATED)

The partial thromboplastin time (PTT) test is used to assess the intrinsic system and the common pathway of clot formation. It evaluates factors I, II, V, VIII, IX, X, XI, and XII. When the amount of any of these factors is inadequate, PTT is prolonged. Heparin has been found to inactivate prothrombin (factor II) and to prevent the formation of thromboplastin, thereby providing therapeutic anticoagulation. The appropriate dose of heparin can be monitored by the PTT.

Recently activators have been added to the PTT test reagents to shorten normal clotting time and provide a narrow normal range. This shortened time is called the activated partial thromboplastin time (APTT). The normal APTT is 30 to 40 seconds.

Peripheral venipuncture is performed, and one or two blue-top tubes are filled to capacity with blood (each tube must be filled to capacity, or the PTT value may be incorrect because of the extra citrate in the tube). The blood samples should be transported on ice to the laboratory as soon as possible.

INDICATIONS

To assess the intrinsic system and the common pathway of clot formation

CONTRAINDICATIONS

None

PATIENT TEACHING

Describe the procedure, and explain to the patient that blood is drawn to assess how quickly it clots.

PLATELET COUNT

The platelet count is an actual count of the number of platelets (thrombocytes) per cubic milliliter of blood. Platelet activity is essential to blood clotting. Because platelets can clump together, automated counting is subject to at least a 10% to 15% error. Counts between 150,000/mm^3 and 400,000/mm^3 are considered normal. Counts below 100,000/mm^3 may indicate thrombocytopenia; counts above 400,000/mm^3 most likely indicate thrombocytosis.

Approximately 7 to 10 ml of peripheral venous blood is collected in a red-top tube and sent to the hematology laboratory for analysis.

INDICATIONS

To detect:
Thrombocytopenia; thrombocytosis; leukemia; malignant disorders; hemorrhage; polycythemia vera; postsplenectomy syndromes

CONTRAINDICATIONS

None

PATIENT TEACHING

Explain the procedure. Advise the patient that although few complications are associated with this procedure, bleeding from the venipuncture site sometimes is seen in patients with thrombocytopenia.

BLEEDING TIME

A bleeding time test is used to evaluate the vascular and platelet factors associated with hemostasis. When injury occurs, the first hemostatic response is a spastic contraction of any lacerated microvessels. Next, platelets adhere to the wall of the vessel in the area of laceration in an attempt to plug the hole. If either process fails, bleeding time is prolonged.

The skin of the inner forearm is cleansed with alcohol or povidone-iodine. A blood pressure cuff is placed on the arm above the elbow and inflated to 40 mm Hg. A small incision 3 mm deep is made into the skin, and the time is recorded. Bleeding ensues, and the blood is blotted clean at 30-second intervals. When no new bleeding occurs, the time is again recorded.

INDICATIONS

To evaluate vascular and platelet factors associated with hemostasis, including:
Decreased platelet counts caused by marrow failure
Infiltration of marrow by primary or metastatic tumor
Consumption of platelets during disseminated intravascular coagulation (DIC)
Increased platelet destruction
Inadequate platelet function caused by aspirin ingestion or by von Willebrand's disease
Increased capillary fragility secondary to collagen-vascular disease, Cushing's disease, or Henoch-Schönlein syndrome
Ingestion of antiinflammatory drugs

CONTRAINDICATIONS

None

PATIENT TEACHING

Explain the procedure. Warn the patient with a factor deficiency that bleeding time may be normal, but that subsequent oozing of blood from the test site may be seen 20 minutes after the bleeding has stopped. If this happens, the patient should apply pressure to the wound with a gauze pad until the oozing stops. This test involves slight discomfort because of the skin laceration.

COAGULATING FACTORS CONCENTRATION

The coagulating factors concentration test measures the concentration of a specific coagulating factor in the blood. Testing is available to measure the quantity of factors I, II, V, VII, VIII, IX, X, XI, and XII. When the concentrations of these factors are below their minimum hemostatic level, clotting time is prolonged. It is important to identify the exact factor or factors involved in the coagulating defect so that appropriate blood component replacement can be administered (Figure 3-5).

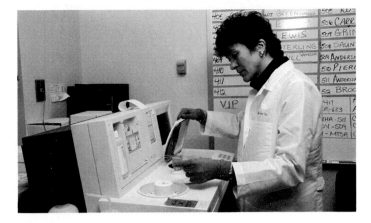

FIGURE 3-5
Laboratory analysis of coagulating factors concentration.

Peripheral venous blood is obtained and placed in a blue-top vacutainer. The blood is sent to the hematology laboratory for bioassay of the desired coagulation factor (in most hospitals the specimen is sent to a commercial laboratory for analysis). The test results usually are available in 1 to 7 days, depending on whether the specimen is tested in the hospital or sent to a commercial laboratory.

INDICATIONS

To detect:
Liver disease; fibrinolysis; congenital deficiency; warfarin ingestion; disseminated intravascular coagulation (DIC); congenital deficiency; heparin administration; autoimmune disease

CONTRAINDICATIONS

None

PATIENT TEACHING

Explain the procedure. Warn the patient with a factor deficiency that bleeding time may be normal, but that subsequent oozing of blood from the test site may be seen 20 minutes after the bleeding has stopped. If this happens, the patient should apply pressure to the wound with a gauze pad until the oozing stops. This involves slight discomfort because of the skin laceration.

FIBRIN DEGRADATION PRODUCTS

Measuring fibrin degradation products (FDPs) provides a direct indication of the activity of the fibrinolytic system. When plasma acts to dissolve fibrin clots, fibrinogen and FDPs (X, D, E, and Y) are formed. These degradation products, which have an anticoagulant effect and inhibit clotting, can be measured. When they are present in large amounts, they indicate increased fibrinolysis, such as occurs in disseminated intravascular coagulation (DIC) and primary fibrinolytic disorders.

Peripheral venous blood is collected in a blue-top tube and taken on ice to the hematology laboratory. The specimen is mixed with a serum containing antifibrinogen degradation fragments A and E, which have been absorbed onto latex particles. If the patient's blood contains the degradation fragments, agglutination occurs; if no degradation fragments are present, agglutination does not occur. Degradation product levels higher than 10 g/ml indicate increased fibrinolysis (DIC or primary fibrinolysis).

INDICATIONS

To determine the activity of the fibrinolytic system
To detect primary fibrinolytic disorders

CONTRAINDICATIONS

None

PATIENT TEACHING

Explain the procedure. Tell the patient that no fasting is required.

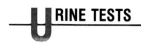RINE TESTS

Urine tests provide valuable information about many aspects of bodily function, including renal status, glucose metabolism, the presence of various normal and abnormal substances, and infection.

URINARY BILIRUBIN

Bilirubin is present in normal urine only in minute amounts that cannot be detected by routine test methods. Because unconjugated bilirubin is not water soluble, it cannot be excreted in the urine when the level is elevated. Conjugated bilirubin, however, is water soluble and can be excreted in the urine when the serum level is abnormally high. Therefore the presence or absence of urinary bilirubin provides important information about the causes of jaundice.

To measure urinary bilirubin, a fresh urine specimen is tested as soon as possible by immersing a Multistix reagent strip or an Icotest tablet into the well-mixed urine. The Multistix strip is immersed and immediately removed. After removal, the dipstick should be tapped to remove excess urine. The strip is held horizontally and compared with a color chart on the bottle at 20 seconds.

Icotest tablets are considered more sensitive. Five drops of urine are placed on a special test mat. The tablet is then placed on this moistened area, and two drops of water are added. The test result is positive if the mat turns blue or purple within 30 seconds.

Many drugs can interfere with test results, particularly phenazopyridine, ethoxazene, chlorpromazine (all associated with false-positive results), indomethacin (associated with either false-negative or false-positive results), and ascorbic acid (associated with false-negative results).

INDICATIONS

Increased levels indicate extrahepatic obstruction caused by:
Tumor; inflammation; stricture; surgical trauma; cirrhosis; hepatitis; gallstones

CONTRAINDICATIONS

None

PATIENT TEACHING

Explain the procedure as described above, emphasizing the need for using a proper urine container and for turning the specimen over to the nurse within 1 hour (bilirubin is not stable in urine, especially when exposed to light).

URINE CULTURE

All urine culture specimens should be clean-catch, midstream collections. First, the patient is asked to wipe the distal urethra with an antiseptic in a front-to-back direction. Then, during voiding, the sterile container is placed into the urine midstream to collect between 5 and 50 ml of urine. The container is removed from the stream, and voiding is completed. The urine can also be collected by suprapubic aspiration or directly from an indwelling catheter. The specimen container is covered, labeled, and transported to the bacteriology laboratory as soon as possible.

It often is helpful to culture the urine of a patient with an indwelling Foley catheter immediately before the catheter is removed. This procedure is called a "terminal urine for culture and sensitivity (C & S)" and usually is more accurate than culturing the tip of the catheter.

Color, appearance, and odor. Normal urine can range in color from pale yellow to amber, darkening according to the degree of concentration and varying with specific gravity. Abnormally colored urine can result from a pathologic condition or from ingestion of certain foods or drugs. Bleeding from the kidney produces dark red urine, whereas bleeding from the lower urinary tract produces bright red urine. Dark yellow urine may indicate the presence of urobilinogen or bilirubin.

The normal odor of fresh urine is caused by the presence of volatile acid. The urine in patients with diabetic ketosis has a strong, sweet smell of acetone. Infections tend to give urine a foul odor, and rectal fistulas can give urine a fecal odor.

RBCs and casts. During a routine urinalysis the urine is checked for blood. Any disruption of the blood-urine barrier, whether at the glomerular or the tubular level, will allow RBCs to enter the urine. This is seen in patients with glomerulonephritis, interstitial nephritis, acute tubular necrosis, pyelonephritis, and renal trauma or tumors. Pathologic conditions involving the mucosa of the collecting system (e.g., tumors, trauma, stones, infection) also cause hematuria. This can easily be detected by routine analysis.

Casts are clumps of material or cells. They are formed in the renal collecting tubule and have the shape of the tubule, thus earning them the name *cast*. RBC casts suggest glomerulonephritis, which may exist in patients with subacute bacterial endocarditis, renal infarct, Goodpasture's syndrome, vasculitis, sickling, and malignant hypertension.

Culture and sensitivity. Urine cultures and sensitivities are done to determine whether pathogenic bacteria are present in patients suspected of having urinary tract infections. All cultures should be performed before antibiotic therapy is started to avoid interrupting the growth of the organism in the laboratory. However, the physician often wants to begin antibiotic therapy for a suspected infection before the culture results can be obtained. In that case, a Gram's stain of a specimen smear is used and can be reported in less than 10 minutes. All forms of bacteria generally can be classified as gram positive (blue staining) or gram negative (red staining); also, determining the shape of the organism is helpful in tentatively identifying it. These findings help the physician institute an appropriate antibiotic regimen.

INDICATIONS

To detect:
RBCs in urine; pathologic conditions (e.g., bleeding from kidney); diabetes insipidus; dehydration; overhydration; jaundice; urinary tract infection; ketonuria; rectal fistula; phenylketonuria; maple sugar urine disease; hepatic failure

CONTRAINDICATIONS

None

PATIENT TEACHING

Explain the procedure for obtaining a clean-catch (midstream) urine collection, as described above.

BENCE JONES PROTEINS

Bence Jones proteins are light weight immunoglobulins commonly found in patients with multiple myeloma. They may also be associated with tumor metastases to the bone and chronic lymphocytic leukemia. These proteins are made by the patient's plasma cells and are rapidly cleared by the kidneys and excreted into the urine.

An early morning specimen of at least 50 ml of uncontaminated urine is collected in a container and taken to the laboratory for immunoelectrophoresis. The specimen should be refrigerated if there will be a delay in taking it to the laboratory. It is important to avoid contamination of the specimen with stool, menstrual blood, prostatic excretions, or semen.

INDICATIONS

To assist in diagnosis of:
Multiple myeloma
Bony metastases
Chronic lymphocytic leukemia

CONTRAINDICATIONS

None

PATIENT TEACHING

Explain the procedure. Assist the patient as needed to obtain a noncontaminated urine specimen.

BONE MARROW EXAMINATION

A bone marrow examination is done to evaluate hematopoiesis, including the number, size, and shape of the RBCs, WBCs, and megakaryocytes (platelet precursors) as these cells evolve through various stages of development in the bone marrow. This aids in diagnosis, evaluation, and monitoring of a wide variety of disorders (see Indications). Samples of the bone marrow are obtained either by aspiration or by surgical removal and then examined under a microscope (Figure 3-6). The examination involves estimating cellularity, determining whether fibrotic tissue or neoplasms (primary or metastatic) are present, and estimating iron storage.

For the estimation of cellularity, the relative quantity of each cell type is determined. This is more accurately done on a biopsy specimen than on an aspirate,

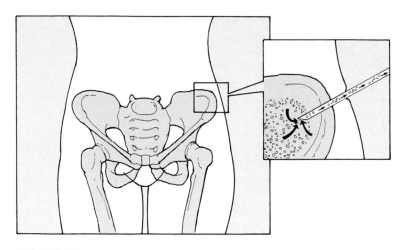

FIGURE 3-6
Aspiration of bone marrow.

because the aspirate may not be truly representative of the entire marrow.

Drug-induced or idiopathic myelofibrosis can be detected by examining the bone marrow. With the use of special stains, iron stores can be estimated by the marrow biopsy. Although fibrosis or neoplasia occasionally can be detected in aspiration studies, biopsy is the best method. Leukemia, multiple myeloma, and polycythemia vera can easily be detected in biopsy specimens. Similarly, diffusely metastatic tumors (as of the breast, kidneys, and lung) can be seen with metastases to the bone marrow.

Bone marrow aspiration is performed on the sternum, iliac crest, anterior or posterior iliac spines, or proximal tibia (in children). Specimens for bone marrow biopsy are taken from the iliac spines or wherever a tumor is suspected. Bone marrow aspiration usually is performed at the patient's bedside using local anesthesia. The preferred site is the posterior iliac crest, with the patient placed prone or on his side. The area overlying the bone is prepared and draped in a sterile manner. The overlying skin and soft tissue, along with the periosteum of the bone, are infiltrated with lidocaine. If aspiration is to be done, a large-bore (14-gauge) needle containing a stylus is slowly advanced through the soft tissues and into the outer table of the bone. Once inside the marrow, the stylus is removed, and a syringe is attached; 0.5 to 2 ml of bone marrow is aspirated, smeared on slides, and allowed to dry. The slides are sprayed with a preservative and taken to the pathology laboratory, where some are stained with Wright's stain and others with a supravital stain.

If a bone marrow biopsy is to be performed, the skin and soft tissues overlying the bone are incised and a core biopsy instrument is screwed into the bone. The biopsy specimen is obtained and sent to the pathology laboratory for analysis.

Aspiration is performed by a nurse or a physician. Removal of a bone marrow biopsy specimen is performed only by a physician. The procedure lasts approximately 10 to 20 minutes. After the needle or core biopsy instrument is removed, pressure is applied to the site, and a sterile dressing is supplied.

INDICATIONS

To diagnose and/or monitor treatment of:
Leukemias or leukemoid reactions; Physiologic marrow compensation for infection; Myelofibrosis; Metastatic neoplasia; Agranulocytosis; Radiation therapy or chemotherapy; Polycythemia vera; Hemorrhagic or hemolytic anemias; Erythroid hypoplasia; Marrow replacement by fibrotic tissue or neoplasms; Acute hemorrhage or some forms of chronic myeloid leukemia; Secondary hypersplenism associated with portal hypertension or other conditions; Neoplastic or fibrotic marrow infiltrative diseases; Aplastic anemia; Infections (such as mononucleosis); Lymphocytic leukemia; Lymphoma; Multiple myelomas; Hodgkin's disease; Hypersensitivity states; Rheumatic fever and other chronic inflammatory diseases; Drug-induced or idiopathic myelofibrosis

CONTRAINDICATIONS

Uncooperative patient

PATIENT TEACHING

Explain the procedure to the patient as described above, and explain the purpose of the study. Encourage the patient to talk about his fears, because many patients are anxious about this study. Provide emotional support.

Explain to the patient that he probably will feel pain during lidocaine infiltration and pressure when the syringe plunger is pulled back for aspiration. Warn him that he may have some apprehension when pressure is applied to the bone for outer table puncture during removal of the biopsy specimen or aspiration.

WOUND CULTURE

Wound infections are most commonly caused by pus. The specimen for a wound culture can best be obtained by aseptically placing a sterile cotton swab into the pus and then putting the swab into a sterile, covered test tube. The specimen is transported to the laboratory as soon as possible. Culturing specimens taken from the skin edge is much less accurate than culturing the suppurative material. If an anaerobic organism is suspected, an anaerobic culture tube is obtained from the microbiology laboratory. Routine wound cultures are also done at the same time.

INDICATIONS
To detect infection

CONTRAINDICATIONS
None

PATIENT TEACHING
Explain the procedure to the patient, as described above.

LIVER SCAN

A liver scan is done to outline and detect structural changes of the liver. An intravenous radionucleotide is given, and 30 minutes later, a gamma-ray detecting device (Geiger counter) records the distribution of the radioactive particles in the liver while the patient is placed in the supine, lateral, and prone positions to visualize all surfaces of the liver (Figure 3-7). The radionucleotide uptake is recorded on either x-ray or Polaroid film.

The spleen can also be visualized this way. Because the scan can demonstrate only filling deficits greater than 2 cm in diameter, false-negative results can occur in patients who have space-occupying lesions (e.g., tumors, cysts, and granulomas) smaller than 2 cm. The

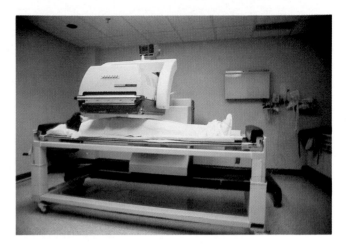

FIGURE 3-7
Patient prepared for liver scan. (From Mourad.)[42]

scan may be incorrectly interpreted as positive in patients who have cirrhosis because of distortion.

Rose bengal radioactive iodine scanning is useful in differentiating intrahepatic cholestasis from extrahepatic obstruction. This isotope normally is taken up and excreted by the hepatocytes. With complete biliary ductal obstruction, the dye will not be detected in the duodenum by the Geiger counter. However, with intrahepatic cholestasis, some isotope may be visualized in the duodenum and small bowel.

This hour-long procedure is performed in the nuclear medicine department by a trained technician, and a physician trained in nuclear medicine interprets the reports. Because only tracer doses of radioisotopes are used, no precautions need be taken against radioactive exposure.

INDICATIONS
To detect:
Tumors; abscesses; hematomas; infiltrative diseases; hepatic cysts; tuberculosis; nonfunctional areas; hepatosplenomegaly

CONTRAINDICATIONS
Pregnancy
Uncooperative patient

PATIENT TEACHING
Explain the procedure, as described above. Encourage the patient to talk about his fears, and provide emotional support. Reassure the patient that the only discomfort is associated with IV injection of the radioisotope. Also reassure him that he will not be exposed to large amounts of radioactivity, because only tracer doses of isotopes are used.

LYMPHANGIOGRAPHY

Lymphangiography involves an x-ray study of the lymphatic system after injection of a contrast medium into a lymphatic vessel in each foot or each hand. Assessment of this system is important, because cancer often spreads via the lymphatic system. When the lymph vessels become obstructed, edema usually results. Lymphangiography aids in evaluating unexplained swelling of an extremity.

Lipid pneumonia may be a complication of lymphangiography if the contrast medium flows into the thoracic duct and causes microemboli in the lungs. These small emboli usually disappear after several weeks or months.

This procedure is performed in the radiology department with the patient lying on his back. A blue dye is injected between each of the first three toes in each foot to outline the lymphatic vessels. (The dye can also be injected into the web of skin between the fingers.) A local anesthetic is injected before a small incision is made in each foot. A lymphatic vessel is identified, and a cannula is inserted to infuse the iodine contrast agent. The dye is infused into the vessels for approximately 1½ hours. An infusion pump usually is used to inject the dye at a slow, continuous rate. The patient must lie very still during injection of the dye. The flow of iodine dye through the body is followed by fluoroscopy (moving x-ray pictures on a television monitor). When the contrast medium reaches a certain level of the lumbar vertebrae, the dye is discontinued. X-ray films are taken of the stomach, pelvis, and upper body to demonstrate the filling of the lymphatic vessels. The patient must return in 24 hours to have additional x-ray studies taken to visualize the lymph nodes. When the injection is given in the hand, the axillary and supraclavicular lymph nodes are evaluated. After the injection is completed, the cannula is removed and the incision is sutured closed.

This procedure is performed by a radiologist and takes approximately 3 hours. Additional x-ray films must be taken again at 24 hours, but these take only about 30 minutes. Because the contrast medium remains in the lymph nodes for 6 months to 1 year, repeat x-ray examinations may be done to follow up on progression of the disease or the patient's response to treatment.

INDICATIONS

Edema
Signs of a tumor (unexplained fever, weight loss, enlarged lymph nodes)

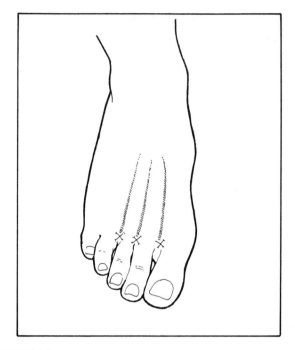

FIGURE 3-8
Lymphangiography. See text for description of procedure.

To evaluate the spread of cancer
To stage a lymphoma (for determining treatment)
To evaluate results of chemotherapy or radiation therapy
To follow up on disease progression or response to therapy

CONTRAINDICATIONS

Allergy to iodine dye
Severe chronic lung disease
Cardiac disease
Advanced liver or kidney disease

PATIENT TEACHING

Explain the procedure to the patient, as described above. Tell him that it is essential that he remain still during the test. Before the study make sure the patient has signed a consent form.

Tell the patient that he may feel discomfort when his toes are anesthetized. The injection of the dye between the toes or the fingers causes transient discomfort. However, the hardest part of this procedure may be lying still on the x-ray table. Inform the patient that the blue dye gives the skin a bluish tinge and may discolor the urine and stool for 2 days. Tell him to report any numbness in the extremity to his physician immediately because of the possibility of nerve damage.

LYMPH NODE BIOPSY

Lymph node biopsy or **excision** generally is performed as a surgical procedure on an outpatient basis using a local anesthetic. The node is removed and evaluated for architectural structure and histologic characteristics. Usually the supraclavicular scalene region is recommended and the inguinal and axillary areas avoided because of the increased risk of local trauma and infection. The Reed-Sternberg cell, polyploid with large nuclei, is indicative of Hodgkin's disease, and may be seen in the biopsy specimen.

INDICATIONS

Staging of malignancies
Tumor diagnosis, such as Hodgkin's disease
To assess immunologic function in immunodeficiency
  disorders

CONTRAINDICATIONS

Bleeding dyscrasias

COMPLICATIONS

Bleeding and infection at the site

NURSING CARE

In conjunction with the physician, obtain written consent. Before the procedure, assess coagulation studies, hematocrit, hemoglobin, and platelets to minimize the risk of bleeding. The patient should have nothing by mouth for 6 to 8 hours before the procedure. Disinfect the skin, and establish a sterile field. After the procedure, monitor the patient for bleeding at the site and check vital signs until stable. Apply a sterile occlusion pressure dressing to the site.

PATIENT TEACHING

Explain the procedure and its purpose. Inform the patient that a local anesthetic will be used and that it may cause a slight sting when injected. Explain that he may feel some discomfort after the procedure when the anesthetic has worn off and that he will be sent home with appropriate analgesic medication. Inform the patient and family that a follow-up visit may be necessary to remove sutures.

HISTOCOMPATIBILITY TESTING

Histocompatibility testing identifies the **human leukocyte antigens (HLA),** which are present on all nucleated cells and most easily detected on lymphocytes. The HLA is the major histocompatibility complex in humans. Two methods are used for histocompatibility testing: tissue typing and cross-matching. Each of these methods encompasses a number of testing approaches that assess specific components of the HLA system. This discussion focuses on the major testing methods.

TISSUE TYPING

There are two primary methods of tissue typing: complement-dependent cytotoxic assay and mixed lymphocyte culture. In the complement-dependent test, the patient's lymphocytes are incubated with antisera to HLA for approximately 30 minutes. This allows time for the antibody to bind to the cell surface. Complement is added for 60 minutes. If the antibody has bound to the antiserum, complement components C1 through C9 will be activated and cause cell lysis. A dye is added to detect cell lysis. If the antibody has not bound to the surface of the cell, the cells will remain intact and appear clear and round under the microscope; this is considered a negative test result. If the antibody has bound to the surface of the cell and complement activation was sufficient to cause cell lysis, the dye will have accumulated in the cells, and they will appear red and swollen; this is considered a positive test result, meaning that 20% or more of the cells have been lysed (are dead). The particular serum that reacts with the cells identifies the HLA antigens on the cell surface.

CROSS-MATCHING

Cross-matching is done before organ transplantation to prevent the risk of rejection after surgery. This test can detect the presence of antibodies in the recipient's serum that are directed against the HLA antigens of the potential donor. A number of testing methods are used to complete this assessment. Patients preparing for organ transplantation undergo four initial cross-matching tests: lymphocyte, T or B lymphocyte–enriched preparations, and preformed antibodies. To differentiate autoantibodies from antidonor antibodies, an auto-cross-match is performed.

The simplest, most common test is the standard cytotoxicity method. (Cytotoxicity is the process of cell lysis by antibody.) In this method the recipient serum is mixed with donor lymphocytes to assess the presence of preformed antibody directed against the donor antigens. If lysis occurs, preformed antibody is present. This is considered a positive reaction, and transplantation is deferred.

INDICATIONS

Organ transplantation; paternity testing; autoimmune disorders

PATIENT TEACHING

Explain to the patient and family why they are undergoing histocompatibility testing and that it requires a blood sample. Tissue typing is so called because blood is considered a tissue.

CYTOGENETIC STUDIES

Chromosomal abnormalities have been found in several types of leukemias, and may serve as prognostic indicators of response to treatment. Most chromosomal changes involve translocations of genetic material from one autosome to another. The symbol *t* indicates a translocation between the two indicated chromosomes at the respective regions or bands symbolized by the letters *p* and *q*. For example, in Burkitt's lymphoma, materials from chromosomes 8 and 14 are rearranged, written as: t [8;14] [q24; q32]. Consistent changes are reported in chromosomes 1 and 17 in a number of hematologic cancers. Changes in chromosome 22 where the long arm is translocated to chromosome 9 are well known in chronic granulocytic leukemia; this is called the Philadelphia chromosome.

Refer to the inside front cover for Expected Normal Laboratory Values

MONOCLONAL ANTIBODIES

Monoclonal antibodies are large numbers of identical antibodies that are active against a specific antigenic target. They are exactly reproducible and their clones are genetically identical. Monoclonal antibody technology provides antibody-producing B lymphocytes that are fused with nonsecreting antibody tumor cells (e.g., myeloma cells) that can replicate indefinitely in a culture medium. These fused, or hybrid, cells are called hybridomas. Clones derived from these cells can survive in cell culture and produce large quantities of identical monoclonal antibodies.

Monoclonal antibodies have now been produced against an array of different antigens, including disease-producing organisms and various types of cancer cells. The availability of these very pure antibodies has been useful in the commercial preparation of diagnostic tests that can be used to identify viruses, bacteria, and even specific cancer cells in the blood or other body fluids. Diagnostic application also includes detection of HLA antigens and lymphocyte subsets.

Monoclonal antibody technology is being used therapeutically in organ transplantation, autoimmune disorders, and antitumor therapy, as well as to treat graft-versus-host disease.

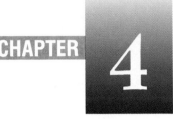
Erythrocytic Disorders

Two basic pathophysiologic states account for all disorders of erythrocytes: (1) an inadequate number of circulating cells or decreased quality or quantity of hemoglobin (**anemia**) and (2) an increased number of circulating cells (**polycythemia**). Anemia results from insufficient production or defective synthesis, increased destruction, loss of erythrocytes, or a combination of these. Polycythemia results from idiopathic causes or as a compensatory mechanism in response to tissue hypoxia.

Although not a disease per se, anemia is the primary manifestation of many abnormal states, including dietary deficiencies of iron, vitamin B_{12}, and folic acid; hereditary disorders; bone marrow damage caused by toxins, radiation, chemotherapy, or renal disease; malignancy; chronic infection; an overactive spleen; or bleeding from a tract or organ. The incidence of anemia is high; as many as 50% of the world's population suffers from anemia at any point in time.

The most common classification of anemias is based on cellular structure (morphology). Terms that refer to cellular size end in the suffix "-cytic," whereas those that describe hemoglobin content end in the suffix "-chromic." Cells of normal size are normocytic, and those with a normal amount of hemoglobin are normochromic. Erythrocytes can be macrocytic (abnormally large) or microcytic (abnormally small); hyperchromic (having an unusually high concentration of hemoglobin in the cytoplasm) or hypochromic (having an abnormally low concentration of hemoglobin). The erythrocytes in some anemias have various shapes (poikilocytosis) or sizes (anisocytosis) (Table 4-1).

The major physiologic effect of anemia is to reduce the oxygen-carrying capacity of the blood; thus the symptoms of anemia are the result of tissue hypoxia. If onset of the anemia occurs gradually, the body's compensation may be such that the person is asymptomatic except during periods of physical exertion. This compensation usually involves the cardiovascular, respiratory, and hematologic systems. The major physiologic effects of polycythemia are increased blood viscosity and blood volume; the symptoms of polycythemia are the result of congestion of tissue and organs with blood.

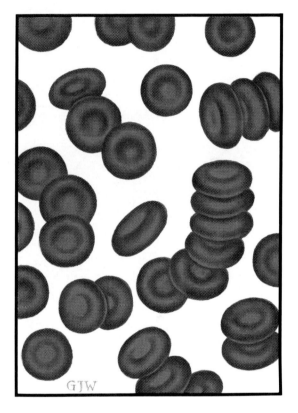

GJW

> **ANEMIA CLASSIFICATION TERMINOLOGY**
>
> Cytic = Refers to cellular size
> Chromic = Describes hemoglobin content

Table 4-1

MORPHOLOGIC CLASSIFICATION OF ANEMIAS

Morphology and cause of reduced oxygen-carrying capacity of the blood	Name and mechanism of anemic condition	Primary cause of associated disorder
Macrocytic-normochromic anemia: large, abnormally shaped erythrocytes but normal hemoglobin concentrations	Pernicious anemia: lack of vitamin B_{12} (cobalamin) for erythropoiesis; abnormal DNA and RNA synthesis in the erythroblast; premature cell death	Congenital or acquired deficiency of intrinsic factor (IF); genetic disorder of DNA synthesis
	Folate-deficiency anemia: lack of folate for erythropoiesis; premature cell death	Dietary folate deficiency
Microcytic-hypochromic anemia: small, abnormally shaped erythrocytes and reduced hemoglobin concentration	Iron-deficiency anemia: lack of iron for hemoglobin production; insufficient hemoglobin	Chronic blood loss; dietary iron deficiency, disruption of iron metabolism or iron cycle
	Sideroblastic anemia: dysfunctional iron uptake by erythroblasts and defective porphyrin and heme synthesis	Congenital dysfunction of iron metabolism in erythroblasts, acquired dysfunction of iron metabolism as a result of drugs or toxins
	Thalassemia: impaired synthesis of alpha- or beta-chain of hemoglobin A; phagocytosis of abnormal erythroblasts in the marrow	Congenital genetic defect of globin synthesis
Normocytic-normochromic anemia: destruction or depletion of normal erythroblasts or mature erythrocytes	Aplastic anemia: insufficient erythropoiesis	Depressed stem cell proliferation, resulting in bone marrow aplasia
	Posthemorrhagic anemia: blood loss	Acute or chronic hemorrhage that stimulates increased erythropoiesis, which eventually depletes body iron
	Hemolytic anemia: premature destruction (lysis) of mature erythrocytes in the circulation	Any condition that increases fragility of erythrocytes
	Sickle cell anemia: abnormal hemoglobin synthesis, abnormal cell shape with susceptibility to damage, lysis, and phagocytosis	Congenital dysfunction of hemoglobin synthesis
	Anemia of chronic disease: abnormally increased demand for new erythrocytes	Chronic infection or inflammation; malignancy

(From McCance and Huether.)[40]

Posthemorrhagic Anemia

Acute posthemorrhagic anemia is a normocytic-normochromic anemia that develops as the result of rapid loss of large quantities of erythrocytes during a hemorrhage, such as occurs with traumatic severance of blood vessels, rupture of an aneurysm, or arterial erosion by a cancerous or ulcerative lesion.

The severity of symptoms and the prognosis depend on the rate and site of bleeding and the volume of blood loss. The rapid loss of less blood is more dangerous than the slower loss of more blood.

In general, 20% loss of total blood volume results in vascular insufficiency; 30% loss causes circulatory failure, shock, and coma; with 40% loss death is imminent unless immediate and extensive blood volume replacement is performed.

PATHOPHYSIOLOGY

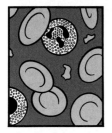

Within 24 hours, to compensate for the reduced blood volume caused by hemorrhage, fluids move from the interstitium into the blood vessels and plasma volume expands. Although this mechanism maintains adequate blood volume, it decreases the viscosity of the blood, which flows faster and with greater turbulence than normal blood. This increased blood flow in the heart can cause ventricular dysfunction, cardiac dilation, and heart valve insufficiency. Hypoxia causes arterioles, capillaries, and venules to dilate, also speeding blood flow. The heart must pump harder and faster to prevent congestion from the rapid venous return. Congestive heart failure may result.

The rate and depth of respiration increase as the body attempts to provide more oxygen to the remaining erythrocytes. Cardiac output increases to handle the increased venous return and to speed the oxygen-carrying erythrocytes to hypoxic tissue cells. The hemoglobin in these erythrocytes releases oxygen faster than usual at the tissue level. If the usual compensatory mechanisms are overcome, the person experiences dyspnea (shortness of breath), palpitations, dizziness, and fatigue.

During the first hours after a hemorrhage, peripheral blood vessels constrict so that available blood flows primarily to the vital organs. The kidneys sense the decrease in blood flow, and in an effort to improve kidney perfusion, the renal renin-angiotensin response is activated, resulting in salt and water retention. Because the hemoglobin concentration has been reduced, the skin, mucous membranes, lips, nail beds, and conjunctivae become pale. Vasoconstriction and loss of plasma volume distort the erythrocyte count, hemoglobin, and hematocrit, which appear high when they are actually quite low. These laboratory tests more accurately reflect the patient's status after intravenous fluids have been infused and extracellular fluid moves into the blood vessels. The red blood cell count usually returns to normal in 4 to 6 weeks, with many reticulocytes observed in the blood. Restoration of a normal hemoglobin level can take 6 to 8 weeks.

Chronic blood loss anemia, which is caused by bleeding peptic ulcers, menstrual disorders, bleeding hemorrhoids, or gastrointestinal neoplasms, results in continuous loss of erythrocytes and iron. The signs, symptoms, and laboratory findings are the same as those for iron-deficiency anemia.

CLINICAL MANIFESTATIONS

A patient with posthemorrhagic anemia shows the signs and symptoms of hypovolemia and hypoxemia. The severity of these conditions correlates with the volume of blood loss. The patient will show weakness, stupor, and irritability, and the skin will be cool and moist. Hypotension and tachycardia will also be present.

Treatment of posthemorrhagic anemia includes restoring blood volume by intravenous administration of saline, dextran, albumin, or plasma. Transfusion of fresh whole blood is the treatment of choice for large blood losses. If the anemia is associated with iron, folate, or cobalamin deficiency, drug therapy is prescribed.

DIAGNOSTIC STUDIES AND FINDINGS

Diagnostic Test	Findings
Erythrocyte count	6.1/mm^3 (initial); 4.7/mm^3 (after fluid volume increase)
Hemoglobin (Hb)	16.5 g/dl (initial); 14.5 g/dl (after fluid volume increase)
Hematocrit (Hct)	50% (initial); 40% (after fluid volume increase)
Reticulocyte count	Increased
Mean corpuscular volume (MCV)	Slightly low

MEDICAL MANAGEMENT

GENERAL MANAGEMENT

Initial IV fluids noncolloid, with electrolytes; followed by plasma and/or packed RBCs as needed to correct cell deficit.

Whole blood may be administered, after typing and cross-matching, to correct fluid volume and cell deficit as needed.

Oxygen by nasal catheter, cannula, or mask to maintain sufficient oxygenation of circulating blood volume.

Sedation and rest to reduce patient's energy expenditure.

Oral fluids as tolerated to maintain adequate tissue hydration and renal perfusion.

Diet high in protein and iron as basis for erythropoiesis.

DRUG THERAPY

Hematinic agents (e.g., ferrous sulfate) to correct iron deficiency.

SURGERY

If indicated to control source of bleeding.

1 ASSESS

ASSESSMENT	OBSERVATIONS
Cardiovascular function	Rapid, thready pulse; hypotension
Sensory function	Restlessness, dizziness, syncope, severe headache
Mental status	Disorientation
Skin	Pallor, diaphoresis, coolness
Respiratory function	Rapid, deep respirations that later become shallow
Fluid and electrolyte balance	Thirst; decreased urinary output

__2__ DIAGNOSE

NURSING DIAGNOSIS	SUBJECTIVE FINDINGS	OBJECTIVE FINDINGS
Decreased cardiac output related to decreased circulating blood volume	Reports dizziness, feeling faint, severe headaches	Rapid, thready pulse; hypotension; rapid, deep respirations that later become shallow; restlessness
Altered peripheral tissue perfusion related to decreased blood volume and vasoconstriction	Reports dizziness, feeling faint, severe headaches	Restlessness; disorientation; pallor, diaphoresis, coolness
Fluid volume deficit related to loss of blood volume	Reports thirst	Decreased urinary output

__3__ PLAN

Patient goals

1. The patient will demonstrate improved cardiac output.
2. The patient will manifest improved tissue perfusion.
3. The patient will have adequate fluid volume.

__4__ IMPLEMENT

NURSING DIAGNOSIS	NURSING INTERVENTIONS	RATIONALE
Decreased cardiac output related to decreased circulating blood volume	Provide rest, and anticipate patient's needs.	To reduce cardiac workload.
	Monitor apical pulse, heart sounds, orthostatic BP, and respirations. Monitor CVP, breath sounds, and PAP as indicated.	To assess cardiopulmonary function. To detect cardiopulmonary failure.
	Instruct patient to avoid stress (e.g., overexertion, fatigue, nonproductive coughing, and straining at stool).	To reduce cardiac workload.
Altered peripheral tissue perfusion related to decreased blood volume and vasoconstriction	Keep patient on bed rest in semi-Fowler's position.	To reduce cardiac workload and enhance systemic circulation.
	Maintain warm environment.	To prevent shivering and vasoconstriction.
	Inspect trunk and extremities; skin should be dry and warm.	To assess adequacy of peripheral circulation.

→ > >

NURSING DIAGNOSIS	NURSING INTERVENTIONS	RATIONALE
	Palpate for arterial pulses.	To determine patency of peripheral arterial circulation.
	Protect patient from injury by maintaining safe environment (e.g., putting up side rails).	To prevent further blood loss.
	Assess level of consciousness and orientation; patient should be alert and oriented to time, place, and person.	To determine adequacy of cerebral circulation.
	Discourage smoking.	Smoking causes vasoconstriction of peripheral vessels.
	Encourage exercise as tolerated.	To promote peripheral circulation.
Fluid volume deficit related to loss of blood volume	Apply ice bag and manual pressure or dressing over site of blood loss as indicated.	To constrict damaged vessels and prevent further blood loss.
	Elevate and immobilize affected body part as indicated.	To promote return of blood to the heart and reduce blood loss at site of damage.
	Estimate blood loss.	To determine need for volume replacement.
	Administer IV fluid, including blood components, as prescribed; monitor for reaction.	To replace lost fluid volume.
	Monitor patient's response to fluid therapy.	To prevent circulatory overload.
	Monitor CVP, breath sounds, and PAP, as indicated.	To assess fluid volume and cardiopulmonary function.
	Measure intake and output; urinary output should be at least 30 ml/hr.	To determine adequacy of renal function.
	Increase oral fluid intake as tolerated.	To maintain tissue hydration and renal perfusion.
	Observe for recurrent bleeding, which may result from dislodgement of clot, increased vascular pressure at site of bleeding, or further pathophysiologic developments.	To prevent further fluid volume loss.

5 EVALUATE

PATIENT OUTCOME	DATA INDICATING THAT OUTCOME IS REACHED
Cardiac output has improved.	Patient's vital signs are stable; erythrocyte count, Hb, and Hct are within normal limits; patient appears rested and not in distress.
Tissue perfusion has improved.	Patient is alert and oriented; arterial pulses are strong and regular; trunk and extremities are dry and warm.
Fluid volume is adequate.	There is no evidence of bleeding; intake is equal to output; patient is taking oral fluids.

PATIENT TEACHING

1. Encourage the patient to avoid overexertion, fatigue, constipation, and smoking, because they put a strain on the cardiovascular system.
2. Discuss the need to report to the physician or nurse such serious signs and symptoms as pain, dyspnea, extreme fatigue, and blood in the urine or feces, because they may signal recurrent internal bleeding.
3. Discuss the importance of regular exercise to maintain adequate peripheral circulation and cardiopulmonary tone.
4. Plan with the patient how to maintain a diet high in iron and protein and an adequate fluid intake.

Iron-Deficiency Anemia

Iron-deficiency anemia, the most prevalent anemia in the world, is caused by inadequate absorption or excessive loss of iron. The disease occurs most frequently in women, young children, and the elderly in underdeveloped countries.

The primary cause of iron-deficiency anemia in adults is acute or chronic bleeding secondary to (1) trauma; (2) menorrhagia (excessive menses); (3) bleeding in the gastrointestinal tract (resulting from a gastric or duodenal ulcer, a hiatal hernia, esophageal varices, cirrhosis, hemorrhoids, ulcerative colitis, diverticulosis, or cancer); (4) pregnancy; or (5) frequent blood donation. A diet lacking in foods high in iron is another cause, as is defective absorption caused by malabsorption syndromes, clay eating (pica), chronic diarrhea, a high intake of cereal products with a low intake of animal protein, and partial or complete gastrectomy. A blood loss of 2 to 4 ml a day is sufficient to cause this anemia.

PATHOPHYSIOLOGY

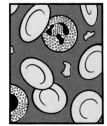

Iron-deficiency anemia is a chronic, microcytic-hypochromic anemia. The erythrocytes are small and pale because the hemoglobin level is low. Although the total erythrocyte count is only moderately reduced, the serum iron level may drop dramatically. This anemia develops slowly through three overlapping stages (see the following box). In stage I the body's stores of iron used for erythropoiesis are depleted; in stage II insufficient iron is transported to the bone marrow, and iron-deficient erythropoiesis begins; in stage III the small, hemoglobin-deficient cells enter the circulation in large numbers, replacing normal erythrocytes as they age and are removed from the circulation. Stage III is also associated with depleted transport of iron stores and diminished production of hemoglobin.

DEVELOPMENT OF ANEMIA

Stage I

Body's iron stores are depleted

Stage II

Insufficient iron is transported to bone marrow

Stage III

Transport of iron stores is depleted; hemoglobin production is diminished

---

CLINICAL MANIFESTATIONS

Because the symptoms of iron-deficiency anemia develop gradually, the individual often does not seek medical attention until the hemoglobin level drops to about 7 to 8 g/dl. Commonly reported symptoms are fatigue, weakness, and shortness of breath. Common signs are pale ear lobes, palms, and conjunctivae.

Epithelial tissue may be structurally or functionally altered. The nails become thin, brittle, and spoon shaped, or concave, as a result of impaired capillary circulation. The tongue may be sore, with redness and burning caused by atrophy of the papillae. Each of these changes can be reversed after 1 to 2 weeks of iron replacement therapy.

The term "angular stomatitis" describes changes in the epithelium at the corners of the mouth that cause soreness and dryness. A "web" of mucus and inflammatory cells at the juncture of the hypopharynx and esophagus may cause difficulty in swallowing.

Because iron is a component of other compounds as well as hemoglobin (e.g., cytochromes, myoglobin, and catalase), iron deficiencies probably alter various tissue enzymes. People with iron-deficiency anemia often experience gastritis, neuromuscular changes, irritability, headaches, numbness, tingling, and vasomotor disturbances. The neurologic symptoms may be caused by hypoxia in already compromised cerebral blood vessels. The elderly may experience mental confusion, memory loss, and disorientation.

Treatment of iron-deficiency anemia requires diagnosis and elimination of sources of blood loss if they are identified as a causative factor. This should precede initiation of drug therapy.

The most conclusive evidence of iron-deficiency anemia is an increase in hemoglobin of 1 to 2 g/dl after initiation of iron therapy. An increase in the reticulocyte count is a useful measure of a positive response to iron therapy. Oral, intramuscular, or intravenous iron preparations may be prescribed. Oral administration of an iron salt (ferrous sulfate, gluconate, or fumarate) that provides 200 mg of elemental iron a day will correct the deficiency.

Patients need to be prepared to deal with the side effects of this therapy, which include a change in stool color to green or black, loose stools, or constipation. Soon after beginning therapy, patients often report a rapid decrease in fatigue, lethargy, and other symptoms. Most of the hemoglobin deficiency is corrected within the first month of therapy, although therapy is continued for 6 to 12 months. Women who are menstruating may need daily therapy until they reach menopause.

DIAGNOSTIC STUDIES AND FINDINGS

Diagnostic Test	Findings
Hemoglobin (Hb)	As low as 3.6 g/dl
Erythrocyte count	Rarely below 3 million/dl
Mean corpuscular hemoglobin (MCH)	<27 pg
Mean corpuscular hemoglobin concentration (MCHC)	20-30 g/dl
Hematocrit (Hct)	Men: <47 ml/dl; women: <42 ml/dl
Serum iron	As low as 10 µg/dl
Iron-binding capacity	Increased
Serum ferritin	Decreased

MEDICAL MANAGEMENT

GENERAL MANAGEMENT

Diet high in iron-rich foods to correct nutritional deficiency, including red meats, organ meats, kidney beans, whole-wheat products, spinach, egg yolks, carrots, and raisins.

DRUG THERAPY

Hematinic agents to increase iron in the blood (e.g., ferrous salts, iron dextran [Imferon]).

1 ASSESS

ASSESSMENT	OBSERVATIONS
Sensory and motor function	Dizziness, headaches, numbness and tingling in limbs, fatigue, sensitivity to cold
Mental status	Irritability, decreased concentration
Cardiovascular function	Tachycardia
Respiratory function	Dyspnea on exertion
Skin	Brittle hair, spoon-shaped nails
Gastrointestinal function	Atrophic glossitis, stomatitis, dysphagia

2 DIAGNOSE

NURSING DIAGNOSIS	SUBJECTIVE FINDINGS	OBJECTIVE FINDINGS
Sensory/perceptual alterations related to tissue hypoxia of the nervous system	Reports dizziness, headaches, numbness and tingling in limbs, decreased concentration, sensitivity to cold	Irritability, decreased concentration
Fatigue related to decreased tissue oxygenation, impaired cardiovascular and respiratory function	Reports shortness of breath on exertion, easy fatigability	Tachycardia

→ > >

NURSING DIAGNOSIS	SUBJECTIVE FINDINGS	OBJECTIVE FINDINGS
Impaired skin integrity related to decreased tissue perfusion	Reports hair loss	Brittle hair, spoon-shaped nails
Altered nutrition: less than body requirements related to inadequate or unbalanced diet	Reports difficulty swallowing	Atrophic glossitis, stomatitis

3 PLAN

Patient goals

1. The patient will demonstrate improved sensory/perceptual function.
2. The patient will have more energy and less fatigue.
3. The patient's skin will be intact.
4. The patient's diet will be improved.

4 IMPLEMENT

NURSING DIAGNOSIS	NURSING INTERVENTIONS	RATIONALE
Sensory/perceptual alterations related to tissue hypoxia of the nervous system	Provide a safe environment (e.g., no smoking or using sharp instruments).	To prevent injury to extremities.
	Assist patient with ambulation and position changes (patient's sense of balance and position may be altered).	To prevent falls and increased dizziness.
	Maintain warm environment.	To decrease patient's exposure to cold.
	Give drugs as prescribed and according to patient's preference when possible.	To treat headaches.
	Anticipate patient's needs, repeat information and instructions, and listen to patient's concerns.	To decrease irritability and counteract altered concentration.
Fatigue related to decreased tissue oxygenation, impaired cardiovascular and respiratory function	Help patient plan periods of activity balanced by periods of rest.	To reduce cardiac and respiratory workload.
	Monitor pulse and respirations.	To identify signs of cardiopulmonary distress.

NURSING DIAGNOSIS	NURSING INTERVENTIONS	RATIONALE
	Explain to patient and loved ones that fatigue will diminish as iron deficiency improves.	To relieve anxiety and frustration.
Impaired skin integrity related to decreased tissue perfusion	Wash hair gently with conditioning shampoo and provide nail care.	To prevent breakage and loss of hair and to avoid damaging fragile nails.
Altered nutrition: less than body requirements related to inadequate or unbalanced diet	Administer hematinic agents as prescribed.	To correct deficiency.
	Encourage diet high in iron.	To correct nutritional deficiency.
	Monitor laboratory reports.	To determine effectiveness of medication and enriched diet.
	Observe for difficulty in swallowing.	To determine the need for changes in diet (texture, route of administration).
	Use frequent mouth care, including oral anesthetics.	To lessen discomfort and treat symptoms of stomatitis.

5 EVALUATE

PATIENT OUTCOME	DATA INDICATING THAT OUTCOME IS REACHED
Sensory/perceptual functioning has improved.	Patient can change position and ambulate without dizziness or damage to limbs; he has no complaints of headache or sensitivity to cold; he seems relaxed and can concentrate on conversations and instructions.
Patient has more energy and less fatigue.	Patient balances activity with rest to prevent fatigue; he reports having more energy.
Skin is intact.	Patient's hair is strong and shiny; nails are firm and well shaped.
Patient's diet has improved.	Patient is taking hematinic drug as prescribed; diet is well balanced and rich in iron; patient has no difficulty swallowing and no complaints of mouth pain.

PATIENT TEACHING

1. Discuss general safety precautions to prevent injury from dizziness or numbness and tingling in limbs.
2. Plan a program of activity balanced with rest.
3. Discuss general hygienic measures, including proper care of hair and nails.
4. Teach the patient how to maintain a diet high in iron.
5. Discuss factors important in taking iron supplements (e.g., proper timing, dilution, and awareness of change in stool color).

Pernicious Anemia

Pernicious anemia is the most prevalent type of vitamin B deficiency anemia in the United States. It is a chronic, progressive, macrocytic (megaloblastic) anemia caused by a deficiency of the intrinsic factor.

The disorder affects adults (primarily men and women over 50 years of age) and people of Scandinavian, English, and Irish origin. In Great Britain and Scandinavia women are more often affected, but in the United States men and women seem to be affected equally.

PATHOPHYSIOLOGY

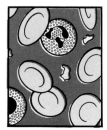 Atrophy of the glandular mucosa of the gastric fundus results in a lack of intrinsic factor. Why this occurs is unknown, but there are several possible explanations: genetic predisposition (the disease tends to run in families); prolonged iron deficiency, which can cause gastric atrophy; or an autoimmune disorder (90% of patients have autoantibodies that react against gastric cells; 40% of patients react against the intrinsic factor). Partial or complete gastrectomy is also a causative factor.

Some evidence suggests that the congenital form of pernicious anemia is an autosomal recessive trait. Siblings of those with the disorder are at highest risk for developing it.

Vitamin B_{12} is necessary for nuclear maturation and DNA synthesis in erythrocytes. Pernicious anemia affects not only erythrocyte precursors in the bone marrow, but also leukocyte and platelet precursors. The number and size of all erythroid cells are increased; enormous leukocytes with large and unusually shaped nuclei are also produced.

Other anemias in this classification result from a lack of vitamin B_{12}, which is caused by inadequate dietary intake (and corrected by daily oral administration and a more balanced diet) or by poor absorption, which is treated with vitamin supplements.

Anemias caused by a deficiency in folic acid (folate) are quite common and usually the result of (1) a poor diet, especially one lacking in green, leafy vegetables, liver, citrus fruits, and yeast; (2) malabsorption syndromes; or (3) the increased need that develops during

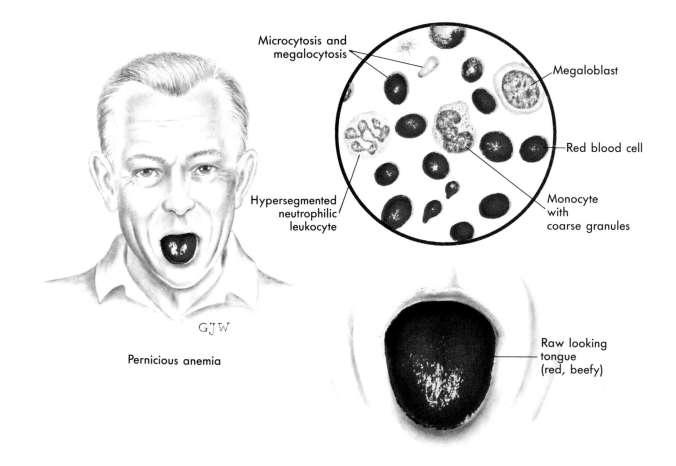

Pernicious anemia

Microcytosis and megalocytosis

Megaloblast

Red blood cell

Hypersegmented neutrophilic leukocyte

Monocyte with coarse granules

GJW

Raw looking tongue (red, beefy)

the third trimester of pregnancy. The signs and symptoms of this anemia resemble those of pernicious anemia except that there are no neurologic manifestations.

Folate deficiency is more common than cobalamin deficiency, especially in chronically malnourished people such as alcoholics. Treatment requires daily administration of oral folate preparations. Parenteral administration can eliminate acute symptoms within 48 hours. Severe cardiac or respiratory distress is treated with blood transfusions.

CLINICAL MANIFESTATIONS

Because pernicious anemia develops slowly, the signs and symptoms usually are severe when it is diagnosed. The patient often ignores such vague early symptoms as infections, mood swings, and gastrointestinal, cardiac, or renal disorders. When the hemoglobin is as low as 7 to 8 g/dl, the person experiences classic symptoms of weakness, fatigue, paresthesia of the fingers and feet, difficulty walking, sore tongue, loss of appetite, abdominal pain, and weight loss.

DIAGNOSTIC STUDIES AND FINDINGS

Diagnostic Test	Findings
Erythrocyte count	<3 million/dl
Hemoglobin (Hb)	Decreased to 4-5 g/dl
Mean corpuscular hemoglobin (MCH)	Decreased
Mean corpuscular volume (MCV)	Increased
Mean corpuscular hemoglobin concentration (MCHC)	Increased
Bone marrow biopsy	Increased number of megaloblasts
Bilirubin	Unconjugated forms; usually elevated
Serum vitamin B	Low
Serum folate	Normal or low
Gastric analysis	Scanty secretions, elevated pH, no free hydrochloric acid
Therapeutic trial with parenteral vitamin B	Large number of reticulocytes in blood 4-5 days after injection

MEDICAL MANAGEMENT

GENERAL MANAGEMENT

Blood transfusions as needed to correct anemia.

Nutritious diet, including fish, meat, milk, and eggs.

Physical therapy to prevent complications from impaired motor function.

DRUG THERAPY

Hematinic agents (e.g., ferrous sulfate).

Vitamins (e.g., cyanocobalamin, folic acid).

Digestants (e.g., hydrochloric acid).

1 ASSESS

ASSESSMENT	OBSERVATIONS
Sensory and motor function	Numbness and tingling of hands and feet; weakness, fatigue; disturbed coordination, including wobbly legs, poor balance
Mental status	Irritability, depression, poor memory, impaired judgment
Skin	Waxy pallor, jaundice, petechiae, purpura
Gastrointestinal tract	Anorexia, weight loss; indigestion; constipation or diarrhea; sore mouth; smooth, red beefy tongue
Cardiovascular function	Tachycardia, wide pulse pressure, palpitations
Respiratory function	Dyspnea

2 DIAGNOSE

NURSING DIAGNOSIS	SUBJECTIVE FINDINGS	OBJECTIVE FINDINGS
High risk for injury related to sensory and motor losses, alteration in mental status	Reports numbness and tingling of hands and feet, weakness, and fatigue; appears depressed	Disturbed coordination, including wobbly legs, poor balance; poor memory, impaired judgment
High risk for impaired skin integrity related to capillary fragility	Reports itching	Waxy pallor; petechiae, purpura
Altered nutrition: less than body requirements related to sore mouth and tongue, constipation, and/or diarrhea	Reports lack of appetite, indigestion, sore mouth	Weight loss; constipation or diarrhea; smooth, red beefy tongue
Impaired gas exchange related to inadequate number and impaired function of erythrocytes	Reports palpitations and shortness of breath	Tachycardia, wide pulse pressure

3 PLAN

Patient goals

1. The patient will avoid injury.
2. The patient's skin will remain intact.
3. The patient's nutritional status will improve.
4. The patient will have adequate gas exchange.

4 IMPLEMENT

NURSING DIAGNOSIS	NURSING INTERVENTIONS	RATIONALE
High risk for injury related to sensory and motor losses, alteration in mental status	Keep patient on bed rest with side rails up and assist with ambulation as needed.	To prevent falls.
	Use bed cradle or foot board.	To prevent pressure on lower extremities.
	Apply heat with extreme caution.	To avoid burning the skin.
	Help patient plan periods of activity followed by periods of rest.	To prevent weakness and fatigue.
	Support patient with patience and reassurance.	To reduce irritability and depression.
	Help patient with verbal and written cues as reminders of things to be remembered and decisions to be made.	To limit impact of poor memory and impaired judgment on patient's self-care.
	Monitor patient's mood, appropriateness of behavior, and orientation; seek expert consultation.	To protect the patient from unnecessary and prolonged depression.
High risk for impaired skin integrity related to capillary fragility	Observe skin for color, warmth, texture, moisture, and intactness.	To detect peripheral and systemic changes.
	Maintain skin hygiene, and apply heat with extreme caution.	To prevent irritation or damage and to prevent burning.
Altered nutrition: less than body requirements related to sore mouth and tongue, constipation, and/or diarrhea	Administer vitamin B and other drugs as prescribed.	To promote erythropoiesis.
	Encourage patient to eat a diet high in vitamins, iron, and protein.	To promote balanced nutrition.
	Provide frequent, thorough oral hygiene; use local anesthetics as needed.	To promote appetite and prevent discomfort.
	Offer small, frequent feedings.	To prevent digestive overload.
	Observe for diarrhea or constipation, and treat as prescribed.	To prevent abdominal or perineal discomfort and to avoid fluid and electrolyte imbalance
Impaired gas exchange related to inadequate number and impaired function of erythrocytes	Provide bed rest with side rails up.	To decrease cardiopulmonary workload.
	Monitor pulse, BP, and respirations.	To assess adequacy of cardiac and respiratory function.
	Assist with self-care activities as needed; increase patient's exercise as tolerated.	To maintain cardiopulmonary fitness.

→ > >

NURSING DIAGNOSIS	NURSING INTERVENTIONS	RATIONALE
	Remind patient to report dyspnea and palpitations.	To determine the need for more frequent monitoring of vital signs and/or modification of activity.
	Monitor laboratory reports.	To determine effectiveness of drug therapy.

5 EVALUATE

PATIENT OUTCOME	DATA INDICATING THAT OUTCOME IS REACHED
Injury has been avoided.	Patient ambulates without difficulty; she is coordinated in carrying out activities and appears calm and in good spirits.
Skin has remained intact.	Skin shows no signs of breakdown or discoloration; color is normal.
Nutrition has improved.	Patient takes vitamins as prescribed; she eats diet high in vitamins, iron, and protein and maintains oral hygiene; she does not complain of sore mouth or tongue and has no reports of constipation or diarrhea.
Gas exchange is adequate.	Vital signs are stable; patient does not report dyspnea or palpitations; laboratory values are within normal limits; patient can tolerate normal activity.

PATIENT TEACHING

1. Discuss with the patient precautions to take when using heat therapy devices such as heating pads or hot compresses, as well as general safety measures.
2. Emphasize skin care and oral hygiene.
3. Discuss the importance of following a nutritious diet and the drug therapy regimen.
4. Practice physical therapy activities and general exercise.

Aplastic Anemia

Aplastic anemia is the term most commonly used to describe a decrease in the number of circulating erythrocytes caused by a failure of the bone marrow. This type of anemia usually is accompanied by agranulocytosis and thrombocytopenia, in which case the condition is called pancytopenia.

In half of all diagnosed cases of aplastic anemia, the cause is unknown. In the other half the disorder results from exposure to a specific toxin. The myelotoxins are (1) agents that always cause damage when given in large doses (e.g., radiation, benzene and its derivatives, alkylating agents, and antimetabolites); (2) agents that sometimes cause failure (e.g., chloramphenicol [Chloromycetin], sulfonamides, and phenytoin); and (3) suspicious agents (e.g., streptomycin, chlorophenothane [DDT], and carbon tetrachloride). The disorder may also be immunologic in origin or the result of a severe disease such as liver failure. Some evidence indicates that this anemia may be a sequela of some viral infections, such as those caused by the Epstein-Barr virus, cytomegalovirus, or the hepatitis B virus.

PATHOPHYSIOLOGY

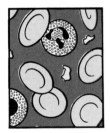

Two theories have been proposed to explain the mechanism that halts erythropoiesis. The seed or stem cell deficiency theory postulates that a common stem cell population is irreversibly altered such that it is incapable of proliferation and differentiation. The microenvironmental deficiency theory proposes that the stem cell environment is altered so as to inhibit erythropoiesis.

If the stem cells or marrow are unable to recover within a few months of the insult, bone marrow aplasia results in death from anemia, infection, or hemorrhage. If only bone marrow hypoplasia results, the individual may live for years with a less severe anemia.

CLINICAL MANIFESTATIONS

A patient with aplastic anemia has the classic cardiovascular and respiratory signs and symptoms of anemia. If the stem cells of leukocytes and platelets have also been damaged or are deficient, thrombocytopenia and leukopenia will ensue.

COMPLICATIONS

Infections
Bleeding

DIAGNOSTIC STUDIES AND FINDINGS

Diagnostic Test	Findings
Erythrocyte count	Usually less than 1 million/mm³
Reticulocyte count	Low
Serum iron	Elevated
Leukocyte count	May be less than 2,000/mm³
Platelet count	<30,000/mm³
Bone marrow biopsy	Fatty marrow with few developing blood cells

---

MEDICAL MANAGEMENT

GENERAL MANAGEMENT

Immediate removal of causative agent and treatment of underlying disorder.

Blood transfusions as needed to replace missing cells.

Prevention or treatment of complications with antibiotics, corticosteroids, and bone marrow transplantation.

1 ASSESS

ASSESSMENT	OBSERVATIONS
Energy level	Progressive fatigue, lassitude
Respiratory status	Dyspnea
Vascular status	Petechiae or ecchymosis; bleeding from gums; hematuria, occult or frank blood in feces
Immune status	Fever, "sniffles," sore throat; anorexia, ulcerations on mucous membranes; pain or burning with urination

2 DIAGNOSE

NURSING DIAGNOSIS	SUBJECTIVE FINDINGS	OBJECTIVE FINDINGS
Activity intolerance related to inadequate tissue oxygenation	Reports progressive fatigue	Lassitude; dyspnea
High risk for infection related to decreased leukocyte count	Reports sore throat, lack of appetite, and pain and burning with urination	Fever, "sniffles," ulcerations on mucous membranes
High risk for fluid volume deficit related to inadequate platelet count and impaired clotting	Reports palpitations	Petechiae or ecchymosis; bleeding from gums; hematuria, occult or frank blood in feces

3 PLAN

Patient goals

1. The patient will demonstrate improved activity tolerance.
2. The patient will have no evidence of infection.
3. The patient will have adequate fluid volume.

4 IMPLEMENT

NURSING DIAGNOSIS	NURSING INTERVENTIONS	RATIONALE
Activity intolerance related to inadequate tissue oxygenation	Place patient in semi-Fowler's or sitting position.	To facilitate breathing.
	Assist with ADLs as needed.	To prevent fatigue.
	Observe respiratory rate, pulse, skin color, and temperature.	To monitor response to activity and determine need for rest periods.

NURSING DIAGNOSIS	NURSING INTERVENTIONS	RATIONALE
	Administer oxygen as needed.	To decrease dyspnea.
High risk for infection related to decreased leukocyte count	Maintain reverse isolation when RBC count is low.	To avoid exposing patient to pathogens.
	Observe for increases in temperature, pulse, and respiration.	To detect signs of infection.
	Observe for other signs or symptoms of infection (e.g., "sniffles," sore throat, anorexia, ulcerations on mucous membranes, pain and burning with urination).	To detect infection of respiratory, GI, or urinary tract.
	Administer antibiotics as prescribed.	To combat specific pathogens.
	Encourage mobility, turning, coughing, deep breathing, and increased fluid intake	To reduce susceptibility to infection.
High risk for fluid volume deficit related to inadequate platelet count and impaired clotting	Protect patient from injury.	To prevent trauma and bleeding.
	Give injections only if necessary; apply pressure at site.	To prevent extravasation.
	Observe patient for signs of bleeding (e.g., petechiae, ecchymoses, hematuria, occult or frank blood in feces).	To detect evidence of intradermal or internal bleeding.
	Monitor laboratory reports (e.g., Hct, Hb).	To detect evidence of internal bleeding.

5 EVALUATE

PATIENT OUTCOME	DATA INDICATING THAT OUTCOME IS REACHED
Activity tolerance is within normal limits.	Patient can carry out ADLs without fatigue or dyspnea; he can exercise for progressively longer periods of time.
Patient shows no evidence of infection.	Patient has no evidence of respiratory, GI, or urinary infection.
Fluid volume is adequate.	There is no evidence of petechiae or ecchymosis; vital signs are stable; there is no observable bleeding; laboratory values are within normal limits.

PATIENT TEACHING

1. Teach the patient how to maintain a balance between rest and activity.
2. Discuss with the patient ways to prevent infection.
3. Discuss with the patient ways to prevent trauma and thus bleeding.
4. Teach the patient how to do self-assessment for signs and symptoms of bleeding, how to determine which to report, and what first-aid measures to implement.

Hemolytic Anemia

Hemolytic anemia is the premature, accelerated destruction of erythrocytes despite normal erythropoiesis. This anemia may be acquired or hereditary.

Acquired hemolytic anemias usually are caused by extrinsic disorders such as trauma (surgery, burns), infection, systemic disease (Hodgkin's lymphoma, leukemia, systemic lupus erythematosus), drugs or toxins, liver or renal disease, or abnormal immune responses. Hereditary forms are caused by such intrinsic abnormalities as structural defects of the erythrocyte, enzyme deficiencies (glycolytic or metabolic enzymes), or defects of globin synthesis or structure. Congenital hemolytic anemias are present at birth and may or may not be hereditary.

PATHOPHYSIOLOGY

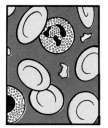 Hemolysis of the erythrocytes in the blood vessels usually is caused by chemicals (drugs or toxins), antibodies, or erythrocyte fragility. Hemolysis that occurs in lymphoid tissues most often is caused by phagocytosis by macrophages of the mononuclear phagocyte system.

Autoimmune hemolytic anemias include:

1. Warm antibody disease, which is mediated by IgG antibody; this antibody can activate the complement cascade, causing intravascular destruction of RBCs; the chronic anemia associated with this disease often is seen in patients with chronic lymphocytic leukemia, lymphoid tumors, and systemic lupus erythematosus (SLE)
2. Cold antibody disease, which is mediated by IgM; this antibody binds to RBCs only at colder temperatures (below 31° C [87.8° F]); it produces pain and tissue destruction in the fingers and toes; if the antibody does not dissociate from the RBCs when the antibody-coated cells warm upon reentering the general circulation, hemolysis of the cell may occur; this disorder is often a complication of infectious mononucleosis, *Myco-plasma pneumoniae* infections, and lymphoid malignancies
3. Drug-induced immune hemolytic anemia, which can be caused in two ways: an immune reaction against a drug may occur, resulting in the formation of antigen-antibody complexes that adhere to the erythrocyte surface, or a drug or its metabolite may bind directly to the erythrocyte's

surface, forming a neoantigen that attracts antibodies; each of these mechanisms activates the complement cascade and hemolysis

Acute conditions develop if the patient also has other diseases, especially viral infection. The peripheral blood hemoglobin level often declines further, and sometimes bone marrow hypoplasia or aplasia may develop.

CLINICAL MANIFESTATIONS

The degree of hemolysis and the outcome of compensatory erythropoiesis determine the presence and severity of signs and symptoms. The spleen becomes enlarged as more and more dead or defective erythrocytes are removed from the circulation. Jaundice develops if heme breakdown exceeds the liver's ability to conjugate and excrete bilirubin.

In severe hemolytic anemia, the bones become deformed and pathologic fractures occur. Cardiovascular and respiratory signs and symptoms vary with the severity of the anemia.

The most effective treatment of hemolytic anemia involves identifying the causative agent or treating the underlying disorder. Hemolytic crisis must be treated with fluid and electrolyte replacement to prevent shock and renal damage from erythrocytes clogging the renal tubules. Transfusions of blood components may be required. Splenectomy is performed if the spleen is identified as the primary site of hemolysis and if splenomegaly is significant.

Corticosteroids are prescribed to treat autoimmune hemolytic anemias. Osmotic diuretics may be administered to prevent acute renal tubular necrosis.

DIAGNOSTIC STUDIES AND FINDINGS

Diagnostic Test	Findings
Erythrocyte count	Low
Hemoglobin (Hb)	Low
Hematocrit (Hct)	Low
Reticulocyte count	High
Erythrocyte fragility	Increased
Erythrocyte life span	Shortened
Serum bilirubin	Increased
Fecal urobilinogen	Increased
Urinary urobilinogen	Increased
Bone marrow biopsy	Erythroid hyperplasia

MEDICAL MANAGEMENT

GENERAL MANAGEMENT

Causative factor is eliminated and underlying disorder is treated.

Fluid and electrolyte balance is maintained.

Transfusions are administered as needed.

DRUG THERAPY

Corticosteroids (e.g., prednisolone).

Osmotic diuretics (e.g., mannitol, urea).

SURGERY

Splenectomy

1　ASSESS

ASSESSMENT	OBSERVATIONS
Fluid and electrolyte balance	Decreased urinary output, fluid loss or overload
Gastrointestinal function	Nausea and vomiting, enlargement of liver and/or spleen, cholelithiasis
Skin	Jaundice
Mobility	Weakness and fatigue
Comfort	Fever and chills, back or abdominal pain

2　DIAGNOSE

NURSING DIAGNOSIS	SUBJECTIVE FINDINGS	OBJECTIVE FINDINGS
Fluid volume deficit related to blood cell hemolysis, impaired renal blood flow	Reports thirst	Decreased urinary output, edema

→ › ›

NURSING DIAGNOSIS	SUBJECTIVE FINDINGS	OBJECTIVE FINDINGS
Altered nutrition: less than body requirements related to liver dysfunction	Reports nausea, abdominal pain	Vomiting, enlargement of liver and/or spleen, cholelithiasis
Impaired skin integrity related to increased serum bilirubin	Reports itching	Jaundice
Impaired mobility related to tissue hypoxia	Reports fatigue	Weakness
Abdominal or back pain related to liver and/or splenic distention	Reports abdominal or back pain	Grimacing, clutching abdomen, or moving with care so as not to strain back

3 ︱ PLAN

Patient goals

1. The patient will have adequate fluid volume.
2. The patient will demonstrate adequate nutrition.
3. The patient will maintain skin integrity.
4. The patient will maintain mobility.
5. The patient will have no pain.

4 ︱ IMPLEMENT

NURSING DIAGNOSIS	NURSING INTERVENTIONS	RATIONALE
Fluid volume deficit related to blood cell hemolysis, impaired renal blood flow	Increase oral fluid intake as tolerated.	To maintain intravascular fluid volume.
	Give small but frequent drinks.	To prevent abdominal distention.
	Monitor intake and output.	To determine fluid needs and prevent fluid overload.
	Observe urine for color, specific gravity, and pH.	To detect renal failure early.
	Assess skin turgor.	To determine adequacy of hydration.
	Administer IV fluids as prescribed.	To correct fluid volume deficit.
	Administer urine alkalizers as prescribed.	To promote renal function.
	Administer blood transfusions as prescribed.	To correct volume deficit.

NURSING DIAGNOSIS	NURSING INTERVENTIONS	RATIONALE
Altered nutrition: less than body requirements related to liver dysfunction	Provide balanced diet rich in iron and protein.	To enhance erythropoiesis.
	Give small, frequent feedings.	To prevent distention.
	Instruct patient to avoid fatty foods.	To decrease discomfort and stress on gallbladder.
	Monitor body weight.	To monitor nutritional status.
	Observe and record food intake.	To assess patient's appetite.
	Observe color of urine.	To assess liver function.
	Monitor laboratory values, especially bilirubin.	To monitor liver function.
Impaired skin integrity related to increased serum bilirubin	Provide frequent skin care, including cool water and lubrication; maintain cool room temperature with adequate humidity.	To maintain comfort and decrease itching.
	Expose skin to sunlight.	To promote warmth and enhance circulation.
	Advise patient not to scratch skin.	To prevent irritation and abrasions.
Impaired mobility related to tissue hypoxia	Assist patient with ambulation.	To compensate for patient's weakness.
	Provide walker, wheelchair, crutches, or cane as needed.	To assist with mobility.
	Observe for weakness and fatigue.	To pace exercise and rest.
	Encourage exercise as tolerated.	To increase strength.
Abdominal or back pain related to liver and/or splenic distention	Place patient in sitting position with support.	To relieve pressure of enlarged liver and/or spleen.
	Provide warmth, prescribed analgesia, and other pain-relief measures as needed.	To relieve discomfort.
	Administer antipyretics as prescribed.	To maintain normal body temperature.
	Have blankets, extra clothing, and external sources of warmth available (e.g., heating pad or lighted bed cradle).	To warm patient when chilling occurs.
	Offer prescribed antiemetics, carbonated beverages, oral care, and other measures of patient's choice.	To reduce nausea and vomiting.

→ › ›

5 EVALUATE

PATIENT OUTCOME	DATA INDICATING THAT OUTCOME IS REACHED
Body hydration is normal.	Skin turgor and color are normal; intake and output are balanced; renal function is adequate.
Nutritional status has improved.	Patient eats a well-balanced diet; weight is returning to normal; no enlargement of liver or spleen is noted.
Skin integrity is maintained.	No abrasions are observed; patient does not scratch skin; skin is warm and dry.
Patient's activity level is normal.	Patient exercises regularly, uses assistive device as needed, and rests when tired.
Patient is free of pain.	Patient has no complaints of back or abdominal pain; temperature is within normal limits.

PATIENT TEACHING

1. Help the patient find a balance between rest and exercise.
2. Discuss with the patient the need for a well-balanced diet with adequate fluids.
3. Remind the patient to maintain skin hygiene and to avoid scratching the skin by using lubricants to relieve itching.
4. Help the patient identify nonprescription comfort measures.

Sickle Cell Disease

Sickle cell disease is a group of disorders characterized by the presence of hemoglobin S (Hb S), an abnormal form of hemoglobin, in the erythrocytes. Hb S is created by a genetic mutation in which one amino acid (valine) replaces another (glutamic acid). The resulting sickle hemoglobin reacts to deoxygenation and dehydration by solidifying and stretching the erythrocyte into an elongated sickle shape.

Sickle cell disease is an inherited, autosomal recessive disorder that is expressed as sickle cell anemia, sickle cell thalassemia, or sickle cell hemoglobin C, depending on the pattern of inheritance. Sickle cell thalassemia and sickle cell hemoglobin C are heterozygous diseases in which the child simultaneously inherits another type of abnormal hemoglobin from one parent. Sickle cell trait, in which the child inherits normal hemoglobin (Hb A) from one parent and Hb S from the other, is a heterozygous carrier state that rarely has clinical manifestations; these occur only when the child experiences extreme stress.

Sickle cell disease is more common in people whose origins are in equatorial countries, including central Africa, the Near East, the Mediterranean area, and parts of India. In the United States the disease is most common among black Americans, with a reported incidence of 1 in every 400 to 500 live births. Sickle cell trait is present in 7% to 13% of black Americans. This trait may provide protection against lethal forms of malaria, which would be a genetic advantage to carriers residing in endemic regions; it is of no advantage in the United States.

Sickle cell anemia is the severest of the sickle cell disorders. It is a homozygous, lifelong disease that has no known cure.

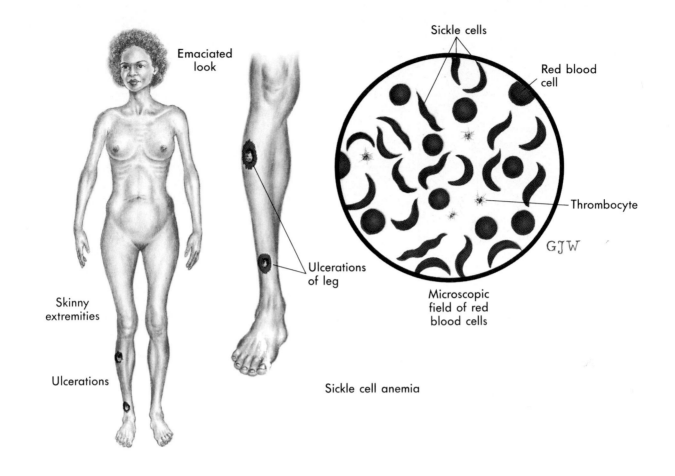

Sickle cell anemia

PATHOPHYSIOLOGY

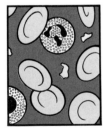

The erythrocytes of people with sickle cell anemia contain more Hb S than Hb A, which causes these cells to assume a sickle or crescent shape when exposed to decreased oxygen tension. The "sickled" cells are then easily destroyed as they enter smaller blood vessels in the body. The exact cause of sickling crises is unknown, but two factors have been identified: (1) hypoxia caused by low oxygen tension in the blood (Po_2), such as that resulting from climbing to high altitudes, exercising strenuously, or inadequate oxygenation during anesthesia; and (2) elevated blood viscosity/decreased plasma volume, increased hydrogen ion concentration (decreased pH), and increased plasma osmolality, caused by a concentration of cells and dehydration resulting from such causes as vomiting, diarrhea, diaphoresis, or diuretics. The microcirculation then becomes occluded, resulting in hypoxia, which causes more sickling. Hypoxemia leads to pain, infarction, and thrombosis in tissues and organs such as the brain, kidneys, bone marrow, and spleen. The resulting anemia triggers erythropoiesis in the marrow and in extreme cases in the liver.

Sickling usually is not permanent in that most sickled erythrocytes regain a normal shape after reoxygenation and rehydration. Irreversible sickling is a consequence of irreversible damage to the plasma membrane caused by the sickling; it is believed that this occurs because the membrane loses its capacity for active transport, permitting an influx of calcium ions.

Many people with sickle cell anemia die during childhood from cerebral hemorrhage or shock. Some individuals survive into their fifties or older. Progressive renal damage, which eventually causes uremia, results in death.

CLINICAL MANIFESTATIONS

The extent, severity, and signs and symptoms of sickling depend to a great extent on the percentage of Hb S. The general manifestations of sickling are those of hemolytic anemia: pallor, jaundice, fatigue, and irritability. Extensive sickling can precipitate four types of crises: a vasoocclusive or thrombotic crisis, an aplastic crisis, sequestration, or, in rare cases, a hyperhemolytic crisis.

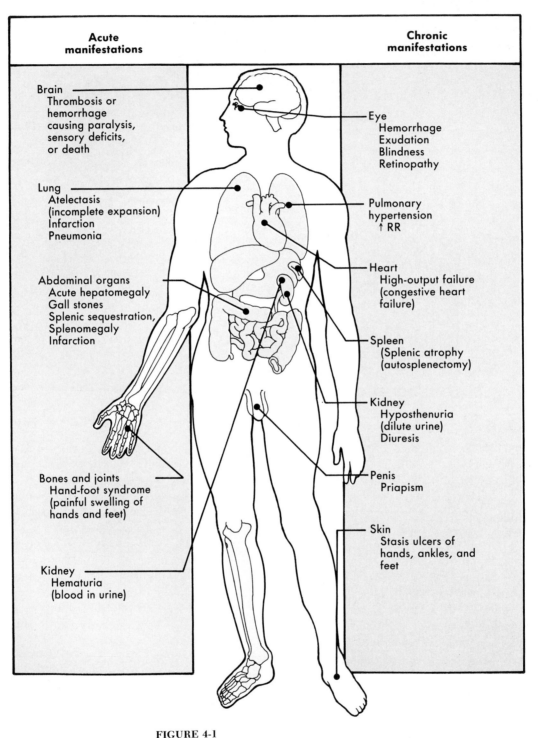

FIGURE 4-1
Clinical manifestations of sickle cell disease.

GENERAL MANIFESTATIONS OF SICKLING
Pallor
Jaundice
Fatigue
Irritability

A **vasoocclusive** crisis begins with sickling in the microcirculation. The resultant vasospasm causes a logjam effect, which brings blood flow through the vessel to a stop. Thrombosis and infarction of local tissue occur. This crisis is extremely painful and lasts an average of 4 to 6 days. It may develop spontaneously or may be precipitated by localized hypoxemia, low P_{O_2}, exposure to cold, dehydration, acidosis (low pH), or infection. Symmetric, painful swelling of the hands and feet (hand-and-foot syndrome) often is the first manifestation of sickle cell disease in infancy. In older children and adults, the large joints and surrounding tissues become swollen and painful. Priapism may occur if penile veins are obstructed. Severe abdominal pain is caused by infarction in abdominal structures. Cerebral vascular accidents may cause paralysis (usually hemiplegia) or other central nervous system deficits.

A **sequestration** crisis, in which large amounts of blood pool in the liver and spleen, is seen only in young children. Death results from cardiovascular collapse.

An **aplastic** crisis develops when a compensatory increase in erythropoiesis is compromised. This results in profound anemia.

A **hyperhemolytic** crisis is rare but may occur with certain drugs or infections. G-6-PD deficiency, when also present, contributes to this type of crisis.

Clinical manifestations of sickle cell disease do not usually appear until an infant is at least 6 months old. Infection is the most common cause of death. Sickle cell hemoglobin C disease usually is milder, with clinical problems related to vasoocclusive crises resulting from higher hematocrit and blood viscosity. In older children obstructive crises cause sickle cell retinopathy, renal necrosis, and aseptic necrosis of the femoral head.

Sickle cell thalassemia has the mildest clinical manifestations. The erythrocytes of those with the disease tend to be microcytic and hypochromic, which makes the cells less likely to clog the microcirculation, even when sickling.

Severe hypoxia in individuals with the sickle cell trait may cause vasoocclusive episodes. The cells in these people form an ivy shape.

The goal of medical management is to prevent the effects of anemia and to avoid crises. Crisis prevention consists of avoiding fever, infection, acidosis, dehydration, constricting clothing, and exposure to cold.

The use of intravenous fluids to correct acidosis and dehydration is critical. Acetaminophen is preferable for antipyretic therapy so as to avoid increased acidosis. The value of blood transfusions must be compared with the risks of hepatitis, hemosiderosis (sequestration of iron complexes in the mitochondria of erythroblasts), and splenic overload.

Genetic counseling and psychologic support are important for both the patient and the family (see Patient Teaching Guide). These interventions help individuals with sickle cell trait or sickle cell disease to make informed decisions about having children.

DIAGNOSTIC STUDIES AND FINDINGS

Diagnostic Test	Findings
Stained blood smear	Sickle cell observed
Sickle cell slide preparation of blood	Sickling noted after deoxygenation
Sickle solubility test	Turbid solution indicates presence of Hb S
Hemoglobin electrophoresis	Presence of Hb S and Hb A indicates sickle cell trait; presence of Hb S only indicates sickle cell anemia
Erythrocyte life span	Decreased (10 to 20 days)

MEDICAL MANAGEMENT

GENERAL MANAGEMENT

Supportive care, including rest, oxygen therapy, IV fluids and electrolytes, analgesics, and sedatives.

Blood transfusions.

Genetic counseling.

DRUG THERAPY

Experimental use of antisickling agents (urea, cyanate, carbamoyl phosphate).

Oral maintenance therapy with folic acid and/or iron.

SURGERY

Splenectomy.

1 ASSESS

ASSESSMENT	OBSERVATIONS
Skin	Jaundice or pallor, ulceration
Skeletal structures	Joint swelling, disproportionately long arms and legs, skeletal fragility
Gastrointestinal function	Enlarged liver and spleen
Comfort	Bone, abdominal pain
Cardiac function	Systolic murmurs, dysrhythmias, cardiac enlargement, hypertension
Respiratory function	Dyspnea, acute respiratory distress
Sensory function	Altered level of consciousness, abnormal pupillary response, abnormal reflexes
Renal function	Decreased urinary output, edema
Sexuality	Delayed sexual maturity

2   DIAGNOSE

NURSING DIAGNOSIS	SUBJECTIVE FINDINGS	OBJECTIVE FINDINGS
Impaired skin integrity related to altered circulation to tissues, resulting in hypoxia and inadequate nutrition	Reports itching, pain	Jaundice, pallor, ulceration
High risk for injury related to joint swelling, bone fragility	Reports pain with movement	Joint swelling, disproportionately long arms and legs, bone fragility
Pain related to bone fragility, joint swelling, and abdominal distention	Reports bone, joint, and/or abdominal pain	Joint swelling, enlarged liver and/or spleen
Altered cardiopulmonary tissue perfusion related to occlusion of microcirculation, increased blood viscosity, and decreased P_{O_2}	Reports palpitations, chest pain, shortness of breath; easily becomes fatigued	Systolic murmurs, dysrhythmias, dyspnea, cyanosis
Altered cerebral tissue perfusion related to increased intracranial pressure	Reports headaches, blurred vision	Decreased level of consciousness, altered pupillary response, altered reflexes
Altered renal tissue perfusion related to occlusion of microcirculation by sickling, dehydration, and increased blood viscosity	Reports difficulty urinating	Decreased urinary output, edema
Sexual dysfunction related to delayed sexual maturity	Reports underdeveloped sexual organs	Small breasts or small penis, sparse body hair

3   PLAN

Patient goals

1. The patient will maintain skin integrity.
2. The patient will retain mobility without injury.
3. The patient will be free of pain.
4. The patient will demonstrate improved cardiopulmonary, cerebral, and renal tissue perfusion.
5. The patient will maintain sexual function.

→ ❯ ❯

4 IMPLEMENT

NURSING DIAGNOSIS	NURSING INTERVENTIONS	RATIONALE
Impaired skin integrity related to altered circulation to tissues, resulting in hypoxia and inadequate nutrition	Remove constrictive clothing, and maintain room and body warmth.	To enhance circulation and prevent chilling and possible sickling.
	Maintain exercise as tolerated, using range-of-motion exercises.	To maintain circulation.
	Inspect extremities.	To detect ulceration early.
	Palpate arterial pulses.	To assess adequacy of arterial circulation.
	Monitor blood studies.	To determine P_{O_2}, blood viscosity, and pH.
	Keep patient on bed rest in semi-Fowler's position if ulceration occurs.	To prevent injury and decrease resistance to peripheral circulation.
	Elevate affected part.	To enhance venous return.
	If ulceration develops, implement wound care procedures.	To remove drainage and necrotic tissue and prevent infection
	Apply sterile dressing or expose affected area to air as appropriate.	To promote healing.
	Apply heat with lamp or lighted cradle.	To enhance circulation and promote healing.
	Observe response of wound to therapy.	To evaluate effectiveness of treatment and modify care as needed.
	Cut patient's fingernails and toenails.	To discourage scratching and prevent injury.
High risk for injury related to joint swelling, bone fragility	Maintain a safe environment.	To prevent falls or other injury.
	Change the patient's position frequently, with joint support.	To prevent trauma.
	Initiate range-of-motion exercises, and encourage patient to do them.	To maintain circulation, joint movement, and muscle tone.
	Encourage patient to eat foods high in calcium, protein, and vitamins.	To prevent possible bone or tissue injury, including fracture.
Pain related to bone fragility, joint swelling, and abdominal distention	Remove restrictive clothing, and change patient's position frequently.	To relieve pressure and enhance comfort.
	Place patient in semi-Fowler's position.	To increase intraabdominal space.
	Give the patient small, frequent feedings.	To prevent abdominal distention.

NURSING DIAGNOSIS	NURSING INTERVENTIONS	RATIONALE
	Auscultate for bowel sounds.	To detect any obstruction.
	Palpate liver.	To monitor liver size.
	Provide analgesics as prescribed, and offer other pain-relief measures as appropriate (e.g., heat, relaxation, imagery, humor).	To relieve pain.
Altered cardiopulmonary tissue perfusion related to occlusion of microcirculation, increased blood viscosity, and decreased P_{O_2}	Encourage patient to rest frequently and to avoid strenuous activity.	To decrease cardiac workload and prevent sickling.
	Have patient stay in semi-Fowler's position when in bed.	To enhance expansion of lungs.
	Advise patient to avoid such stimulants as caffeine and smoking.	To prevent vasoconstriction.
	Auscultate apical pulse.	To detect dysrhythmias.
	Monitor BP.	To assess cardiac function and peripheral resistance to blood flow.
	Monitor respirations.	To assess pulmonary function and detect onset of respiratory failure.
	Notify physician if patient complains of chest pain or increasing dyspnea, cyanosis, and restlessness.	To allow quick intervention.
	Monitor blood studies.	To assess adequacy of blood flow and tissue perfusion.
Altered cerebral tissue perfusion related to increased intracranial pressure	Keep patient on complete bed rest with head of bed elevated.	To reduce energy expenditure and lower intracranial pressure.
	Decrease environmental stimuli.	To promote rest and prevent stress.
	Change patient's position slowly.	To prevent trauma.
	Discourage stimulants such as caffeine and smoking.	To prevent vasoconstriction.
	Monitor neurologic signs (e.g., level of consciousness, pupillary response, reflexes).	To detect changes indicating increasing intracranial pressure.
	Observe for changes in pulse, BP, and respirations.	To detect changes in patient's status.

→ 〉 〉

NURSING DIAGNOSIS	NURSING INTERVENTIONS	RATIONALE
Altered renal tissue perfusion related to occlusion of microcirculation by sickling, dehydration, and increased blood viscosity	Provide adequate fluid intake (oral or IV).	To maintain fluid balance and enhance renal perfusion.
	Monitor intake and output.	To maintain balance between the two.
	Test urine for protein.	Protein in the urine is a sign of renal dysfunction.
	Monitor body weight.	To assess for fluid retention.
	Inspect for edema of face and extremities.	To detect evidence of impaired renal function and fluid retention.
	Monitor blood studies for abnormal electrolytes and increased blood viscosity, and monitor urine studies.	To evaluate adequacy of renal function.
	Monitor vital signs, especially BP.	To determine adequacy of blood flow.
Sexual dysfunction related to delayed sexual maturity	Encourage patient to describe current sexual interactions and behavior patterns.	To identify problem areas.
	Provide privacy when discussing sexual topics.	To avoid embarrassing patient.
	Help patient obtain information needed to improve sexual interactions.	To help patient change or modify current actions and behavior.

5   EVALUATE

PATIENT OUTCOME	DATA INDICATING THAT OUTCOME IS REACHED
Skin integrity has been maintained.	Patient's skin is warm, dry, and of natural color; there is no evidence of ulceration.
There is no evidence of injury.	Patient ambulates without assistance; there are no signs of swelling or abnormal alignment; patient has no joint or bone pain.
Patient does not complain of pain.	Patient does not report joint, bone, or abdominal pain; he monitors his diet and activity to prevent abdominal distention or trauma.
Perfusion of cardiopulmonary, cerebral, and renal tissues is adequate.	Patient has normal vital signs, pupillary responses, and reflexes; he is alert and has no headaches; intake and output are balanced.
Sexual function is normal.	Patient reports satisfaction with sexual activity.

PATIENT TEACHING

1. Provide genetic counseling as appropriate.
2. Discuss ways to avoid sickle cell crisis (e.g., maintain hydration, keep warm, use stress-reduction techniques).
3. Practice range-of-motion exercises with the patient, and encourage regular physical activity. Explain the need for balance between rest and activity.
4. Discuss the principles of good nutrition and the value of avoiding stimulants such as caffeine and smoking.
5. Teach the patient and family the signs and symptoms of cardiopulmonary dysfunction, increasing intracranial pressure, and renal impairment, which need to be reported to the physician or nurse.
6. Discuss ways to deal with delayed sexual maturity in particular and the impact of chronic disease in general.

Thalassemias

The **alpha-** and **beta-thalassemias** are inherited, autosomal recessive disorders that impair the rate of synthesis of one of the two chains of normal hemoglobin (Hb A). Alpha-thalassemia is most common among Chinese, Vietnamese, Cambodians, and Laotians. Beta-thalassemia is more prevalent among Greeks, Italians, and some Arabs and Sephardic Jews. Both of these thalassemias are common among black Americans.

Both thalassemias can be major or minor, depending on (1) whether the defects are inherited homozygously (thalassemia major) or heterozygously (thalassemia minor) and (2) how many of the genes that control alpha- or beta-chain synthesis are defective.

PATHOPHYSIOLOGY

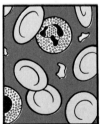

The pathophysiologic effects of the thalassemias range from mild microcytosis to death in utero; the anemic manifestation of thalassemia is microcytic-hypochromic hemolytic anemia.

The hemoglobin abnormality most often consists of the substitution of a single amino acid for another; other possible molecular abnormalities are two amino acid substitutions, amino acid deletions or fusions, and synthesis of elongated chains.

There are four types of alpha-thalassemia (see box): (1) alpha trait (the carrier state), in which one of the four genes that form the alpha chain is defective; (2) alpha-thalassemia minor, in which two genes are defective; (3) hemoglobin H disease, in which three genes are defective; and (4) alpha-thalassemia major, a fatal disorder in which all four alpha-chain–forming genes are defective (without alpha chains, oxygen cannot be released to the tissues).

In beta-thalassemia the fundamental defect is the uncoupling of alpha- and beta-chain synthesis. Beta-chain production is moderately depressed in beta-thalassemia minor and severely depressed in beta-thalassemia major (also called Cooley's anemia). Depression of beta-chain synthesis causes production of erythrocytes with a reduced amount of hemoglobin and accumulation of free alpha chains, which are unstable and easily precipitate in the cell. Most erythroblasts containing precipitates are destroyed by mononuclear phagocytes in the bone marrow, which results in ineffective erythropoiesis and anemia. Some of these cells do mature and enter the bloodstream, but they are destroyed prematurely in the spleen.

FOUR TYPES OF ALPHA-THALASSEMIA

Alpha trait (the carrier state)
   One alpha-chain–forming gene is defective.
Alpha-thalassemia minor
   Two genes are defective.
Hemoglobin H disease
   Three genes are defective.
Alpha-thalassemia major (fatal disorder)
   All four genes are defective.

Beta-thalassemia is more common than alpha-thalassemia. In rare cases synthesis of gamma or delta polypeptide chains is defective, resulting in gamma- or delta-thalassemia.

CLINICAL MANIFESTATIONS

Individuals who inherit the alpha trait usually are asymptomatic, with possible mild microcytosis. Alpha-thalassemia minor has signs and symptoms almost identical to those of beta-thalassemia: mild microcytic-hypochromic anemia, enlargement of the liver and spleen, and bone marrow hyperplasia.

Alpha-thalassemia major causes hydrops fetalis and fulminant intrauterine congestive heart failure; the fetus has a grossly enlarged heart and liver, edema, and massive ascites. The disorder usually is diagnosed post mortem. Prenatal screening can be done through chorionic villus sampling; the cells can be analyzed and a DNA genetic map constructed and evaluated.

Beta-thalassemia minor causes mild to moderate microcytic-hypochromic anemia, mild splenomegaly, bronze coloring of the skin, and hyperplasia of the bone marrow. Skeletal changes depend on the degree of reticulocytosis, which in turn depends on the severity of the anemia.

People who have beta-thalassemia minor usually are asymptomatic, whereas those with beta-thalassemia major may become very ill. In beta-thalassemia major the anemia is severe, resulting in a great cardiovascular burden, with high-output congestive heart failure. Blood transfusions can increase the person's life span by a decade or two (death usually is caused by hemochromatosis). People with beta-thalassemia major have an enlarged liver and spleen, and growth and maturation are retarded. A characteristic deformity (chipmunk deformity) develops on the face as the bones expand to accommodate hyperplastic marrow.

Both alpha- and beta-thalassemia major are life threatening. Children with thalassemia major usually are weak, fail to thrive, show poor development, and experience cardiovascular compromise with high-output failure; if the condition goes untreated, these children die by 6 years of age.

Blood transfusions can return hemoglobin and hematocrit to normal levels, alleviating the anemia-induced cardiac failure. Iron overload and hemochromatosis, which are complications of transfusion therapy, are treated with chelating agents.

Splenectomy can lessen the need for transfusions by eliminating a site of hemolysis, thus prolonging erythrocyte survival.

Two possible treatment techniques are under investigation. One involves iron chelation therapy combined with hypertransfusion (to a hematocrit of 35); the other involves neocyte transfusion, in which young erythrocytes in a unit of blood are separated from old erythrocytes by centrifugation and then infused.

DIAGNOSTIC STUDIES AND FINDINGS

Diagnostic Test	Findings
Blood smear	Target cell and other strangely shaped erythrocytes; pale, nucleated RBCs
Erythrocyte count	Decreased
Serum bilirubin	Elevated
Serum iron	Slightly elevated
Fecal urobilinogen	Greatly elevated
Urinary urobilinogen	Greatly elevated
Fetal hemoglobin (Hb F)	Elevated; may be as high as 90%
Hemoglobin A (Hb A)	Elevated; may be as high as 6%

MEDICAL MANAGEMENT

GENERAL MANAGEMENT

Supportive therapy, including blood transfusions.

Prenatal diagnosis and genetic counseling.

DRUG THERAPY

Chelating agents (e.g., deferoxamine mesylate).

SURGERY

Splenectomy.

1   ASSESS

ASSESSMENT	OBSERVATIONS
Skin	Jaundice, pallor, leg ulcers
Gastrointestinal function	Enlarged liver and spleen, fat intolerance
Cardiovascular function	Dysrhythmias, heart failure, bleeding tendency

2   DIAGNOSE

NURSING DIAGNOSIS	SUBJECTIVE FINDINGS	OBJECTIVE FINDINGS
Impaired skin integrity related to peripheral hypoxia	Reports itching and pain	Jaundice, pallor, leg ulcers
Altered nutrition: less than body requirements related to enlarged liver and spleen, altered metabolism	Reports intolerance of fatty foods and abdominal distention and discomfort	Enlarged spleen and liver, mahogany-colored urine, clay-colored stool
Altered cardiopulmonary tissue perfusion related to high-output cardiac failure	Reports palpitations, shortness of breath, and weakness	Dysrhythmia, tachycardia and tachypnea, edema

3   PLAN

Patient goals

1. The patient will maintain skin integrity.
2. The patient will maintain adequate nutritional status.
3. The patient will demonstrate improved cardiopulmonary tissue perfusion.

4   IMPLEMENT

NURSING DIAGNOSIS	NURSING INTERVENTIONS	RATIONALE
Impaired skin integrity related to peripheral hypoxia	Assess color, tone, temperature, and moistness of skin.	To gather baseline data for detecting changes.
	Provide skin care, using cool water and lubrication.	To promote hygiene and prevent itching.

→ ❯ ❯

NURSING DIAGNOSIS	NURSING INTERVENTIONS	RATIONALE
	Advise patient not to scratch skin.	To prevent injury.
	Keep patient on bed rest if leg ulcer develops.	To rest affected extremity.
	Elevate affected extremity.	To enhance peripheral circulation.
	Implement wound care as prescribed.	To remove drainage and necrotic tissue and to prevent infection.
	Apply sterile dressing, or expose affected area to air as appropriate; apply heat with lamp or lighted cradle.	To promote healing.
	Observe wound's response to treatment.	To evaluate effectiveness of therapy and determine whether procedure needs to be modified.
Altered nutrition: less than body requirements related to enlarged liver and spleen, altered metabolism	Help patient into semi-Fowler's position for eating.	To lessen abdominal pressure.
	Provide low-fat, high-calorie, high-protein, iron-rich diet.	To prevent indigestion and maintain energy while restoring erythrocytes.
	Give small, frequent feedings.	To prevent abdominal distention.
	Offer antiflatulence medication and warmth as indicated.	To reduce abdominal bloating.
	Remove constrictive clothing.	To relieve abdominal pressure and increase comfort.
	Auscultate for bowel sounds.	To detect obstruction.
	Palpate liver.	To monitor its size and location.
Altered cardiopulmonary tissue perfusion related to high-output cardiac failure	Encourage patient to rest frequently and to avoid strenuous activity.	To reduce cardiac workload.
	Tell patient to avoid oral stimulants such as caffeine and smoking.	To prevent vasoconstriction.
	Auscultate apical pulse.	To assess cardiac function and detect dysrhythmias.
	Monitor arterial pulses.	To assess peripheral circulation.
	Monitor BP and respirations.	To assess peripheral resistance and pulmonary status.
	Monitor blood studies, such as enzymes, erythrocyte count, and ABGs.	To assess cardiac status.

NURSING DIAGNOSIS	NURSING INTERVENTIONS	RATIONALE
	Observe patient for signs of cardiac failure, including edema.	To ensure quick intervention.

5 EVALUATE

PATIENT OUTCOME	DATA INDICATING THAT OUTCOME IS REACHED
Skin integrity has been maintained.	Patient's skin is warm, dry, and normal in color; there is no evidence of ulceration.
Nutrition is adequate.	Patient is eating a well-balanced, protein-rich diet; she has no complaints of abdominal distention; liver and spleen are within normal limits.
Tissue perfusion has improved.	Patient can tolerate ADLs; she has no complaints of palpitations or dyspnea; vital signs are within normal limits.

PATIENT TEACHING

1. Help the patient maintain skin hygiene and prevent injury, especially to the extremities.
2. Discuss the value of a diet low in fat and high in protein, calories, and iron.
3. Explain to the patient the need to avoid oral stimulants such as caffeine and smoking.
4. Advise the patient to seek genetic counseling (see Patient Teaching Guide).

Polycythemias

Polycythemia (myeloproliferative red cell disorders) is a term used to describe an increase in the number of circulating erythrocytes and the concentration of hemoglobin in the blood. In response to exogenous (radiation, drugs) or endogenous (physiologic compensatory response, immune disorder) factors, the bone marrow stimulates the production of excessive numbers of cells.

Polycythemia vera (primary polycythemia) usually develops in middle age, particularly among Jewish men. The etiology is unknown, but the overproduction of erythrocytes, leukocytes, and thrombocytes increases blood viscosity, blood volume, and congestion of tissues and organs with blood.

Secondary polycythemia, the more commonly seen form of the disorder, is a compensatory response to tissue hypoxia found with chronic obstructive lung disease, congenital heart disease, and prolonged exposure to high altitudes (10,000 feet or higher).

Relative polycythemia is just that, a relative increase in erythrocyte concentration found with plasma loss caused by fluid loss and dehydration. Specific causes may include insufficient fluid intake, diarrhea, vomiting, burns, or excessive diuretics.

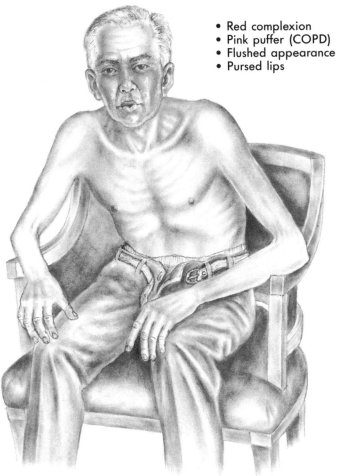

- Red complexion
- Pink puffer (COPD)
- Flushed appearance
- Pursed lips

GJW

Polycythemia (COPD)
(Clinical appearance)

PATHOPHYSIOLOGY

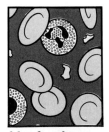

Polycythemia vera is caused by excessive proliferation of erythrocyte precursors in the bone marrow. The presence of increased numbers of circulating platelets and granulocytes suggests an abnormality of the pluripotential stem cell.

Erythrocytosis causes increased blood volume and viscosity because of the increased erythrocyte count. The liver and spleen become increasingly congested with RBCs as viscosity slows blood flow. Eventually the thick, sticky, slow-moving blood becomes an ideal environment for acidosis and clotting. Tissue or organ infarction results when thrombi obstruct blood vessels.

CLINICAL MANIFESTATIONS

The signs of polycythemia vera are plethora (ruddy color of the face, hands, feet, ears, and mucous membranes), engorgement of retinal and sublingual veins, and splenomegaly and hepatomegaly. Symptoms include headaches, a feeling of fullness in the head, dizziness, weakness, fatigue on exertion, visual disturbances, hypertension, sweating, itching, weight loss, epigastric distress, and backache.

The patient might have bloodshot eyes. Pruritus after bathing may cause the patient to avoid warm water (the cause of this pruritus is unknown, and it does not respond to antihistamines).

Clinical manifestations of vascular disease may be the most prevalent symptoms. These include angina pectoris, intermittent claudication (calf pain associated with walking-induced vasospasm), thrombotic disease, and cerebral insufficiency. Ulcers and mesenteric pain can result from thrombosis of gastric vessels. Hoarseness and respiratory infections are common. Some patients tend to bleed, especially from the genitourinary and gastrointestinal tracts. A syndrome resembling disseminated intravascular coagulation may occur.

The goal of medical management of polycythemia is to reduce erythrocytosis and blood volume, control symptoms, and prevent thrombosis. Phlebotomy involves venipuncture and removal of blood.

Patients who smoke should be urged to stop, and those with congestive heart failure and chronic obstructive pulmonary disease require appropriate drug therapy and other supportive measures.

Although myelosuppressive drugs (antineoplastic agents) may be of some value, their side effects often are worse than the disease. Likewise, radioactive phosphorus may cause general suppression of hematopoiesis, with resultant anemia, leukopenia, or thrombocytopenia.

Without proper treatment, half of those with polycythemia die within 28 months of the onset of the disease; the major cause of death is thrombosis or hemorrhage.

DIAGNOSTIC STUDIES AND FINDINGS

Diagnostic Test	Findings
Erythrocyte count	As high as 8-12 million/mm^3
Mean corpuscular hemoglobin concentration (MCHC)	Decreased
Leukocytes	Increased
Thrombocytes	Increased
Total blood volume	Increased

MEDICAL MANAGEMENT

GENERAL MANAGEMENT

Venesection (phlebotomy with removal of 300-500 ml two or three times a week until Hct drops sufficiently; every 3-4 months thereafter).

Smoking cessation.

DRUG THERAPY

Antineoplastic agents to suppress bone marrow function (may include busulfan, chlorambucil, and mechlorethamine).

Radioactive phosphorus (^{32}P) PO or IV.

1 ASSESS

ASSESSMENT	OBSERVATIONS
Cardiopulmonary function	Hypertension with headaches, dizziness, sense of fullness in head; congestive heart failure with shortness of breath, orthopnea, fatigue on exertion, weakness; angina pectoris; respiratory infection, hoarseness; ruddy complexion; dusky redness of mucosa, hands, feet, and ears; intermittent claudication
Cerebrovascular function	Altered level of consciousness; altered pupillary response; weakness in extremities; visual disturbances
Gastrointestinal function	Enlargement of liver and spleen; weight loss; epigastric distress; backache; bleeding
Skin	Sweating, itching

2 DIAGNOSE

NURSING DIAGNOSIS	SUBJECTIVE FINDINGS	OBJECTIVE FINDINGS
Altered cardiopulmonary tissue perfusion related to increased arterial pressure, blood volume, and blood viscosity	Reports dizziness, headaches, sense of fullness in head, shortness of breath, difficulty in breathing while lying down, chest pain, weakness, fatigue on exertion, intermittent pain in extremities	Ruddy complexion; redness of mucous membranes, hands, feet, and ears; hypertension; respiratory infection; hoarseness

→ > >

NURSING DIAGNOSIS	SUBJECTIVE FINDINGS	OBJECTIVE FINDINGS
Altered cerebrovascular tissue perfusion related to increased intracranial pressure	Reports weakness in arms and legs, and visual disturbances	Altered level of consciousness, altered pupillary response
Pain related to abdominal distention and ulceration	Reports backache, upset stomach	Enlarged liver and spleen, weight loss, bleeding (e.g., occult or frank blood in stool, hematemesis)
Impaired skin integrity related to itching and sweating secondary to pruritus	Reports itching	Sweating, gangrene of the feet

3 PLAN

Patient goals

1. The patient will have adequate cardiopulmonary function.
2. The patient will have adequate cerebrovascular function.
3. The patient will be free of pain.
4. The patient will maintain skin integrity.

4 IMPLEMENT

NURSING DIAGNOSIS	NURSING INTERVENTIONS	RATIONALE
Altered cardiopulmonary tissue perfusion related to increased arterial pressure, blood volume, and blood viscosity	Encourage rest and quiet.	To decrease cardiac workload.
	Discourage use of oral stimulants such as caffeine and smoking.	To prevent vasoconstriction.
	Tell patient to avoid emotional stress.	Stress increases systemic BP and decreases cardiac output.
	Administer medication as prescribed.	To promote vasodilatation and/or diuresis.
	Monitor BP.	To assess effectiveness of therapy.
	Tell patient to avoid sodium-rich foods.	To reduce fluid retention.
	Change patient's position frequently, and maintain in semi-Fowler's position as tolerated.	To enhance pulmonary function.
	Encourage coughing and deep breathing.	To maintain open airway and prevent infection.

NURSING DIAGNOSIS	NURSING INTERVENTIONS	RATIONALE
	Ambulate as tolerated, and assist with ambulation.	To prevent venous stasis and enhance cardiac function; assistance helps prevent injury resulting from dizziness.
	Observe respiratory rate, and auscultate breath sounds.	To monitor cardiopulmonary status.
	Provide medications as prescribed and nonpharmacologic interventions as appropriate.	To relieve headaches and feeling of fullness in head.
	Report complaints of angina to physician.	To determine need for immediate assessment and intervention.
	Observe color of face, hands, feet, ears, and mucous membranes.	To monitor disease status.
Altered cerebrovascular tissue perfusion related to increased intracranial pressure	Monitor level of consciousness, pupillary response, and reflexes.	To detect increasing pressure early.
	Monitor vital signs and BP.	To detect intracranial bleeding.
	Keep patient on bed rest in semi-Fowler's position.	To improve cerebrovascular circulation.
	Assist patient with ADLs and with ambulation if visual disturbance or weakness in extremities is present.	To prevent injury.
Pain related to abdominal distention and ulceration	Auscultate for bowel sounds.	To detect obstruction.
	Observe feces and emesis for evidence of blood.	To detect GI bleeding.
	Assess complaints of abdominal and back pain, and use prescribed medications, positioning, heat, and nonpharmacologic interventions as appropriate.	To relieve pain.
	Place patient in semi-Fowler's position.	To relieve pressure on abdomen.
	Place antacids at bedside for patient to use prn.	To relieve epigastric distress.
	Encourage adequate nutrition.	To maintain or regain weight.
	Palpate liver.	To monitor size and location.

→ > >

NURSING DIAGNOSIS	NURSING INTERVENTIONS	RATIONALE
Impaired skin integrity related to itching and sweating secondary to pruritus	Maintain skin hygiene, including use of cool water for bathing and lubrication.	To prevent and/or relieve itching.
	Observe color, temperature, and moistness of skin.	To monitor response to disease and treatment.
	Inspect feet frequently.	To detect early evidence of gangrene.

5   EVALUATE

PATIENT OUTCOME	DATA INDICATING THAT OUTCOME IS REACHED
Cardiopulmonary tissue perfusion has improved.	Patient's vital signs are stable; he has no complaints of dyspnea, orthopnea, angina, dizziness, or headache.
Cerebrovascular tissue perfusion has improved.	Patient is alert; pupillary response is normal and equal; reflexes are normal; patient has no complaints of visual disturbances or weakness in extremities.
There is no evidence of abdominal or back pain.	Patient can walk without pain or nurse's assistance; there is no evidence of bleeding; Bowel sounds are normal.
Skin integrity has been maintained.	Skin is warm, moist, and normal in color; there are no signs of gangrene; patient maintains skin hygiene and does not scratch.

PATIENT TEACHING

1. Discuss with the patient and family the signs and symptoms of cardiac failure, pulmonary distress, bleeding, and thrombus formation; identify appropriate interventions, including the need to call the physician or nurse.

2. Encourage the patient to stop smoking and to avoid caffeine.
3. Remind the patient to maintain skin hygiene, to inspect his feet regularly, and to avoid injury.
4. Encourage the patient to balance rest with activity and to handle stress in healthy ways.

CHAPTER 5

Leukocytic Disorders

Diseases and abnormalities of the white blood cells can be classified in various ways, such as by the nature of the abnormality, by etiologic origin, by the progression of symptoms and outcome, and by cell lineage. The nature of the abnormality may be described as quantitative or qualitative. Quantitative classification is based on the number of cells in the bone marrow or peripheral blood, or both (leukocytopenias or leukocytoses); qualitative classification is based on a defect or deficiency in a cell component, that is, a morphologic defect, a functional defect, or a combination of the two. The etiologic origin may be hereditary, acquired, or idiopathic, and the progression of symptoms and outcome may be acute or chronic. Cell lineage describes the cell line most obviously affected (see the box on the next page).

Leukocytosis

Leukocytosis is the term used to describe an increase in the number of white blood cells in the peripheral blood.

Neutrophilia is an increase in peripheral blood neutrophils (more than 7,500 per microliter), which occurs in such stressful situations as vigorous exercise, stimulation of catecholamine secretion, administration of certain drugs (especially steroids), and response to infections. A leukemoid reaction is a neutrophilic response that resembles leukemia in that the number of granulocytes increases (50,000 to 100,000 per microliter) and a degree of relative immaturity is evidenced as a "shift to the left." Most of these changes are transient, reflecting movement of polymorphonuclear leukocytes (PMNs) among bone marrow storage, circulating, and tissue compartments.

The number (concentration) and stages (degree of immaturity) of neutrophils are proportional to the severity of a bacterial infection. White cell responses to inflammatory and infectious processes such as leukemia usually are differentiated by the bone marrow. Leukemic cells have features that the normal precursors of a leukemoid reaction lack, such as Auer rods, chromosome abnormalities, and enzyme and cell membrane markers.

CLASSIFICATION APPROACHES FOR DISORDERS OF WHITE BLOOD CELLS

Classification by nature of abnormality
1. Quantitative: based on number of cells in marrow, peripheral blood, or both
   a. Leukocytopenias: decreased number of cells (e.g., neutropenia)
   b. Leukocytoses: increased number of cells (e.g., reactive lymphocytosis)
2. Qualitative: based on a defect or deficiency in a cell component
   a. Morphologic: defect is observed primarily as a structural abnormality (e.g., Pelger-Huët anomaly)
   b. Functional: defect is primarily functional (e.g., myeloperoxidase deficiency)
   c. Combined: most disorders involve structural and metabolic changes (e.g., lipid storage diseases)

Classification by etiologic origin
1. Hereditary: genetically passed as an allele from generation to generation
   a. Recessive: disease expressed in homozygous and hemizygous conditions (e.g., Chediak-Higashi syndrome)
   b. Dominant: disease expressed in heterozygous as well as homozygous conditions (e.g., May-Hegglin anomaly)
2. Acquired: disorder occurs to individual, not included in genome
   a. Congenital: present at birth, often involves developmental abnormalities; some of these may have a genetic basis that has not yet been demonstrated (e.g., DiGeorge's syndrome)

b. Postnatal: acquired during childhood or as an adult; may be primary, attributable to an environmental agent (e.g., drug-induced cytopenia) or secondary to another disease process (e.g., myeloid displacement caused by a metastatic carcinoma)
3. Idiopathic: cause unknown; although a number of different factors have been investigated as potential causative agents for different leukemias, most cases cannot be attributed to specific environmental or hereditary origins

Classification by progression of symptoms and outcome
1. Acute: onset of symptoms and rate of disease progress is rapid; morphologic changes in the blood cell picture often are dramatic (e.g., immature cells seen in acute leukemias)
2. Chronic: onset of symptoms may be gradual, sometimes insidious (unrecognized), progression may occur over many years, and morphologic changes may be slight to moderate (e.g., chronic leukemias)

These manifestations are not mutually exclusive; they may undergo transitions from chronic to acute or back as a result of therapy or relapse following failure of therapy (e.g., many of the myeloproliferative disorders begin as chronic disorders but may terminate as acute leukemias)

Classification by cell lineage
Disorders are classified on the basis of the cell line most obviously affected; several diseases involve precursors of more than one cell line (e.g., pluripotential stem cells), so that abnormalities appear in two or more of the myeloid and erythroid elements

From Powers.[46]

LYMPHOCYTOSIS

Lymphocytosis may be relative (caused by a decrease in granulocytes) or absolute. Benign increases in lymphocytes can be categorized as those dominated by small, mature lymphocytes and those involving a significant number of reactive lymphocytes (large cells with increased cytoplasm and "monocytoid" and/or other immature features). These cells have been referred to as Downey cells, virocytes, and atypical lymphocytes. There is a recognized association between reactive lymphocytes and viral infections. The immature features of the lymphocytes indicate blast transformation, which heralds a response to antigen.

Increases in mature lymphocytes are especially evident in children with pertussis, adults with disseminated forms of tuberculosis or brucellosis, acute infectious lymphocytosis, and hyperthyroidism. Reactive lymphocytoses are seen in many viral infections, with the classic example of a moderate to marked increase in reactive cells occurring in patients (especially the immunocompromised) infected with the Epstein-Barr virus (EBV), cytomegalovirus (CMV), and human immunodeficiency virus (HIV) infections (see box on the next page).

Infectious mononucleosis, a reactive lymphocytosis, is caused by the Epstein-Barr virus, which infects B lymphocytes. Signs and symptoms include mild to severe adenopathy, hepatosplenomegaly, fever, malaise, and pharyngitis; also, reactive lymphocytes make up more than 10% of the total differential WBC count. This disease is more likely to strike healthy adolescents and young adults as the "kissing disease." In most cases it is self-limiting.

LYMPHOCYTOSIS

Mature cells dominate		Reactive cells dominate	
Mild	Moderate to marked	Upper respiratory	Epstein-Barr virus
Early chronic lympho-	Advanced chronic	infections	(infectious
cytic leukemia	lymphocytic	Inflammatory	mononucleosis)
Hyperthyroidism	leukemia	processes	Cytomegalovirus in-
	Acute infectious lym-	Viral hepatitis	fections (CMV)
	phocytosis (children)	Mumps, measles,	*Toxoplasma* infections
	Pertussis (children)	chickenpox	Human immunodefi-
	Disseminated tuber-		ciency virus (HIV)
	culosis (adults)		

(From Powers p. 339, 1989.)

AGRANULOCYTOSIS

Also called granulocytopenia or malignant neutropenia, agranulocytosis is an acute, potentially fatal blood disorder characterized by the absence of neutrophils or severe neutropenia and an extremely low granulocyte count. The onset usually is rapid, and prompt treatment is required. When the condition is drug induced, it may develop slowly depending on drug dosage and duration of effect, such as in response to cancer chemotherapy.

PATHOPHYSIOLOGY

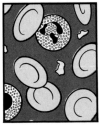 The usual cause of agranulocytosis is interference with hematopoiesis in the bone marrow or increased cell destruction in the circulation. This most often is the result of drug toxicity or hypersensitivity caused by large-dose, long-duration drugs (e.g., nitrogen mustard, radiation, and benzenes) and drugs that produce individual sensitivity, such as certain tranquilizers (chlorpromazine [Thorazine]), antithyroid drugs (propylthiouracil), anticonvulsants (phenytoin), and antibiotics (chloramphenicol). Agranulocytosis may also develop during the course of such diseases as tuberculosis, uremia, aplastic anemia, multiple myeloma, and overwhelming infection.

CLINICAL MANIFESTATIONS

The signs and symptoms of granulocytopenia include infection (particularly of the respiratory tract), fever, tachycardia, general malaise, and ulcers in the mouth and colon. If untreated, sepsis will result in death in 3 to 6 days.

DIAGNOSTIC STUDIES AND FINDINGS

Diagnostic test	Findings
Leukocyte count	500-3,000 WBCs/mm^3 with PMN cell count of 0% to 2%
Bone marrow biopsy	Absence of PMN cells; immature young cells

MEDICAL MANAGEMENT

GENERAL MANAGEMENT

Reverse isolation.

High-protein, high-calorie diet.

Granulocyte transfusions.

DRUG THERAPY

Broad-spectrum antibiotics.

Specific antibiotics.

1   ASSESS

ASSESSMENT	OBSERVATIONS
Energy level	Severe fatigue and weakness, high fever, severe chills, prostration
Cardiac function	Weak, rapid pulse
Gastrointestinal function	Sore throat, dysphagia, ulcerative lesions of buccal and pharyngeal mucosa
Immune function	Increased susceptibility to infection

2   DIAGNOSE

NURSING DIAGNOSIS	SUBJECTIVE FINDINGS	OBJECTIVE FINDINGS
Activity intolerance related to effects of infection on energy level, cardiac function	Complains of severe fatigue and weakness and rapid heart beat	High fever, severe chills, prostration; weak, rapid pulse
Altered oral mucous membranes related to ulceration	Complains of sore throat and difficulty swallowing	Ulcerative lesions of pharyngeal and buccal mucosa
High risk for infection related to granulocytopenia	Complains of chills, warmth, and restlessness	Fever, tachycardia, dyspnea, hypertension

3   PLAN

Patient goals

1. The patient will be able to tolerate moderate activity, including activities of daily living (ADLs).

2. The patient will have intact oral mucous membranes.
3. The patient will be free of infection.

4   IMPLEMENT

NURSING DIAGNOSIS	NURSING INTERVENTIONS	RATIONALE
Activity intolerance related to effects of infection on energy level, cardiac function	Anticipate the patient's needs; place objects within reach while patient is confined to bed.	To prevent excess energy expenditure and to decrease need for reaching or getting out of bed.
	Encourage a balance between rest and activity.	To maintain energy level.
	Assess pulse rate and strength.	To monitor cardiac function.

NURSING DIAGNOSIS	NURSING INTERVENTIONS	RATIONALE
Altered oral mucous membranes related to ulceration	Give frequent mouth care.	To maintain hygiene and ensure comfort.
	Apply ice collar.	To reduce pharyngeal swelling.
	Offer anesthetic lozenges, analgesics, and sedatives as prescribed.	To provide comfort.
	Offer soft, bland foods and protein concentrates.	To reduce buccal irritation and increase ease of swallowing.
High risk for infection related to granulocytopenia	Enforce reverse isolation.	To protect patient from pathogens.
	Provide high-protein, high-calorie diet.	To maintain nutritional status.
	Encourage patient to take fluids.	To promote hydration.
	Monitor pulse, respirations, BP, and temperature; observe for restlessness and irritability, and monitor WBC count for marked change.	To assess for signs of infection.
	Use cooling measures (alcohol rub and tepid baths).	To reduce fever.
	Administer antibiotics as prescribed.	To combat specific pathogens.
	Use enemas and stool softeners as needed.	To prevent intestinal stasis as site for infection.
	Provide perineal care.	To maintain hygiene and prevent infection.

5 EVALUATE

PATIENT OUTCOME	DATA INDICATING THAT OUTCOME IS REACHED
Patient can tolerate moderate activity.	Patient can exercise and carry out ADLs.
Oral mucous membranes are intact.	There is no evidence of irritation.
There is no evidence of infection.	Patient has normal vital signs; patient is calm, and skin is dry and cool to touch; WBCs are within normal limits.

PATIENT TEACHING

1. Discuss with the patient the need for frequent, thorough oral hygiene to treat or prevent mouth and pharyngeal infection.
2. Explain the need for a diet high in protein and calories with soft, bland foods.
3. Discuss the need to avoid self-medication because of the danger of hypersensitivity.
4. Encourage a balance between rest and activity to prevent fatigue.
5. Advise the patient to avoid crowds, people with infectious diseases, and cold or hot environments.
6. Review the signs and symptoms of infection and appropriate measures the patient can take.

Lymphocyte Deficiency Disorders

Lymphocyte deficiencies range from the absence of such organs as the thymus, spleen, and lymph nodes to impaired immunoglobulin synthesis (see box).

B cells, T cells, or both may be involved. The disorder may manifest itself in infancy with recurrent infections. In addition, Ig production is decreased, and vaccines fail to achieve immunization. Combined B- and T-cell deficiencies (severe combined immunodeficiency, or SCID) cause severe, recurrent infections that usually are fatal in infancy or early childhood unless a bone marrow transplant is successful.

Acquired immunodeficiency can occur as a result of chemotherapy, radiation exposure, and viral infections; the best known example of the latter is acquired immunodeficiency syndrome (AIDS).

LYMPHOCYTE DEFICIENCIES	
B-cell deficiency	
Sex-linked agammaglobulinemia (Bruton's)	Absence of B-cell production and tissue
Common variable hypogammaglobulinemia	Deficiency of immunoglobulin production
Selective IgA deficiency	Deficiency of IgA production
T-cell deficiency	
Congenital thymic hypoplasia (DiGeorge's)	Absence of thymus, T-cell production
B- and T-cell deficiency	
Severe combined immunodeficiency (SCID)	Several types: decreased or absent B- and T-cell production

(From Powers, p. 340, 1989.)

Leukemia

The **leukemias** are disorders of uncontrolled proliferation of leukocytes and their precursors in the bone marrow, with infiltration of lymph nodes, spleen, liver, and other body organs.

Although the cause or causes of the leukemias are unknown, the currently accepted theory is that they begin with the development of a single malignant clone of cells. However, several predisposing factors have been identified: ionizing radiation; occupational exposure to the chemical benzene; exposure to certain drugs such as the alkylating agents (especially melphalan) and the nitrosoureas used in cancer chemotherapy; chloramphenicol and phenylbutazone, which cause bone marrow depression and aplasia; genetic and congenital disorders such as Down's syndrome, Fanconi's syndrome, and ataxia telangiectasia; and viruses.

The specific type of leukemia a patient develops depends on which stem cell line is affected (myeloid or lymphoid) and the point of maturation at which growth is arrested. Acute leukemias are the result of arrest of immature leukocytes, whereas chronic leukemias involve more mature cells.

PATHOPHYSIOLOGY

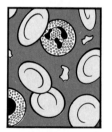

Nonfunctional WBCs accumulate in the bone marrow or lymph tissue, then spill into the peripheral blood and infiltrate other organs, thus interfering with normal function. Leukemic cell infiltration of the bone marrow impairs hematopoiesis through overcrowding of the marrow space or release of unknown inhibitory factors. This impaired hematopoiesis is responsible for anemia and thrombocytopenia. Other common signs of leukemic cell infiltration are enlargement of the lymph nodes and hypertrophy of the liver and spleen.

Leukemia is classified according to the type and maturation of aberrant WBCs. It may arise as an acute or chronic disease (see box on page 100). An international effort by the French-American-British (FAB) Cooperative Group resulted in the publication of a scheme for classifying acute leukemias based on morphologic characteristics (Table 5-1).

In acute lymphocytic leukemia, the aberrant cells are lymphoblasts produced in the bone marrow, lymph

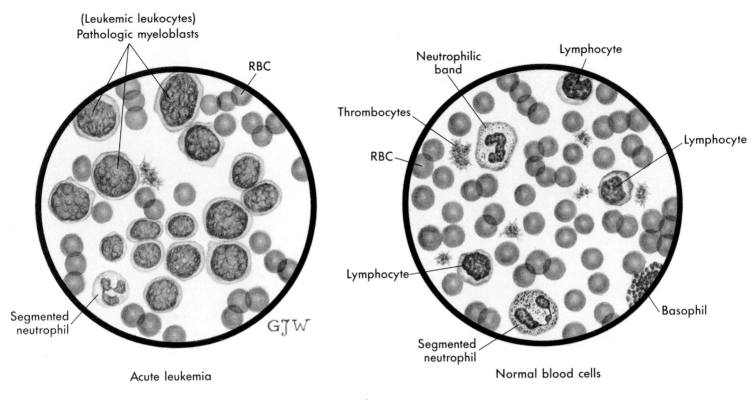

Acute leukemia

Normal blood cells

Leukemia

Table 5-1

FAB* CLASSIFICATION OF ACUTE LEUKEMIA

FAB number	Name
M1	Acute myeloblastic leukemia without maturation
M2	Acute myelocytic leukemia with differentiation
M3	Hypergranular promyelocytic leukemia
M4	Myelomonocytic leukemia
M5	Monocytic leukemia
	M5a Monoblastic (poorly differentiated)
	M5b Promonocyticmonocytic (differentiated)
M6	Erythroleukemia (erythroblastic)
M7	Megakaryocytic leukemia
L1	Acute lymphoblastic leukemia, small blast
L2	Acute lymphocytic leukemia, heterogenous
L3	Acute lymphocytic leukemia, Burkitt type

(From Powers.)[46]
French-American-British Cooperative Group.

MANIFESTATIONS OF LEUKEMIA

Acute leukemia

Acute myelogenous leukemia (AML) (acute nonlymphoid, ANLL)
  Undifferentiated leukemia (stem cell; acute myeloblastic)
  Acute myelocytic leukemia (differentiated AML)
  Promyelocytic leukemia (hypergranular promyelocytic; progranulocytic)
  Myelomonocytic
  Monocytic
  Erythroleukemia (erythroblastic; DiGuglielmo's disease)
  Megakaryocytic
Acute lymphocytic leukemia (ALL)
  T-cell ALL
  B-cell ALL
    Pre-B-cell ALL
  Null cell ALL (non-T-, non-B-cell ALL)
    Acute lymphoblastic leukemia of childhood
    Null cell ALL of adults

Chronic leukemia

Chronic myelogenous leukemia (CML)
    Granulocytic leukemia (CGL)
    Eosinophilic leukemia
    Basophilic leukemia
    Myelomonocytic leukemia
  Chronic lymphocytic leukemia (CLL)
  T-cell CLL
  B-cell CLL
  Hairy cell leukemia (HCL) (leukemic reticuloendotheliosis)
  Plasma cell leukemia (PCL) (see multiple myeloma in Chapter 8)

Other leukemia

Mast cell leukemia (systemic mastocytosis)

From Powers.

---

nodes, and other lymphoid organs. In acute nonlymphocytic leukemia (ANLL; also called granulocytic or myelogenous leukemia), the cells are myeloblasts, monoblasts, erythroblasts or, in rare cases, megakaryoblasts produced in the bone marrow. Acute leukemias involve immature cells that tend to divide and proliferate quickly, whereas chronic leukemias involve mostly mature cells and some immature cells that exist in a steady state until the blast crisis phase develops.

Lymphoid leukemia includes acute lymphoblastic leukemia (ALL), chronic lymphocytic leukemia (CLL), prolymphocytic leukemia (PPL), plasma cell leukemia (PCL), and hairy cell leukemia (HCL). Acute lymphoblastic leukemia (see Table 5-1 for subtypes L1, L2,

and L3) is characterized by an increased number of immature lymphocytes in the peripheral blood and infiltration of these cells into the bone marrow. These lymphoblasts typically cannot be distinguished as T cells or B cells. ALL is the most prevalent cancer in children, with a peak incidence at ages 3 to 7 years. (Although ALL in adults usually occurs in the third or fourth decades of life, it is much less common than ANLL.) Eighty-five percent of diagnosed cases of ALL occur in children. L1 (ALL small blast) is the most common subtype and the one with the most favorable prognosis. Monoclonal antibody tests have characterized pre-B-cell leukemia as a separate entity; it is one of the forms included in the null cell category (L1 and L2). Considerable progress has been made in chemotherapeutic remission of ALL over the past 20 years, but the mortality rate has remained at 30% to 70%. Regardless of the subtype, the outcome of ALL has correlated in most studies with the following clinical findings: remissions maintained for 3 years or longer were most prevalent in children who were at least 2 but under 10 years of age; white children fared better than black children; patients with WBC counts below 10,000/μl responded best, and those with WBCs over 50,000/μl did poorly. Other indicators for a poor prognosis included early central nervous system (CNS) involvement, the presence of a mediastinal mass, or a greatly enlarged liver or spleen. The poorer prognosis of both T-cell and B-cell leukemia may be due to the origin of these cancers outside the bone marrow. About 10% of acute leukemias in adults are lymphoid in origin, whereas 80% of leukemias in children are ALL. With treatment about 90% of children survive at least 5 years, whereas about 50% of adults survive at least 5 years. Chronic lymphocytic leukemia is characterized by proliferation of small lymphocytes in the bone marrow, lymph nodes, and spleen, with their eventual appearance in the peripheral blood. CLL is primarily a cancer of older adults (over age 40); it is rare in children or adolescents. B cells represent the abnormal clone in more than 90% of cases. The T-cell form, although rare, is more malignant, progresses rapidly, and responds poorly to chemotherapy. Most patients have increased leukocyte counts; more than 90% exceed 10,000/μl. Smudge cells, fragile lymphocytes that are ruptured during preparation of the wedge smear, are typical in CLL. The median survival time after first diagnosis is about 10 years. Prolymphocytic leukemia is characterized by large numbers of small lymphocytes in the peripheral blood with scant cytoplasm and the immature features of prolymphocytes. Plasma cell leukemia may be the fulminant conclusion of multiple myeloma, since it is characterized by the appearance of large numbers of plasma cells in the bone marrow and peripheral blood. Patients with PCL often display a hypergammaglobulinemia composed of IgD and IgE. Hairy cell leukemia is a chronic lymphoid cancer characterized by cells with fine, irregular pseudopods and immature nuclear features, with a proliferation of B cells in 90% of cases. The delicate cytoplasmic projections that give this leukemia its name can be seen by staining with Janus green. "Hairy" cells can be found in the peripheral blood, bone marrow, spleen, liver, and lymph nodes. HCL is seen only in adults with a median age of 50 to 60 years, with a slow and relatively benign clinical course. Most patients die from secondary or unrelated causes.

Myelogenous leukemia refers to cancers that are not lymphoid in origin. The term *acute nonlymphocytic leukemia (ANLL)* has attained widespread use in recent years. ANLL is characterized by the appearance of blasts and other early precursors in the peripheral blood and excess amounts of the cells in the bone marrow. It can appear suddenly and progress rapidly, or it may have a slower onset with progression through a chronic phase before terminating in a blast crisis. Moderate to severe normocytic-normochromic anemia and thrombocytopenia develop as leukemic cells displace normal blood cell precursors. There are seven major types (see Table 5-1; M1, M2, M3, M4, M5, M6, and M7). ANLL accounts for about 20% of leukemias in children; in adults it is more common than ALL, typically appearing between ages 30 and 60. Even with treatment, the prognosis is poor in both children and adults. Chronic myelogenous leukemia (CML) is diagnosed with WBC counts of 50,000 to more than 500,000/μl. CML has a longer clinical course than AML, with a chronic phase typically lasting 1 to 4 years and an acute phase (blast crisis) that is invariably fatal within 3 to 6 months. About 90% to 95% of CML patients possess a somatic cell mutation commonly referred to as the Philadelphia chromosome (Ph^3), a translocation t(9;22). The Philadelphia chromosome initially is present in the myeloid precursors but is expressed in other cell lines as the leukemia progresses. CML is less common than the acute forms and usually occurs in older adults.

CLINICAL MANIFESTATIONS

Acute lymphoblastic leukemia manifests as a rapid onset of fatigability, infection with fever, and such signs as bleeding gums, easy bruising, petechial hemorrhage, and bone or joint pain. The patient often has an enlarged liver or spleen (or both), lymphadenopathy, and manifestations of bleeding and anemia (Table 5-2). A patient with chronic lymphoblastic leukemia initially complains of fatigability or enlarged lymph nodes, although 25% are asymptomatic individuals who are diagnosed on routine physical examination or routine laboratory work. Most patients die of complications of infec-

tion or other chronic conditions associated with the elderly. Patients with prolymphocytic leukemia have very severe splenomegaly and a rapidly progressive disease that does not respond well to chemotherapy. Patients with plasma cell leukemia display signs of anemia and bleeding manifestations. Splenomegaly usually is marked in patients with hairy cell leukemia; lymphadenopathy is an infrequent finding.

In patients with acute nonlymphocytic leukemia, a common finding is recurrent infections unresponsive to standard oral antibiotics. Easy bruising, epistaxis, or gingival bleeding are reported. Splenomegaly is a common finding in patients with chronic myelogenous leukemia. The increased rate of cell production and turnover produces a hypermetabolic state characterized by night sweats, fever, weight loss, and fatigability. Anemia and bleeding result from disease progression.

DISEASE-RELATED COMPLICATIONS

Leukostasis is likely to occur in patients with extremely high circulating blast counts. This syndrome results when leukemic blasts aggregate and invade capillary walls, causing rupture and bleeding. This "sludging syndrome" occurs most commonly in the brain and lungs. Leukostasis is a medical emergency that requires immediate reduction of circulating leukocytes. High doses of hydroxyurea or other chemotherapy may be used; leukapheresis with a filtered continuous-flow cell separator may be helpful.

Disseminated intravascular coagulation (DIC) is likely to occur in patients with promyelocytic leukemia (M3) after chemotherapy is initiated, since granules from the promyelocytes are released and initiate the coagulation cascade (see Chapter 6 for discussion of DIC).

Typhlitis, or inflammation of the cecum, may develop in a neutropenic patient as a result of clostridial sepsis or infection with other bacteria. The patient develops severe abdominal pain with bloody diarrhea, absence of bowel sounds, rebound tenderness, and fever. An abdominal x-ray may reveal a soft tissue mass in the right lower quadrant, a dilated colon, or pericecal edema. The pathogen that is identified is treated with antibiotics.

Renal failure may result from urate nephropathy, aminoglycoside toxicity, sepsis, or leukemic infiltration of the kidneys.

MANAGEMENT

Chemotherapy, the treatment of choice for acute leukemia, involves three phases: induction, consolidation, and maintenance. The induction phase, an intensive course with drugs, aims to achieve complete remission. The consolidation phase then begins to eliminate remaining occult disease. The maintenance phase consists of low-dose combinations of drugs administered every 3

Table 5-2

CLINICAL FINDINGS IN ACUTE LEUKEMIAS

System	Manifestation
HEENT	Retinal capillary hemorrhage Fundic leukemic infiltration Papilledema Oropharyngeal infections Periodontal infections Gingival hypertrophy (ANLL) Dry mucous membranes Dysphagia Cervical adenopathy
Cardiovascular/ Pulmonary	Possible tachycardia, tachypnea Conduction defects Murmurs Pericarditis Congestive heart failure Abnormal lung sounds
Abdomen	Splenomegaly (ALL) Enlarged, tender kidneys (more common in pediatric ALL) Hepatomegaly
Genitourinary	Renal failure or anuria
Rectal	Perirectal abscesses
Extremities	Skin pallor Ecchymosis, petechiae Leukemic skin infiltrates: small, raised, pinkish nodules Swollen joints or tenderness (most common in pediatric ALL)
Neurologic	Headache Visual disturbances Cranial nerve VI, VII palsy

(From Otto.)[45]

or 4 weeks to prevent possible relapse.

In acute lymphocytic leukemia, induction therapy and postremission therapy are used, with prophylactic treatment to prevent central nervous system disease incorporated into both parts. The primary drugs used to induce remission are vincristine and prednisone; these agents alone induce remission in 36% to 67% of patients. The addition of daunorubicin increases the remission rate to 80%. Other drugs may be added but do not appear to increase response rates.

The central nervous system (CNS) may serve as a "sanctuary" for leukemic cells. This finding is more common in children than in adults at diagnosis; however, if the cerebrospinal fluid (CSF) is not treated, up to 40% of adults will develop CNS involvement. Repeated treatment with intrathecal methotrexate is the standard preventive therapy. An Ommaya reservoir may be inserted in high-risk patients for ease of access to CSF, and higher and more predictable levels of the drug may be used in ventricular CSF.

ALL almost certainly will recur without postremission therapy of some type. The most widely used therapies are consolidation/intensification and maintenance. Consolidation/intensification therapy may include high-dose chemotherapy or repetition of the drugs used in induction. An extended program of low-dose maintenance therapy using weekly 6-mercaptopurine and methotrexate is effective in preventing relapse and improving survival in children, but there is insufficient evidence of the most effective regimen in adults.

Up to half of patients who relapse (usually within 2 years of remission) can achieve a second remission by repeating their original induction regimen. Those who relapse after completing maintenance therapy have a better chance of attaining a second remission than do those who relapse while receiving treatment. Patients who fail to achieve a first remission may respond to intermediate- to high-dose methotrexate and leucovorin rescue or L-asparaginase. Bone marrow transplantation

(BMT) may induce long-term survival for as many as 50% of patients after a second relapse and 10% to 20% after a third relapse.

In patients with acute nonlymphocytic leukemia, complete remission is defined as less than 5% marrow blasts and less than 5% progranulocytes in a normocellular marrow. Peripheral blood cell counts must return to normal, and preexisting organomegaly and adenopathy must be absent. The most effective induction agents are cytarabine with an anthracycline (either daunorubicin or doxorubicin). Daunorubicin usually is preferred, because it is less cardiotoxic and less irritating to the gastrointestinal (GI) tract. It is not yet known whether the addition of vincristine, corticosteroids, or 6-thioguanine increases response rates.

A positive response to induction therapy, determined by a bone marrow examination the second week after treatment, is evidenced by a hypocellular, aplastic marrow. At the 14-day nadir, peripheral blood studies reflect marrow aplasia with profound neutropenia and thrombopenia. The bone marrow examination is repeated as the peripheral counts begin to recover. If evidence of leukemia persists 3 to 4 weeks after initiation of induction, the patient is reinduced with the same drugs and dosages. Remissions achieved after reinduction are less durable. Current induction regimens produce complete response in 65% to 80% of patients, of whom 15% to 30% may be cured.

Most patients relapse in 6 to 8 months if further chemotherapy is not administered. Consolidation therapy involves using induction drugs either at a slightly lower dosage or given over fewer days. One to three courses of this therapy may be given on an outpatient or inpatient basis, depending on the extent of immunosuppression.

Maintenance therapy involves monthly courses of outpatient chemotherapy given for a minimum of 6 months. The efficacy of consolidation therapy alone or accompanied by an extended maintenance program currently is being studied. Maintenance therapy may be combined with intensification therapy.

BMT may be the treatment of choice in some ANLL patients in first remission. Achieving remission after relapse is difficult, and these remissions rarely last longer than a year. Retreatment with Ara-C and daunorubicin gives patients a 30% to 50% chance of attaining a second remission. Patients with resistant disease may respond to high-dose Ara-C with or without daunorubicin, L-asparaginase, amsacrine, or mitoxantrone.

The goal of therapy for a patient with chronic myelogenous leukemia is to alleviate symptoms during the chronic phase, since there is no evidence to suggest that maintaining the WBC count in a normal range prolongs survival. Chemotherapy includes administration of busulfan or hydroxyurea, which improve marrow cellularity and decrease splenomegaly but do not eliminate the Philadelphia chromosome (Ph^3). Even though these agents control the disease for an average of 3 years, all patients progress to the acute and blastic phases. Intensive multidrug regimens are used for the blastic phase, but overall response rates are low. Biotherapy, specifically alpha-2B interferon, has been shown to partially suppress the expression of Ph^3; however, many patients still progress from chronic to blastic phase.

BMT is being studied for use in the chronic phase. Radiation therapy or splenectomy may be used to relieve painful splenomegaly. Leukapheresis may be performed to lower the WBC count quickly; however, the effects are temporary.

The inevitably fatal outcome of CML has researchers evaluating biologic response modifiers, growth factors, tumor necrosis factor, colony-stimulating factors, combinations of chemotherapy and biologic response modifiers, and reinfusion of autologous peripheral or marrow stem cells in the chronic phase of the disease.

Chronic lymphocytic leukemia requires the difficult decision of when to treat. Therapy does not prolong survival in early-stage patients. Indications for treatment are disease-related symptoms (fever, sweats, weight loss, fatigue, lymphadenopathy, or organomegaly); progressive anemias or thrombocytopenia; and repeated infections. A high WBC count alone is not an indication for therapy. The alkylating drug chlorambucil is most commonly used and best tolerated. A response rate of 60% is common. A pulse program involves less toxicity than does a high drug dose administered once every 2 to 4 weeks. Patients unresponsive to chlorambucil may benefit from cyclophosphamide. Corticosteroids are used to control leukocytosis and to treat immune-mediated hemolytic anemia and thrombocytopenia. They may also be used to treat patients with extensive disease before chemotherapy is initiated.

Combination chemotherapy with cyclophosphamide, vincristine, and prednisone has been used in patients with advanced disease; the addition of doxorubicin has resulted in a survival advantage that requires confirmation in a randomized trial.

Splenectomy may be indicated for autoimmune anemia or thrombocytopenia refractory to systemic therapy or persistent symptomatic splenic enlargement in a patient who is responsive to chemotherapy.

Radiation may be beneficial in hypersplenism, progressive splenomegaly, or lymphocytosis. Nodal radiation may be used to palliate symptoms or relieve organ dysfunction. Total body irradiation is used infrequently, because it is less effective than chemotherapy for disease control and it induces more profound cytopenias.

DIAGNOSTIC STUDIES AND FINDINGS

Diagnostic test	Findings
Acute lymphoblastic leukemia	
WBC	Usually >10,000/µl; 25% of cases are aleukemic (counts <5,000/µl); lymphocytes predominate; marked increase in lymphoblasts; neutropenia
Platelets	Normal to moderately decreased
Hematocrit	30%-35%
Bone marrow aspiration	50% lymphoblasts, hypercellularity
Cerebrospinal fluid	Presence of leukemic cells
Uric acid	Elevated
Lactate dehydrogenase	Elevated
Chronic lymphocytic leukemia	
WBC	Increased; 20% of cases exceed 100,000/µl; more than 90% exceed 10,000/µl; percentage of lymphocytes is 60% to 85%
Platelets	Decreased
Red blood cells	Decreased
Direct Coombs test	Positive
Bone marrow aspiration	Hypercellularity, diffuse lymphocytes
Lymph node biopsy	Diffuse lymphoma
Plasma cell leukemia	
Plasma cells	Large numbers in marrow and blood
Gamma-globulin	Hypergammaglobulinemia of IgD, IgE
Acute nonlymphocytic leukemia	
WBC	Increased blasts and other early precursors in blood and marrow; count may be normal, decreased, or increased
Red blood cells	Normocytic-normochromic anemia
Platelets	Decreased
Peripheral blood smear	Auer bodies (rods)
Bone marrow aspiration	Myeloblasts at least 50% of nucleated cells; hypercellularity ("packed," 90%-100%)
Chronic myelogenous leukemia	
WBC	50,000 to more than 500,000/µl; greatly expanded buffy coat; blasts less than 10%; myelocytes and later forms of neutrophils predominate; relative percentage of eosinophils and basophils is increased
Red blood cells	Nucleated with anisocytosis and basophilic stippling
Bone marrow	Generalized hyperplasia of granulocytic series; hypercellularity
Chromosomes	Presence of Philadelphia chromosome

MEDICAL MANAGEMENT

GENERAL MANAGEMENT

Transfusions.

Reverse isolation.

Antibiotics.

Parenteral fluids.

Leukapheresis.

SURGERY

Splenectomy.

DRUG THERAPY

Acute lymphoblastic leukemia
   Induction therapy: vincristine, weekly for 3-5 weeks; prednisone, daily for 3-5 weeks; daunorubicin; L-asparaginase; cyclophosphamide; methotrexate; 6-mercaptopurine; cytosine arabinoside.
   Consolidation/intensification therapy: repetition of vincristine and prednisone or other high-dose agents.
   Maintenance therapy: 6-mercaptopurine weekly; methotrexate weekly.

Acute nonlymphocytic leukemia
   Induction therapy: cytarabine (Ara-C), 100-200 mg/m^2 continuous IV infusion for 7 days; daunorubicin, 45-70 mg/m on days 5, 6, and 7.
   Consolidation therapy: induction regimen drugs at slightly lower dose or given over fewer days.
   Maintenance therapy: cytarabine, SC q6h for 5-10 days; prednisone, vincristine, doxorubicin, or 6-thioguanine.
   Intensification therapy: in combination with maintenance therapy.

Chronic myelogenous leukemia
   Busulfan, 4-6 mg PO daily; hydroxyurea, 0.5-2 g PO daily in divided doses; for blast crisis, Ara-C; programs with anthracyclines, amsacrine, 6-thioguanine, hydroxyurea; high doses of Ara-C with anthracyclines and mitoxantrone.
   Interferon.

Chronic lymphocytic leukemia
   Chlorambucil, 6-14 mg PO daily; cyclophosphamide; corticosteroids; cyclophosphamide, vincristine, and prednisone (CVP); cyclophosphamide, vincristine, prednisone, and doxorubicin (CHOP).

ADJUNCT THERAPY

Radiation therapy (RT)
   Cranial radiation for CNS leukemia
   Local RT for bulky mediastinal infiltration, testicular infiltration
   Total body irradiation
Bone marrow transplantation (BMT)

1 ASSESS

ASSESSMENT	OBSERVATIONS
Energy level	Easy fatigability, weakness, malaise, fever
Vascular integrity	Bleeding gums, easy bruising, petechiae, ecchymoses, purpura, epistaxis
Cardiopulmonary function	Tachycardia, tachypnea, shortness of breath on exertion, palpitations, pallor
Gastrointestinal function	Anorexia, nausea, vomiting, dysphagia, esophagitis, weight loss, splenomegaly, hepato-megaly, abdominal distension and discomfort
Tissue integrity	Swollen joints or tenderness, leukemic skin infiltrates, perirectal abscesses, mediastinal mass with tenderness
Sensory and motor function	Headache, visual disturbances, lethargy, irritability, syncope, hemiparesis

2 DIAGNOSE

NURSING DIAGNOSIS	SUBJECTIVE FINDINGS	OBJECTIVE FINDINGS
High risk for infection related to inadequate number of and immature leukocytes	Complains of easy fatigue, weakness	Fever, perirectal abscesses
Altered peripheral tissue perfusion related to decreased platelet count and bleeding	Complains of easy bruising, bleeding from gums	Bleeding from gums, petechiae, ecchymoses
Altered cardiopulmonary tissue perfusion related to blood loss and side effects of chemotherapy	Complains of rapid heart beat, shortness of breath	Tachycardia, tachypnea, pallor, abnormal lung sounds, murmurs
Altered nutrition: less than body requirements related to organ enlargement and side effects of chemotherapy	Complains of lack of appetite, feeling of distension	Hepatomegaly, splenomegaly, abdominal distension
Pain related to infusion of leukocytes into joints, bones, liver, spleen, or lymph nodes	Complains of joint and bone pain, abdominal pain, site-specific pain	Swollen joints, abdominal distension, swollen lymph nodes (e.g., inguinal, cervical)

NURSING DIAGNOSIS	SUBJECTIVE FINDINGS	OBJECTIVE FINDINGS
Altered cerebral tissue perfusion related to diffusion of leukocytes into central nervous system	Complains of headache, blurred vision, weakness in arms and legs	Lethargy, difficulty with walking and ADLs, visual disturbances, decreased pupillary response
High risk for altered pattern of urinary elimination related to uric acid nephropathy and side effects of chemotherapy	Complains of difficulty voiding	Hematuria, decreased output

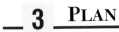

3 PLAN

Patient goals

1. The patient will be free of infection.
2. The patient will have no bleeding episodes.
3. The patient will demonstrate adequate cardiopulmonary function.
4. The patient will maintain adequate nutrition.
5. The patient will be free of pain.
6. The patient will have adequate cerebral tissue perfusion.
7. The patient will demonstrate adequate urinary elimination.

4 IMPLEMENT

NURSING DIAGNOSIS	NURSING INTERVENTIONS	RATIONALE
High risk for infection related to inadequate number of and immature leukocytes	Teach patient and family proper handwashing; screen visitors. Place patient in reverse isolation. Require handwashing with povidone-iodine scrub for all personnel and visitors before entering room. Ensure that no fresh fruits, vegetables, plants, or cut flowers are taken into patient's room.	To protect patient from pathogens.
	Encourage rest and limited activity.	To prevent fatigue.
	Maintain warm, clean environment.	To prevent chilling.
	Encourage increased intake of fluids and food high in protein.	To enhance production of antibodies and prevent dehydration.
	Maintain oral and perineal hygiene.	To prevent infection.
	Monitor vital signs, since changes, particularly in temperature, may signal infection.	To assess for infection.

→ › ›

NURSING DIAGNOSIS	NURSING INTERVENTIONS	RATIONALE
	Check blood and urine studies.	To assess for evidence of specific pathogens.
	Administer antibiotics as prescribed.	To treat infection.
	Use cool sponge baths, alcohol rubs, and antipyretic drugs as needed.	To reduce fever.
	Administer granulocyte transfusions as prescribed.	To replace defective WBCs and to fight infection.
	Administer gamma-globulin as prescribed.	To provide exogenous protein for antibody formation.
Altered peripheral tissue perfusion related to decreased platelet count and bleeding	Handle patient carefully, and assist with ambulation.	To prevent injury and possible bleeding.
	Avoid injections, constrictive clothing, razors, or other items that impair circulation or cause trauma.	To prevent trauma.
	If an injection is necessary, apply pressure over the site.	To prevent extravasation.
	Observe patient's gums, nose, skin, urine, and feces.	To detect evidence of bleeding.
	Prevent constipation by using stool softener, fiber in diet, and increased fluids.	To prevent anal trauma.
	Observe the skin for petechiae, ecchymoses, and purpura.	To detect signs of bleeding.
	Monitor vital signs.	To detect blood loss early.
	Monitor blood studies.	To detect decreased Hct, Hb, and platelets—indicators of actual or potential bleeding.
	Observe patient for restlessness or confusion.	To detect outward signs of bleeding.
	Administer blood component therapy as prescribed.	To replace blood loss and enhance clotting.
Altered cardiopulmonary tissue perfusion related to blood loss and side effects of chemotherapy	Encourage balance between rest and activity.	To reduce cardiopulmonary workload.
	Monitor vital signs.	To assess adequacy of cardiopulmonary function.
	Observe patient for dyspnea on exertion; ask about palpitations.	To determine whether tissue perfusion is adequate.

NURSING DIAGNOSIS	NURSING INTERVENTIONS	RATIONALE
Altered nutrition less than body requirements related to organ enlargement and side effects of chemotherapy	Provide balanced diet, with emphasis on protein and calories.	To restore nutritional balance.
	Monitor caloric intake.	To ensure sufficient nutrition.
	Give small, frequent meals.	To enhance appetite and prevent distension.
	Encourage patient to make specific food requests.	To increase intake.
	Provide oral hygiene before meals.	To increase likelihood patient will eat.
	Eliminate factors predisposing to anorexia and nausea and vomiting (e.g., unpleasant odors, perfume, disturbing sights or sounds).	To decrease likelihood of these symptoms.
	Serve foods cold or at room temperature.	To eliminate odors.
	Provide high-protein drinks to supplement patient's diet.	To stimulate appetite.
	Discourage smoking and oral stimulants.	To prevent altering taste or appetite.
	Measure body weight at least weekly.	To monitor nutritional status.
	Encourage patient to take frequent fluids.	To maintain hydration.
	Administer antiemetics as prescribed and as requested by patient.	To decrease nausea and vomiting.
	Administer NG tube feedings or total parenteral nutrition (TPN) as prescribed.	To ensure sufficient nutrition if patient is unable to eat.
Pain related to infusion of leukocytes into joints, bones, liver, spleen, or lymph nodes	Position patient comfortably in semi-Fowler's position.	To decrease abdominal pressure.
	Support joints and extremities with pillows or pads.	To prevent discomfort.
	Remove constrictive clothing; use bed cradle or foot board; handle patient gently.	To relieve pressure and to prevent irritation or injury.
	Provide soothing baths and back care, warm or cold applications.	To relax patient and relieve discomfort.
	Discuss characteristics of pain and ways to relieve it.	To individualize interventions.

NURSING DIAGNOSIS	NURSING INTERVENTIONS	RATIONALE
Altered cerebral tissue perfusion related to diffusion of leukocytes into central nervous system	Keep patient on bed rest with quiet, dim environment.	To reduce stimulation.
	Provide safety (e.g., side rails up).	To protect patient from injury.
	Provide emergency equipment (e.g., padded tongue blade).	To be ready for an emergency, such as convulsion.
	Observe for increased intracranial pressure: vital signs, pupillary response, level of consciousness, reflexes, and orientation.	To assess need for intervention.
	Assess range of motion, strength, and ability to communicate.	To detect cerebrovascular accident.
	Give patient drugs for headaches as prescribed and as requested by patient.	To relieve pain.
	Assist patient with ambulation and ADLs as needed.	To compensate for blurred vision.
High risk for altered pattern of urinary elimination related to uric acid nephropathy and side effects of chemotherapy	Ambulate patient as tolerated, and change patient's position frequently.	To enhance circulation and elimination.
	Encourage patient to take fluids such as carbonated beverages and urine-alkalinizing juices.	To maintain normal pH and prevent crystallization.
	Inspect for blood in urine and flank pain.	To assess signs of possible irritation or obstruction.
	Test pH of urine.	To assess effectiveness of interventions.
	Administer allopurinol as prescribed.	To inhibit uric acid biosynthesis.
	Observe urine and blood studies.	To assess renal function, and to detect elevated levels of minerals.

5   EVALUATE

PATIENT OUTCOME	DATA INDICATING THAT OUTCOME IS REACHED
Patient has no signs of infection.	Vital signs are within normal limits; skin is cool and dry; patient is calm and comfortable in environment; urine is clear; there is no evidence of lung congestion; previous sites of infection are healing.
Perfusion of peripheral tissues is adequate.	There is no evidence of bleeding; vital signs are within normal limits; there is no discoloration of the skin.

PATIENT OUTCOME	DATA INDICATING THAT OUTCOME IS REACHED
Perfusion of cardio-pulmonary tissue is adequate.	Vital signs are within normal limits; patient has sufficient energy to carry out ADLs.
Patient is taking nutritious foods and liquids.	Weight has stabilized; bowel elimination has returned to normal pattern and consistency.
Patient acknowledges feelings of increased comfort.	Patient has no complaints of pain; patient alternates other pain control methods with medication and arranges rest and activity without difficulty.
Perfusion of cerebral tissues is adequate.	Vital signs are within normal limits; patient is alert and oriented; reflexes are normal.
Patient maintains adequate urinary elimination.	Patient voids without difficulty or discomfort; urine is clear; pH is within normal limits; blood studies indicate normal levels of minerals.

PATIENT TEACHING

1. Advise the patient to avoid situations in which there is likelihood of contact with pathogens (e.g., inclement weather or crowds).
2. Instruct the patient to observe for and report to the physician signs and symptoms of infection, bleeding, or anemia.
3. Discuss ways to avoid tissue damage (e.g., use a soft toothbrush, blow nose gently, and avoid constipation).
4. Plan with the patient a well-balanced diet especially high in protein, fiber, and fluids.
5. Encourage the patient to take antibiotics as prescribed.
6. Discuss nonpharmacologic pain-relief measures (e.g., relaxation and guided imagery).
7. Encourage the patient to avoid smoking and oral stimulants.
8. Be sure that the patient is aware of support resources available: financial, treatment related, and psychosocial.

CHAPTER 6

Thrombocytic Disorders

Platelet disorders are classified as quantitative or qualitative. Thrombocytopenia (a decrease in the number of circulating platelets) and thrombocytosis (an increase in the number of circulating platelets) are the quantitative abnormalities. Qualitative disorders (thrombocytopathy), which affect the structure or function of individual platelets, usually prevent platelet adherence and aggregation; as a result, no platelet plug forms at the site of blood vessel damage. The two types of disorders may be present simultaneously (see the box below).

Coagulation disorders tend to cause more serious bleeding and usually are due to a deficiency of one or more clotting factors. Thromboembolic disease includes those disorders in which coagulation proceeds unnecessarily; these tend to result from vascular abnormalities that stimulate clotting.

Thrombocytosis is a secondary increase in platelet concentration caused by increased production, which may arise from conditions such as splenectomy or the use of such drugs as epinephrine, antifungal agents, and *Vinca* alkaloids. Rebound thrombocytosis occurs after resolution of thrombocytopenia caused by cytotoxic drugs, alcohol abuse, surgery, or vitamin deficiency. It is also associated with iron-deficiency states, chronic inflammatory diseases, Hodgkin's lymphoma, and breast, lung, stomach, and ovarian cancer. The platelet concentration in the peripheral blood may exceed 10 million/μl. This produces a paradoxic combination of thromboembolic and hemorrhagic episodes. Bleeding manifestations are related to the many qualitative abnormalities found in the platelets, including decreased adhesion.

Thrombocytopathies include those disorders associated with interaction with vascular tissue; abnormalities involving platelet adhesion and aggregation; and abnormalities involving coagulation factor receptors (see the box on pages 112-113).

CLASSIFICATION OF PLATELET DISORDERS

Quantitative abnormalities: Changes in platelet numbers

A. Thrombocytopenia: decrease in circulating platelets
  1. Impaired or decreased production of platelets
    a. Resulting from damage to marrow cells by acquired agents
    b. Resulting from marrow replacement by other cells
    c. Resulting from congenital conditions
      1. Fanconi's syndrome with megakaryocyte hypoplasia
      2. Intrauterine exposure to drugs or infections
      3. Wiskott-Aldrich syndrome
      4. Thrombocytopenia with absent radii (TAR baby syndrome)
    d. Resulting from ineffective thrombopoiesis
      1. Defective DNA synthesis associated with megaloblastic anemia
      2. Thrombopoietin deficiency
  2. Increased destruction of circulating platelets
    a. Resulting from immunological mechanisms
      1. Drug induced: protein-drug-platelet complexes

CLASSIFICATION OF PLATELET DISORDERS—cont'd

2. Idiopathic (autoimmune) thrombocytopenic purpura (ITP)
3. Neonatal isoimmune thrombocytopenia
4. Secondary autoimmune thrombocytopenia
5. Posttransfusion purpura
   b. Resulting from increased platelet use or damage
      1. Thrombotic thrombocytopenic purpura (TTP)
      2. Disseminated intravascular coagulation (DIC)
      3. Interaction with nonendothelial surfaces (e.g., artificial heart valve)
      4. Hemolytic-uremic syndrome (HUS)
3. Disorders related to distribution or dilution
   a. Resulting from increased splenic sequestration accompanying splenomegaly
   b. Resulting from hepatic sequestration during hypothermia
   c. Resulting from dilution after massive transfusion with stored blood
B. Thrombocytosis and thrombocythemia: increase in circulating platelets
   1. Reactive thrombocytosis: secondary to other conditions
      a. In association with iron deficiency
      b. In association with inflammation, especially chronic diseases
      c. In association with certain malignancies
      d. Following splenectomy
      e. As a transient response to epinephrine, some drugs
      f. As a transient rebound after thrombocytopenia
   2. Thrombocytosis associated with myeloproliferative disorders
      a. Increased megakaryocyte mass associated with polycythemia vera and myeloid metaplasia
      b. Increased megakaryocyte number (decreased volume) associated with chronic myelogenous leukemia
   3. Thrombocythemia: essential or autonomous thrombocytosis

Qualitative abnormalities: Changes in platelet function (thrombocytopathy)

A. Abnormalities involving platelet interaction with vascular tissue
   1. Ehlers-Danlos syndrome
   2. Hereditary hemorrhagic telangiectasia
   3. Acquired defects
      a. Scurvy (vitamin C or ascorbic acid deficiency)
      b. Amyloidosis
B. Abnormalities involving platelet adhesion
   1. Bernard-Soulier syndrome: vWF receptors (GP I) deficient
   2. von Willebrand's disease: various hereditary forms of factor VIII deficiency

3. Acquired defects
   a. Autoimmune form of von Willebrand's disease (antibodies to VII:vWF)
   b. Uremia, metabolite accumulation
   c. Drug induced (especially, antithrombotic drugs)
C. Abnormalities involving primary aggregation
   1. Glanzmann's thrombasthenia: impaired binding of fibrinogen
   2. Acquired defects
      a. Resulting from increased fibrin degradation products
      b. Resulting from dysproteinemias
      c. Drug induced (especially synthetic penicillins and dextran)
D. Abnormalities involving secondary aggregation (release reaction)
   1. Storage pool deficiencies
      a. Gray platelet syndrome: absence of alpha granules
      b. Hereditary dense granule deficiencies
      c. Anomalies associated with other abnormalities
         1. Hermansky-Pudlak syndrome: albinism, ceroid deposits
         2. Chédiak-Steinbrinck-Higashi syndrome: albinism, abnormal WBC granules
         3. Wiskott-Aldrich syndrome: abnormal glycolysis, infections, eczema
         4. Thrombocytopenia with absent radii (TAR baby syndrome)
   2. Prostaglandin pathway deficiencies: "aspirinlike defects"
      a. Cyclooxygenase deficiency
      b. Thromboxane synthetase deficiency
   3. Defects in nucleotide metabolism
      a. Glycogen storage disease
      b. Fructose-1,6-diphosphate deficiency
   4. Acquired defects
      a. Viral infections
      b. Drug induced
         1. Aspirin
         2. Other nonsteroidal antiinflammatory drugs
      c. Ethyl alcohol, especially acute bouts of consumption
      d. Primary bone marrow disease (dyspoiesis) and myeloproliferative disorders
      e. Autoimmune diseases (e.g., AIHA, SLE)
      f. During open heart surgery: alpha-granule depletion
E. Abnormalities involving coagulation factor receptors (procoagulant activity)
   1. Congenital deficiency of platelet factor 3 (factor V_m receptor)
   2. PF-3 nonavailability, secondary to defects in aggregation and release reaction

From Powers.

Thrombocytopenia

Thrombocytopenia generally is diagnosed when the platelet count falls below 100,000/mm^3.

With a count of 50,000 or less, the likelihood of hemorrhage with minor trauma increases. Spontaneous bleeding can occur with counts between 10,000 and 20,000; the individual will have petechiae, ecchymoses, larger purpuric spots, or frank bleeding from mucous membranes. With a count below 10,000, severe bleeding may occur; this can be fatal if the bleeding is in the gastrointestinal tract, respiratory system, or central nervous system.

PATHOPHYSIOLOGY

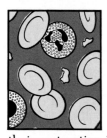

Three mechanisms can precipitate thrombocytopenia: defective platelet production, disordered platelet distribution, and accelerated platelet destruction or consumption. Defective platelet production in the bone marrow occurs if too few platelet stem cells proliferate or if their maturation is defective. This usually is caused by drugs or malignancies that suppress or replace normal stem cells in the bone marrow. Some of these drugs are the myelosuppressive drugs used in cancer treatment; thiazide diuretics; ethanol or its acetyldehyde metabolites; antibiotics such as chloramphenicol; and estrogens. Malignancies that may have this effect include acute and chronic leukemia, Hodgkin's disease, various lymphomas, metastatic cancers, multiple myeloma.

Disordered platelet distribution is related to splenomegaly, in which an abnormally large number of platelets (as much as 90% of the total) is sequestered in the spleen; this alteration usually is not sufficient to cause hemorrhage. Causes include various lymphomas, portal hypertension, and hypothermia during open heart surgery.

Accelerated platelet destruction or consumption is the most common cause of thrombocytopenia; it can be precipitated by antibody-mediated injury or such non-immunologic causes as mechanical injury resulting from infectious processes or damaged blood vessels.

Immune-related platelet destruction is most often caused by drugs or their metabolites, which combine with albumin or other plasma proteins to form antigens. The patient produces antibodies to the drug-protein complex, which adheres to platelet surfaces. Cells of the mononuclear phagocyte system of the liver and spleen recognize and remove the coated platelets. If IgM, IgG1, or IgG3 is involved, complement may also be activated and affixed to platelet surfaces, resulting in intravascular lysis of platelets. Once the drug has been discontinued, continuance of the thrombocytopenia depends on the rate at which the drug-protein complex is cleared by the bone marrow's compensating platelet production. A return to normal platelet concentration may take days to months. Second exposure can produce marked thrombocytopenia and bleeding in less than 24 hours. Causative drugs include quinine, quinidine, digitoxin, gold salts, rifampicin, alpha-methyldopa (Aldomet), morphine, and heroin. Heparin is also suspect.

Destruction from mechanical damage or consumption is caused by hemolytic-uremic syndrome, platelet thrombosis syndrome, and thrombotic thrombocytopenic purpura (TTP). TTP affects young adults and manifests as microangiopathic hemolytic anemia, thrombocytopenia, fever, renal abnormalities, and neurologic changes. Platelet thrombi form in small blood vessels throughout the circulation, resulting in organ damage and death. Factors released from the damaged vessels may be responsible for inducing platelet thrombus formation. Red blood cells, attempting to negotiate the thrombosed vessels, become fragmented and are called *schistocytes*; they are diagnostic of microangiopathies and characteristic of TTP. Many cases occur secondary to other conditions such as pregnancy or immediately post partum; the condition can also develop with neoplasms and connective tissue disorders (especially systemic lupus erythematosus), after a viral infection or bacterial endocarditis, and after administration of penicillin and other drugs.

Thrombocytopenia may be acute or chronic, idiopathic or secondary. Idiopathic thrombocytopenic purpura (ITP) is believed to be an autoimmune response to disease-related antigens. Chronic ITP may occur in women 20 to 40 years of age. The onset is gradual, with less severe bleeding, but platelet transfusions generally are futile. Splenectomy ultimately is necessary in most patients.

The acute form is seen most often after upper respiratory infections or such childhood diseases as measles, rubella, mumps, and chickenpox. Platelet survival is measured in hours rather than days, and remission usually is spontaneous. It appears that virus-viral antibody complexes attach to the platelets. Complement is further activated, resulting in lysis of platelets or removal of cells by splenic and hepatic macrophages.

Secondary thrombocytopenia develops as a result of conditions associated with drug hypersensitivities that produce antibodies; viral, bacterial, fungal, and parasitic infections; and some autoimmune disorders. Vi-

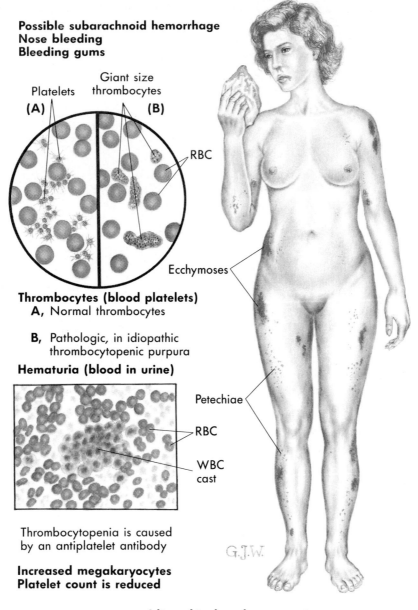

Possible subarachnoid hemorrhage
Nose bleeding
Bleeding gums

Platelets (A) Giant size thrombocytes (B)

RBC

Thrombocytes (blood platelets)
A, Normal thrombocytes

B, Pathologic, in idiopathic thrombocytopenic purpura
Hematuria (blood in urine)

Petechiae

RBC

WBC cast

Thrombocytopenia is caused by an antiplatelet antibody

Increased megakaryocytes
Platelet count is reduced

Ecchymoses

Idiopathic thrombocytopenic purpura

ruses involve the megakaryocytes and inhibit platelet production, destroy circulating platelets, or form viral antigen-antibody complexes. Platelets from septic patients often are found to be coated with IgG antibody.

In recent years low platelet counts have been identified as a common manifestation of infection with HIV. In addition, patients with adult respiratory distress syndrome (ARDS) have manifested increased platelet deposition in the lungs. These patients do not respond to platelet transfusions, since the transfused platelets may be deposited in the lung and fail to circulate.

CLINICAL MANIFESTATIONS

Patients with thrombocytopenia may have easy bruising, with petechiae or ecchymoses or both, especially over body prominences; bleeding from the nose or gums; or blood in the urine, emesis, or stool. When examining these patients, the nurse will observe ecchymoses, purpura, petechial rash, and oozing from puncture sites. Purpura is the term used to describe diffuse internal hemorrhage that is visible through the skin. This discoloration occurs when there are not enough normal platelets to plug damaged blood vessels or to prevent leakage from the multiple minute tears that occur each day in normal capillaries.

There may also be subconjunctival hemorrhages and hemorrhagic blisters (bullae) on the tongue and oral mucous membranes. Other findings such as renal failure or increased intracranial pressure may be the result of bleeding in these areas or related disease processes. Splenic enlargement occurs when platelets are trapped in the spleen.

Plasmapheresis and plasma transfusions have been found to be lifesaving in TTP and should be initiated as soon as the disorder is suspected. Although the reason for their effectiveness is unknown, it is believed that plasmapheresis may remove substances that cause platelet thrombosis; the plasma may provide natural antithrombotic agents. Platelet transfusions are contraindicated, because the infused platelets may aggravate the vascular occlusion.

Corticosteroids usually are effective in the treatment of ITP. It is hypothesized that steroids inhibit the removal of sensitized platelets by the reticuloendothelial system. If the condition does not respond to steroids, or if unacceptable side effects develop, other treatments such as splenectomy or immunosuppressive drugs may be considered. High-dose intravenous immunoglobulin recently has been shown to have temporary therapeutic value. It works by competing with the platelet antibodies for macrophage receptors.

DIAGNOSTIC STUDIES AND FINDINGS

Diagnostic test	Findings
Platelet count	$<100,000/mm^3$
Bleeding time	Prolonged
Coagulation time	Normal
Capillary fragility	Increased
Bone marrow biopsy	Decreased megakaryocytes

MEDICAL MANAGEMENT

GENERAL MANAGEMENT

Plasmapheresis.

Plasma transfusion.

SURGERY

Splenectomy.

DRUG THERAPY

Corticosteroids.

1   ASSESS

ASSESSMENT	OBSERVATIONS
Vascular integrity	Petechiae, ecchymoses, easy bruising, epistaxis, bleeding from gums and nose, subconjunctival hemorrhages, oozing from puncture sites
Female reproductive function	Heavy menses, bleeding between periods
Sensory and motor function	Signs and symptoms of increased intracranial pressure, nerve pain, anesthesia of extremities and/or paralysis
Gastrointestinal tract	Hematemesis, melena
Renal function	Hematuria
Cardiac function	Tachycardia
Respiratory function	Dyspnea, tachypnea

2   DIAGNOSE

NURSING DIAGNOSIS	SUBJECTIVE FINDINGS	OBJECTIVE FINDINGS
Impaired skin integrity related to intradermal bleeding	Complains of easy bruising	Petechiae, ecchymoses, hematomas
Impaired tissue integrity, nasal mucous membranes, related to bleeding	Complains of nasal irritation, stuffiness	Bleeding from nose
Impaired tissue integrity, oral mucous membranes related to bleeding	Complains of sore mouth	Bleeding from gums
Impaired gynecologic tissue integrity related to bleeding	Complains of frequent, heavy periods	Heavy menstrual flow
Altered cerebral tissue perfusion related to bleeding	Complains of headache and confusion	Altered pupillary response; increased pulse, respirations, and BP; decreased level of consciousness; sluggish reflexes
Pain related to pressure and altered sensations or loss of sensation in joints and extremities due to bleeding	Complains of pain, numbness, and tingling	Decreased mobility; increased frequency of falls and other trauma
Impaired gastrointestinal tissue integrity related to bleeding	Complains of nausea, abdominal distention, rectal pain, or irritation	Hematemesis, melena
Altered renal tissue perfusion related to bleeding	Complains of flank pain	Hematuria
Altered cardiopulmonary tissue perfusion related to bleeding	Complains of rapid heart beat and shortness of breath	Tachycardia, tachypnea

3   PLAN

Patient goals

1. The patient's skin, nasal and oral mucous membranes, and gynecologic and gastrointestinal tracts will be intact.

2. The patient will demonstrate improved cerebral, renal, and cardiopulmonary tissue perfusion.
3. The patient will be free of pain.

4 IMPLEMENT

NURSING DIAGNOSIS	NURSING INTERVENTIONS	RATIONALE
Impaired skin integrity related to intradermal bleeding	Avoid injections or use of straight razor.	To prevent bleeding.
	Apply ice bag and/or manual pressure over any puncture site.	To control bleeding.
	Handle patient gently; assist with ambulation, and remove environmental hazards and barriers.	To prevent trauma and injury.
	Observe patient's skin for petechiae, ecchymoses, or hematomas; report to physician.	To determine need for further therapy.
Altered nasal mucous membranes related to bleeding	Position patient with head forward and elevated.	To stop bleeding.
	Observe color, amount, and consistency of discharge.	To monitor blood loss.
	Encourage patient to blow nose gently and to press nostrils together.	To control irritation and subsequent bleeding.
	Maintain moisture in environment.	To reduce nasal membrane dryness.
Altered oral mucous membranes related to bleeding	Remove dentures, and provide mouth care with soft toothbrush.	To prevent irritation and minimize tissue trauma.
	Give soft foods and iced liquids.	To decrease oral irritation.
	Observe for bleeding from gums; report precipitating factor, amount, and character to physician.	To determine treatment.
Impaired gynecologic tissue integrity related to bleeding	Provide frequent perineal hygiene.	To promote comfort.
	Count perineal pads used.	To determine amount of bleeding.
	Observe color, consistency, and frequency of discharge.	To monitor blood loss and determine need for treatment.
Altered cerebral tissue perfusion related to bleeding	Observe for signs and symptoms of increasing intracranial pressure (headache, confusion, decreasing level of consciousness, decreased pupillary response and reflexes, change in vital signs), and intervene according to findings.	To prevent permanent damage.
	Instruct patient to avoid Valsalva maneuver (i.e., coughing or straining at stool).	To decrease potential for bleeding.

NURSING DIAGNOSIS	NURSING INTERVENTIONS	RATIONALE
Pain related to pressure and altered sensations or loss of sensation in joints and extremities due to bleeding	Position patient comfortably.	To minimize pain and pressure.
	Assist patient with ambulation.	To prevent falls or other injury.
	Handle patient gently, massaging tense muscles.	To promote relaxation.
	Apply bed cradle, lightweight clothing, and blanket.	To relieve pressure on lower extremities.
	Apply heat lamp, hot water bottle, warm or cool compresses as requested by patient.	To relieve pain.
	Encourage patient to use relaxation, imagery, and other pain-relief alternatives.	To enhance or replace traditional analgesic therapy.
	Administer analgesics as prescribed.	To relieve pain.
Impaired gastrointestinal tissue integrity related to bleeding	Observe amount, color, consistency, and frequency of hematemesis and melena.	To monitor blood loss.
	Offer patient frequent oral care and perianal hygiene.	To maintain comfort.
	Do not use a rectal thermometer, enema tube, or other instruments that might precipitate rectal bleeding.	To prevent rectal bleeding.
	Encourage patient to eat high-fiber foods and drink carbonated beverages.	To prevent constipation and control nausea.
	Test stool and emesis for occult blood.	To detect evidence of internal bleeding.
	Place patient in semi-Fowler's position.	To relieve abdominal pressure.
Altered renal tissue perfusion related to bleeding	Observe color, amount, and presence of red blood cells in urine; record and report to physician.	To determine need for treatment
	Encourage patient to drink fluids.	To maintain renal blood flow
Altered cardiopulmonary tissue perfusion related to bleeding	Keep patient in semi-Fowler's position.	To enhance cardiopulmonary function.
	Dress patient warmly, and maintain warm environment.	To enhance tissue perfusion.
	Remove constrictive clothing.	To facilitate chest expansion.
	Discourage smoking and oral stimulants.	To prevent increased cardiopulmonary workload.
	Monitor vital signs and laboratory studies.	To determine adequacy of cardiac and respiratory function.
	Report complaints of palpitations or dyspnea to physician.	To implement further treatment.

→ 〉 〉

5 EVALUATE

Skin integrity is maintained.	Skin shows no signs of discoloration or irritation.
Nasal and oral mucous membranes and gynecologic and gastrointestinal membranes are intact.	There is no evidence of bleeding from the nose, mouth, vagina, or rectum.
	Stools and emesis test negative for occult blood.
Urinary elimination is normal.	There is a balance between intake and output.
Cerebral and cardiopulmonary tissue perfusion is stable.	Patient is alert and oriented; reflexes are normal.
Patient is comfortable.	Patient has no complaints of pain; patient alternates rest and activity without difficulty.

PATIENT TEACHING

1. Help the patient avoid mechanical trauma that might cause bleeding: explain general safety precautions, use of a soft toothbrush, gentle nose blowing, stool softeners, and maintenance of a diet high in fiber and fluids.
2. Discuss with the patient the need to detect and report signs and symptoms of bleeding; focus on assessment of skin, mucous membranes, urine, and feces.
3. Explain the need to stop smoking and to decrease the use of oral stimulants such as caffeinated coffee or tea.

Disseminated Intravascular Coagulation Syndrome

Disseminated intravascular coagulation syndrome (DIC), although rare, is life threatening and associated with such states of physiologic disequilibrium as hemorrhagic shock, crush syndrome, leukemia, carcinoma, abruptio placentae, septic abortion, incompatible blood transfusion, and endotoxic shock.

Venomous snake bites are a common cause of the syndrome. The disease is characterized by inappropriate systemic activation and acceleration of normal clotting mechanisms.

PATHOPHYSIOLOGY

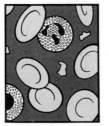

DIC is initiated when the extrinsic pathway of coagulation is activated, which occurs when tissue thromboplastin is liberated by tissue destruction or when endothelial damage activates the intrinsic pathway. Widespread coagulation consumes clotting factors and platelets, which in turn activates the fibrinolytic system, resulting in diffuse fibrinolysis. Fibrin degradation products (FDP)

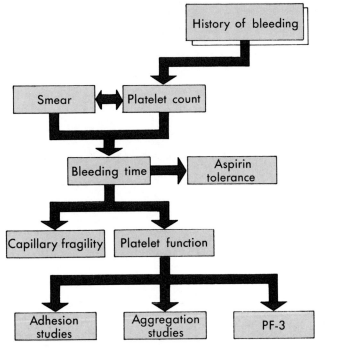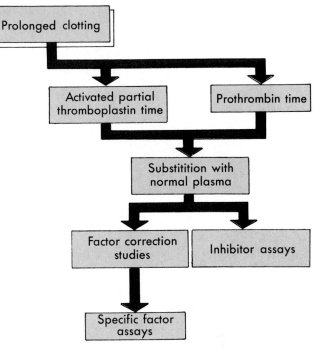

FIGURE 6-1
Laboratory study algorithm for bleeding disorders.

combine with the fibrin monomer, preventing the laying of fibrin threads and inhibiting platelet aggregation. A self-perpetuating vicious cycle of bleeding, clotting, and fibrinolysis is created by the failure of normal compensatory processes. The outcome is determined by the interplay among the various pathologic processes and compensatory mechanisms, such as fibrin deposition versus fibrinolysis; depletion versus repletion of clotting factors and platelets; production versus clearance of fibrin, FDP, and other coagulation products (Figure 6-1).

CLINICAL MANIFESTATIONS

DIC can be either acute or gradual in onset. The predominant problem is bleeding from numerous sites. Oozing or frank bleeding occurs from mucous membranes, deep tissues, injured tissues, sites of venipuncture or injection, and every natural orifice. Patients commonly have petechiae and ecchymoses. Often pulmonary, renal, hepatic, and central nervous system dysfunction ensues, caused by vascular obstruction by microthrombi.

The role of heparin in treating DIC remains controversial. Heparin is known to inhibit the coagulation process by preventing tissue thromboplastin from activating the extrinsic pathway, thus slowing the consumption of coagulation factors and deposition of fibrin, but it does not stop bleeding that is already occurring.

DIAGNOSTIC STUDIES AND FINDINGS

Diagnostic test	Findings
Prothrombin time (PT)	Prolonged
Partial thromboplastin time (PTT)	Prolonged
Platelet count	$<100,000/mm^3$
Fibrinogen level	Decreased
Antithrombin III level	Decreased
Thrombin time	Prolonged
Fibrin degradation products	Elevated
Plasminogen levels	Decreased

MEDICAL MANAGEMENT

GENERAL MANAGEMENT

Elimination of the causative factor; may require correction of hypovolemia, hypotension, hypoxia, acidosis, or hemostatic deficiencies; treatment of septic shock may be necessary.

Administration of depleted factors such as whole blood or fresh frozen plasma, cryoprecipitate (factor VIII), platelets, and erythrocytes.

DRUG THERAPY

Heparin (controversial).

Antineoplastic drugs.

Antibiotics.

1 ASSESS

ASSESSMENT	OBSERVATIONS
Vascular integrity	Bleeding from the nose, gums, and sites of injury; petechiae, purpura, and ecchymoses
Respiratory function	Tachypnea, dyspnea, cyanosis or pallor, basilar rales
Cardiac function	Dysrhythmias, tachycardia, hypotension, gallop rhythm
Renal function	Decreased urinary output
Sensory and motor function	Altered level of consciousness, orientation, and pupillary reaction Decreased movement and strength of extremities
Mental status	Fear, anxiety, restlessness

2 DIAGNOSE

NURSING DIAGNOSIS	SUBJECTIVE FINDINGS	OBJECTIVE FINDINGS
Fluid volume deficit related to bleeding	Complains of thirst and dizziness	Altered level of consciousness; disorientation; bleeding from nose, gums, and injury sites; petechiae, ecchymoses, purpura
Impaired gas exchange related to arterial hypotension	Complains of shortness of breath, decreased activity tolerance	Tachypnea, cyanosis or pallor, basilar rales

NURSING DIAGNOSIS	SUBJECTIVE FINDINGS	OBJECTIVE FINDINGS
Decreased cardiac output related to altered cardiac tissue perfusion	Complains of rapid heart beat	Dysrhythmias, tachycardia, hypotension, gallop rhythm
Altered patterns of urinary elimination related to decreased renal blood flow	Complains of difficulty urinating	Decreased urinary output
Sensory/perceptual kinesthetic alterations related to arterial hypotension	Complains of dizziness and weakness in arms and legs	Altered level of consciousness, disorientation, decreased pupillary response, decreased movement of extremities
Fear related to dyspnea, palpitations, bleeding, dizziness, and weakness	Expresses fear about symptoms and outcome	Anxious facies, restlessness, rigid posturing

__3__ PLAN

Patient goals

1. The patient will demonstrate improved fluid volume.
2. The patient will demonstrate improved gas exchange and cardiac output.
3. The patient will demonstrate normal urinary elimination.
4. The patient will manifest normal sensory/perceptual function.
5. The patient will express a positive attitude toward prognosis.

__4__ IMPLEMENT

NURSING DIAGNOSIS	NURSING INTERVENTIONS	RATIONALE
Fluid volume deficit related to bleeding	Monitor vital signs and behavior for evidence of hemorrhage; assess amount, consistency, and frequency of bleeding from nose, mouth, and other body orifices.	To determine need for replacement therapy.
	Assess skin for presence, size, and color of petechiae, ecchymoses, and purpura.	To determine extent of bleeding into tissues.
	Check stool, urine, emesis, and sputum for occult and observable blood.	To detect internal bleeding.
	Administer blood component and IV fluids as prescribed.	To replace fluid loss.

→ ❯ ❯

NURSING DIAGNOSIS	NURSING INTERVENTIONS	RATIONALE
	Administer heparin as prescribed.	To control bleeding.
	Monitor results of laboratory tests.	To determine degree of blood loss and impact of therapy.
	Apply ice pack and manual pressure over site of bleeding.	To prevent respiratory distress caused by nasal bleeding.
	Place patient in semi-Fowler's position.	To promote clotting and retard bleeding.
	Avoid using injections or straight-edge razor.	To prevent further bleeding.
	Provide gentle care to skin, oral mucosa, nose, fingernails, and toenails.	To prevent injury.
	Assist patient with ambulation and other activities of daily living (ADLs).	To prevent trauma.
Impaired gas exchange related to arterial hypotension	Position patient to facilitate breathing (semi-Fowler's position).	To reduce pressure on diaphragm and promote chest expansion.
	Encourage patient to take deep breaths.	To reduce hyperventilation.
	Provide oxygen therapy as prescribed.	To reduce cardiopulmonary workload and enhance tissue oxygenation.
	Help patient maintain a balance between rest and activity.	To decrease oxygen requirement.
	Monitor respiratory rate and breath sounds.	To identify pulmonary dysfunction.
	Assess skin color and temperature.	To determine adequacy of tissue oxygenation.
Decreased cardiac output related to altered cardiac tissue perfusion	Keep patient in semi-Fowler's position with legs elevated.	To enhance cardiac output and venous return.
	Administer antiarrhythmic drugs as prescribed.	To correct dysrhythmias.
	Administer cardiotonic and vasoconstricting drugs as prescribed.	To strengthen pumping action of the heart and increase vascular tone.
	Help patient avoid stress by balancing rest and activity, using relaxation techniques.	To decrease cardiac workload.
	Assess skin color and temperature.	To determine adequacy of tissue perfusion.
	Monitor results of laboratory tests, including blood pH.	To detect acidosis.

NURSING DIAGNOSIS	NURSING INTERVENTIONS	RATIONALE
	Monitor apical, brachial, carotid, radial, femoral, and tibial pulses.	To determine adequacy of tissue perfusion.
Altered patterns of urinary elimination related to decreased renal blood flow	Monitor intake and output, color and consistency of urine, and frequency of voiding.	To assess renal function.
	Use Foley catheter and drainage bag as prescribed.	To monitor urine production.
	Monitor results of laboratory studies, including electrolytes.	To determine adequacy of renal function.
	Monitor IV and PO fluids.	To detect early signs and symptoms of fluid overload.
	Report shortness of breath, restlessness, confusion, hypertension, and edema.	To determine presence of renal failure.
Sensory/perceptual kinesthetic alterations related to arterial hypotension	Keep patient on bed rest with head elevated.	To enhance oxygenation.
	Decrease environmental stimuli.	To lessen stress on central nervous system.
	Discourage use of oral stimulants such as cigarettes and caffeine.	To avoid decreased cardiac output and consequent cerebral hypoxia.
	Monitor neurologic signs (e.g., level of consciousness, orientation, and pupillary responses and reflexes).	To detect changes early.
	Assess range of motion and strength of extremities.	To monitor neurologic status.
	Monitor vital signs for evidence of cerebral hypoxia.	To detect evidence of impaired or inadequate blood flow.
	Assist patient with ambulation.	To prevent injury.
Fear related to dyspnea, palpitations, bleeding, dizziness, and weakness	Encourage patient to talk about specific fears.	To deal with each fear realistically.
	Have patient describe her perceptions of danger, isolation, and so on.	To reduce degree of fear.
	Orient patient to critical care environment, as needed.	To reduce fear of the unfamiliar.
	Assure patient of constant monitoring by nurses.	To reduce fear of abandonment.

NURSING DIAGNOSIS	NURSING INTERVENTIONS	RATIONALE
	Tell patient what to expect and when.	To avoid startling her.
	Teach patient ways of maintaining some degree of control (e.g., having access to call light or bell, asking about test results).	To reduce fear of dependence.

5 EVALUATE

PATIENT OUTCOME	DATA INDICATING THAT OUTCOME IS REACHED
Fluid volume is within normal limits.	Vital signs are within normal limits; laboratory values are normal; there is no evidence of bleeding.
Gas exchange and cardiac output have improved.	Vital signs are within normal limits; laboratory values are normal; patient can carry out ADLs; skin color and temperature are appropriate; peripheral pulses are regular and strong.
Urinary elimination is normal.	Intake and output show appropriate balance.
Kinesthetic sense has improved.	Patient can ambulate without difficulty; range of motion and strength of extremities are within normal limits.
Patient expresses confidence in prognosis.	Patient shows no evidence of anxiety and describes fears in realistic terms.

PATIENT TEACHING

1. Discuss with the patient and family the signs and symptoms of disseminated intravascular coagulation, which should be reported immediately to the nurse or physician.

2. Teach the patient how to administer heparin therapy as prescribed (see Patient Teaching Guide).
3. Teach the patient how to prevent mechanical trauma (e.g., use a soft toothbrush, blow nose gently, avoid contact sports).

Hemophilia

Until 1952 the term *hemophilia* described a deficiency of factor VIII (antihemophilic factor); since that time, factor IX (plasma thromboplastin component [PTC]) and factor XI (plasma thromboplastin antecedent [PTA]) have been identified. A congenital deficiency of one of these clotting factors accounts for 90% to 95% of the hemorrhagic bleeding disorders collectively called hemophilia.

Hemophilia A (classic hemophilia) is a result of factor VIII deficiency and is the most common form. The incidence rate is 1 per 10,000 male births. It is inherited as an X-linked recessive disorder that affects males and is transmitted by females. A family history of the disorder confirms the diagnosis.

Hemophilia B (Christmas disease) is a result of factor IX deficiency. It too is transmitted as an X-linked recessive trait, and clinically it is the same as factor VIII deficiency. Hemophilia A and hemophilia B occur with varying degrees of severity, depending on the concentrations of clotting factor VIII or IX in the blood. With severe hemophilia (a concentration of clotting factors less than 1% of normal), bleeding occurs spontaneously; with moderate hemophilia (1% to 5% of normal concentration), bleeding usually occurs as a result of trauma; with mild hemophilia (5% to 50% of normal concentration), bleeding occurs only after severe trauma or surgery.

Hemophilia C (factor XI deficiency) is an autosomal recessive disease with equal incidence in males and females. Bleeding usually is less severe than that seen with hemophilia A or hemophilia B.

Von Willebrand's disease is an inherited factor VIII deficiency with an autosomal dominant trait. Infusion of plasma causes factor VIII activity to increase for several days, because infusion of factor VIII temporarily induces endogenous synthesis of factor VIII. This is the most common genetic defect involving hemostasis.

PATHOPHYSIOLOGY

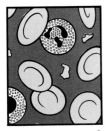

Coagulation factor disorders are characterized by deep tissue bleeding, including intraarticular bleeding with resultant crippling hemarthrosis (bleeding into the joints), deep intramuscular bleeding with resultant compression syndromes and, at times, intracranial bleeding. Patients may also suffer moderate to severe mucosal membrane hemorrhages involving gastrointestinal, gen-

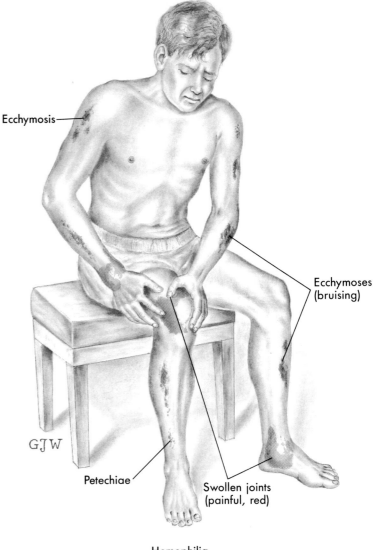

Hemophilia

itourinary, and intrapulmonary tissues and the paranasal sinuses. The bleeding may manifest as diffuse, bilateral epistaxis.

CLINICAL MANIFESTATIONS

Spontaneous bleeding caused by hemophilia is infrequent during the first few years of life, although abnormal bleeding may occur in the newborn period, particularly after circumcision (however, many hemophilic infants are circumcised without excessive bleeding). Because clotting is activated through the extrinsic coagulation cascade, which does not involve factors VII, IX, or XI, normal hemostasis is achieved.

Hematomas may form as a result of injections or holding the infant firmly. Easy bruising, hemarthrosis, or both occur when the child begins to walk. By 3 to 4 years of age, 90% of hemophilic children have experienced persistent bleeding from minor trauma, such as lacerations of the lip or tongue, which usually is the first sign of hemophilia. Hemorrhage into the elbows, knees, and ankles causes limited joint movement and pain and predisposes the child to crippling, degenerative joint changes. Early signs of hemarthrosis are a feeling of stiffness and tingling or ache in the joint, followed by decreased ability to move the affected joint. Spontaneous hematuria and epistaxis are minor but bothersome complications.

Recurrent bleeding is a chronic problem, with many hemophiliacs having phases or cycles of spontaneous bleeding episodes. Intracranial hemorrhage and bleeding into the neck, mouth, or thorax; hematomas in the spinal cord; and gastrointestinal hemorrhage are life-threatening emergencies.

DIAGNOSTIC STUDIES AND FINDINGS

Diagnostic test	Findings
Clotting time	Prolonged
Prothrombin time (PT)	Normal
Partial thromboplastin time (PTT)	Prolonged
Fibrinogen	Normal
Bleeding time	Prolonged in von Willebrand's disease

MEDICAL MANAGEMENT

GENERAL MANAGEMENT

Local pressure and/or topical application of hemostatic agents.

Replacement of deficient factor: For hemophilia A, cryoprecipitate containing 8-100 U of factor VIII per bag at 12-hour intervals until bleeding ceases. For hemophilia B, plasma or factor IX concentrate (Konyne or Proplex) given q 24 h until bleeding ceases. Treatment for the development of antibody inhibitors against the specific coagulation factor (e.g., plasmapheresis, prothrombin complexes).

DRUG THERAPY

Immunosuppressive agents

Synthetic product DDAVP (1-deamino 8-D arginine vasopressin), administered IV to increase factor VIII activity level.

Antifibrinolytic agent (tranexamic acid or epsilon-aminocaproic acid [EACA]).

---

1   ASSESS

ASSESSMENT	OBSERVATIONS
Vascular integrity	Bleeding from nose, gums, lips, tongue, and sites of trauma; petechiae, purpura, ecchymoses; menorrhagia; hemarthrosis; hematuria; melena
Cardiopulmonary function	Hypotension, tachycardia, hyperpnea
Sensory, motor, and mental function	Disorientation, confusion, convulsions, decreased reflexes

2 DIAGNOSE

NURSING DIAGNOSIS	SUBJECTIVE FINDINGS	OBJECTIVE FINDINGS
Fluid volume deficit related to bleeding	Complains of easy bruising, nasal stuffiness, sore mouth, heavy menstrual periods, pain in joints	Bleeding from nose, gums, lips, tongue, and sites of trauma; petechiae, purpura, and ecchymoses; hemarthrosis; hematuria
Altered cardiopulmonary tissue perfusion related to bleeding	Complains of dizziness, rapid heart beat, shortness of breath	Hypotension, tachycardia, hyperpnea
Altered cerebral tissue perfusion related to bleeding	Complains of confusion, headache	Disorientation, convulsions, decreased reflexes

3 PLAN

Patient goals

1. The patient will have intact skin, nasal and oral mucous membranes and gynecologic and urinary tracts, and full range of motion.
2. The patient will demonstrate normal fluid volume.
3. The patient will demonstrate improved cerebral and cardiopulmonary tissue perfusion.

4 IMPLEMENT

NURSING DIAGNOSIS	NURSING INTERVENTIONS	RATIONALE
Fluid volume deficit related to bleeding	Assess amount, consistency, and frequency of bleeding (include facies, mouth, nose, skin, joints, stool, and urine).	To determine need for replacement therapy.
	Do pad count during menstrual period.	To determine extent of bleeding.
	Monitor vital signs for evidence of acute hemorrhage.	To detect hemorrhage early.
	Administer blood component therapy as ordered.	To control bleeding.
	Monitor results of laboratory tests.	To determine degree of blood loss and effect of therapy.
	Help patient prevent such trauma as falls, bumps, and injections.	To prevent bleeding.
	Apply ice pack to affected joint or traumatized area.	To control bleeding.
	Casting (e.g., non-weight-bearing sling or lightweight splint) may be used.	To protect and rest affected joints.

➜ ❯ ❯

NURSING DIAGNOSIS	NURSING INTERVENTIONS	RATIONALE
Altered cardiopulmonary tissue perfusion related to bleeding	Assess patient's complaints of dizziness by monitoring BP.	To detect hypotension related to blood loss or cardiac failure.
	Monitor pulse and respirations, as well as patient's complaints of palpitations or dyspnea.	To detect changes indicating increased cardiopulmonary workload related to decreasing blood volume.
	Administer oxygen, blood component therapy, and other interventions as prescribed.	To support cardiopulmonary function.
Altered cerebral tissue perfusion related to bleeding	Keep patient on bed rest with head elevated.	To reduce intracranial pressure and lower activity level.
	Protect head with helmet, and use padded side rails if patient is restless.	To prevent injury, particularly if convulsion occurs.
	Discourage oral stimulants such as caffeine.	To prevent an increase in intracranial pressure.
	Monitor neurologic signs (e.g., level of consciousness, orientation, pupillary response, and reflexes); report changes to physician.	To detect evidence of intracranial bleeding.

5 EVALUATE

PATIENT OUTCOME	DATA INDICATING THAT OUTCOME IS REACHED
Fluid volume is within normal limits.	Vital signs are within normal limits; laboratory values are normal; there is no evidence of bleeding.
Cerebral and cardiopulmonary tissue perfusion are stable.	Vital signs are within normal limits; patient is alert and oriented; reflexes are normal.

PATIENT TEACHING

1. Teach the patient how to prevent mechanical trauma, which might cause bleeding (e.g., observe general safety precautions, use a soft toothbrush, blow nose gently, use stool softeners, and adopt a diet high in fiber and fluids).
2. Discuss with the patient the need to detect and report signs and symptoms of bleeding; focus on assessment of skin, mucous membranes, urine, and feces.
3. Explain the need to stop smoking and to decrease the use of oral stimulants.
4. Encourage the patient to obtain genetic counseling.

CHAPTER 7

Myelodysplastic Syndromes

The myelodysplastic syndromes (MDS) are a group of hematologic disorders caused by a clonal disorder of certain stem cells in the bone marrow. In the past these syndromes were referred to as preleukemic states, but they do not always develop into malignancies.

In MDS the bone marrow is normocellular, hypocellular, or hypercellular in the presence of peripheral cytopenias. The cause is unknown, but the diversity of manifestations results from a clonal disorder of the pluripotent hematopoietic stem cell. The stem cells still differentiate, but the differentiation is not effective, resulting in anemia, thrombocytopenia, and neutropenia, which develop simultaneously or as separate entities. Approximately 30% of myelodysplastic syndromes develop into acute myelogenous leukemia (AML). The incidence of MDS is unknown, but therapy-related MDS that does not progress to acute leukemia may represent 30% to 40% of all myeloid disorders associated with cancer chemotherapy.

Most patients who develop MDS are over 60 years of age; however, the incidence of the disorder in younger patients is increasing as a result of prolonged treatment with radiotherapy, chemotherapy, or both for cancer. This is referred to as secondary MDS, as opposed to idiopathic, or primary, MDS.

PATHOPHYSIOLOGY

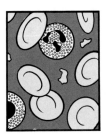

MDS probably results from neoplastic transformation in the stem cell, which often manifests as an increased number of circulating blast cells. These clonal cells always display some degree of differentiation, with slower disease progression than is seen in AML. The cells have characteristic morphologic abnormalities, and functional deficiencies are common. The bone marrow is replaced partly or wholly by the clone of stem cells.

CLINICAL MANIFESTATIONS

Most cases of MDS are diagnosed as a result of complications of anemia, thrombocytopenia, or neutropenia, but some patients are asymptomatic, and the diagnosis is made from an incidental blood test. Infections and bleeding are common; respiratory infections and gram-negative septicemias are frequently seen, with neutropenia as the usual antecedent. However, some patients become infected secondarily because they have an adequate number of circulating granulocytes, but the cells function ineffectively. Likewise, some patients with an adequate number of circulating platelets have episodic bleeding because the cells function poorly.

Table 7-1

FRENCH-AMERICAN-BRITISH (FAB) CLASSIFICATION OF MYELODYSPLASTIC DISORDERS

Type	Abbreviation	% Blasts in bone marrow	% Blasts in peripheral blood
Refractory anemia	RA	<5%	<1%
Refractory anemia with ringed sidero-blasts	RARS	<5%*	<1%
Refractory anemia with excess blasts	RAEB	5%-20%	<5%
Chronic monomyelocytic leukemia	CMML	5%-20% (plus monocytes)	<5%
Refractory anemia with excess blasts in transition	RAEB-T	20%-30%	>5%

*At least 15% of all erythroblasts identified are ringed sideroblasts.
(From Cain, Hood-Barnes, and Spangler.)[9]

As the disorder progresses, general bone marrow failure may develop. These patients often are resistant to the transfusion of blood products. The patterns of disease progression are delineated in the box at right.

The French-American-British (FAB) classification of myelodysplastic disorders is based on several characteristics found in bone marrow and the peripheral blood (Table 7-1). The relationship between the number of peripherally circulating blast cells and the number of blast cells in the bone marrow serves as the primary prognostic indicator.

In general, refractory anemia with excess blasts (RAEB) and refractory anemia with excess blasts in transition (RAEB-T) correlate with short survival. Refractory anemia (RA) and refractory anemia with ringed sideroblasts (RARS) correlate with long survival. Chronic monomyelocytic leukemia (CMML) falls between these two categories. Progression to AML is a significant cause of mortality.

PATTERNS OF DISEASE PROGRESSION IN MYELODYSPLASTIC SYNDROMES

Gradual increase in bone marrow blasts, usually with increasing pancytopenia (most of these patients progress to acute leukemia).

Some patients with relatively stable disease manifest an abrupt transformation to acute leukemia.

Many patients have stable disease that may persist for 10 years or longer without an increase in bone marrow blasts.

DIAGNOSTIC STUDIES AND FINDINGS

Diagnostic test	Findings
Bone marrow aspirate	Increased percentage of blasts
Peripheral blood	Increased percentage of blasts

Table 7-2

SIDE EFFECTS/TOXICITIES OF TREATMENTS FOR MYELODYSPLASTIC SYNDROMES

Treatment	Side effects/toxicities
Supportive blood therapy	Anemia, thrombocytopenia, leukopenia, blood transfusion reaction
Hormonal therapy	Moon face, fragile skin, increased risk of infection
Differentiation-inducing agents	Dry skin, dry lips (cheilitis), myalgia, lethargy, hypercalcemia
Biologic response modifiers	Flulike symptoms: fever, fatigue, rigors
Colony-stimulating factors	Bone pain, chills or rigors, fever, leukocytosis

(From Cain, Hood-Barnes, and Spangler).[9]

MEDICAL MANAGEMENT

Supportive therapy

Antibiotic therapy.

Transfusions with blood products.

Hormonal therapy

Androgens.

Corticosteroids.

Differentiation-inducing drugs

Retinoic acid and 13-cisretinoic acid.

Chemotherapy

Low-dose cytarabine.

6-Thioguanine.

Bone marrow transplantation

Biologic response modifiers.

Alpha-interferon.

Gamma-interferon.

Colony-stimulating factors

Granulocyte-macrophage colony-stimulating factor (GM-CSF).

Granulocyte colony-stimulating factor (G-CSF).

SUPPORTIVE THERAPY

Supportive therapy is the treatment of choice for less aggressive types of MDS. It includes hematologic monitoring, antibiotic therapy, and transfusions with blood products. Neutropenic patients require close monitoring and prompt treatment with broad-spectrum antibiotics; prophylactic antiviral, antifungal, and antibiotic agents may be prescribed to prevent superinfections. Erythrocyte transfusions are administered to patients with anemia and associated cardiopulmonary symptoms. Platelet transfusions are prescribed for uncontrolled active bleeding or when the platelet count falls between 10,000 to 20,000.

HORMONAL THERAPY

The response has been disappointing with both androgen therapy and corticosteroid therapy. Patients receiving androgens have not shown either improved bone marrow function or extended survival. With corticosteroids, response occurs in only 10% of patients with markedly elevated RBC counts secondary to enhanced clonal growth. Corticosteroid treatment should be used only in patients with RA and RARS.

DIFFERENTIATION-INDUCING DRUGS

If effective, differentiation-inducing drugs can transform nonfunctional, immature blasts and promyelocytes into functional mature granulocytes. Retinoic acid is a promising treatment for MDS, because it does not suppress bone marrow and may potentiate differentiation-inducing and antiproliferative agents. Toxicities include dry skin, cheilitis, myalgia, and lethargy.

CHEMOTHERAPY

The antileukemic and bone marrow–suppressive properties of low-dose cytarabine are beneficial. The drug can be administered as a continuous infusion or as daily subcutaneous injections with equal efficacy. One third of patients will respond with partial or complete remission, but the response is brief and has not been shown to prolong survival.

Low-dose 6-thioguanine is well-tolerated and achieves a partial response in about half of these patients. Low-dose combination therapy (daunomycin, cytarabine, and 6-thioguanine) has shown promising results in phase II clinical trials. Aggressive antileukemic chemotherapy generally has been unsuccessful.

BONE MARROW TRANSPLANTATION

Allogeneic bone marrow transplantation (BMT) is a potentially curative therapy; the prognosis is better when transplantation occurs early in the course of the disease. Most studies on the efficacy of BMT have involved patients aged 50 or younger.

BIOLOGIC RESPONSE MODIFIERS

Alpha-interferon also is a potentially effective treatment; it is known to suppress myeloid proliferation and to induce differentiation of certain myeloid cell lines. Gamma-interferon has produced minor responses in patients with MDS by inducing both monocytic differentiation and the release of granulocyte-macrophage colony-stimulating factor (GM-CSF) and interleukin-3.

COLONY-STIMULATING FACTORS

GM-CSF and granulocyte colony-stimulating factor (G-CSF) are being tested in phase I and phase II studies of patients with MDS; G-CSF shows greater potential for eliciting a response in myeloid cell differentiation. It may also play a role in increasing the number of neutrophil precursors and actual circulating mature neutrophils.

Each type of treatment presents the patient and the nurse with a variety of side effects and toxicities that must be managed (Table 7-2; bone marrow transplantation is described in Chapter 10).

1 ASSESS

ASSESSMENT	OBSERVATIONS
Energy level	Progressive fatigue, lassitude
Respiratory status	Dyspnea
Vascular status	Petechiae or ecchymoses, bleeding from gums, hematuria, occult or frank blood in feces
Immune status	Fever, nasal discharge, sore throat, anorexia, ulcerations on mucous membranes, pain or burning with urination

2 DIAGNOSE

NURSING DIAGNOSIS	SUBJECTIVE FINDINGS	OBJECTIVE FINDINGS
Activity intolerance related to inadequate tissue oxygenation due to decreased erythrocyte count	Reports progressive fatigue, shortness of breath	Lassitude, dyspnea
High risk for infection related to decreased leukocyte count	Reports sore throat, loss of appetite, pain and burning with urination	Fever, nasal discharge, ulcerations on mucous membranes
High risk for fluid volume deficit related to inadequate platelet count and impaired clotting	Reports rapid heart beat, dry mouth	Petechiae or ecchymoses, bleeding from gums, hematuria, occult or frank blood in feces

3 PLAN

Patient goals

1. The patient will demonstrate improved activity tolerance.
2. The patient will have no evidence of infection.
3. The patient will demonstrate adequate fluid volume.

4 IMPLEMENT

NURSING DIAGNOSIS	NURSING INTERVENTIONS	RATIONALE
Activity intolerance related to inadequate tissue oxygenation due to decreased erythrocyte count	Place patient in semi-Fowler's or sitting position.	To facilitate breathing.
	Assist with ADLs as needed.	To prevent fatigue.
	Observe respiratory rate, pulse, skin color, and temperature. Administer oxygen as needed.	To monitor response to activity and determine need for rest. To decrease dyspnea.
High risk for infection related to decreased leukocyte count	Maintain reverse isolation when WBC is low.	To prevent exposure to pathogens.
	Observe for increases in temperature, pulse, and respirations.	To detect signs of infection.

➔ ❭ ❭

NURSING DIAGNOSIS	NURSING INTERVENTIONS	RATIONALE
	Observe patient for other signs or symptoms of infection (nasal discharge, sore throat, anorexia, ulceration of mucous membranes, pain and burning with urination).	To detect infection of respiratory, GI, or urinary tracts.
	Administer antibiotics as prescribed.	To combat specific pathogens.
	Encourage patient to move about; also turning, coughing, deep breathing, and increased fluid intake as tolerated.	To reduce susceptibility to infection.
High risk for fluid volume deficit related to inadequate platelet count and impaired clotting	Protect patient from injury.	To prevent trauma and bleeding.
	Give injections only if necessary; apply pressure at site.	To prevent extravasation.
	Observe for increased pulse and respirations.	To detect bleeding.
	Observe for evidence of bleeding (petechiae, ecchymoses, hematuria, occult or frank blood in feces, bleeding gums).	To detect intradermal or internal bleeding.
	Monitor laboratory reports (e.g., Hct and Hb).	To detect evidence of internal bleeding.

5 EVALUATE

PATIENT OUTCOME	DATA INDICATING THAT OUTCOME IS REACHED
Activity tolerance is within normal limits.	Patient can carry out ADLs without fatigue or dyspnea and can exercise for progressively longer periods.
Patient has no infection.	There is no evidence of respiratory, GI, or urinary infection.
Fluid volume is adequate.	Patient has no petechiae or ecchymoses; vital signs are stable: there is no observable bleeding; laboratory values are within normal limits.

PATIENT TEACHING ■■■■■■■■■■■■■■■■■■■■■■■■■■■■■■■■■■■

1. Teach the patient how to maintain a balance between rest and activity.
2. Discuss with the patient ways of avoiding infection.
3. Discuss with the patient how to avoid trauma and prevent bleeding.
4. Teach the patient self-assessment for signs and symptoms of bleeding, which conditions to report to the physician, and what first aid measures to take.

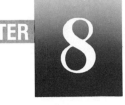

Multiple Myeloma

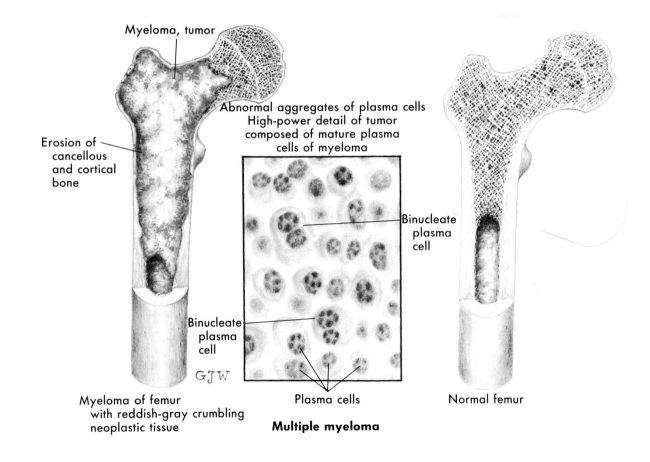

Myeloma, tumor

Abnormal aggregates of plasma cells
High-power detail of tumor
composed of mature plasma
cells of myeloma

Erosion of
cancellous
and cortical
bone

Binucleate
plasma
cell

Binucleate
plasma
cell

GJW

Myeloma of femur
with reddish-gray crumbling
neoplastic tissue

Plasma cells

Multiple myeloma

Normal femur

Multiple myeloma, a disseminated neoplasm of B cells and mature plasma cells that invade the bone marrow, used to be relatively rare, but the incidence has doubled in the past two decades.

The disorder strikes about 10,000 people each year, mostly men 50 to 69 years of age. The rate in blacks is at least twice that in whites. Although the cause is unknown, some studies suggest that multiple myeloma reflects an inappropriate response to an antigen or a viruslike particle, specifically, chronic stimulation of the mononuclear phagocyte system by chemicals, bacteria, or viruses. This theory is supported by the increased frequency of plasma cell neoplasms in people with long-standing chronic infections such as tuberculosis, osteomyelitis, or pneumonitis. Genetic factors have also been suggested as a possible cause, because tumors occur in specific strains of mice and in human siblings and other near relatives.

The prognosis usually is poor, because the diagnosis often is made after the disease has already infiltrated the vertebrae, pelvis, skull, ribs, clavicles, and sternum. Most patients die within 2 years of diagnosis after developing such complications as infection, renal failure, hematologic imbalance, fractures, hypercalcemia, hyperuricemia, or dehydration.

PATHOPHYSIOLOGY

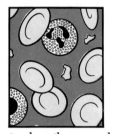
Malignant plasma cells arise from one clone of B cells, proliferate within the hematopoietic tissue of the bone marrow, and then infiltrate the rest of the bone to produce osteolytic lesions. Subsequent bone destruction leads to hypercalcemia and pathologic fracture, most often in the ribs, vertebrae, femora, skull, and pelvis.

The proliferation of plasma cells in the bone marrow crowds the marrow space, usually inhibiting production of RBCs. Also, plasma cells synthesize and secrete an abnormally small number of immunoglobulins, increasing the risk of infection. In rare cases a marked increase in a single immunoglobulin (usually IgG, occasionally IgA) increases blood viscosity, leading to occlusion of small blood vessels, especially those of the brain, retina, and glomeruli.

The hallmark of multiple myeloma is the production of an abnormal immunoglobulin (the M component), indicated by elevated blood levels and the presence of Bence Jones protein in the urine in 60% to 80% of patients.

CLINICAL MANIFESTATIONS

The onset of the disease usually is gradual and often insidious. Many patients have a presymptomatic period that lasts 5 to 20 years, during which some suffer from recurrent bacterial infections, especially pneumonia.

The symptoms usually involve the skeletal system, especially the pelvis, spine, and ribs, and include backache or bone pain that worsens with movement. Some patients sustain a pathologic fracture that causes severe

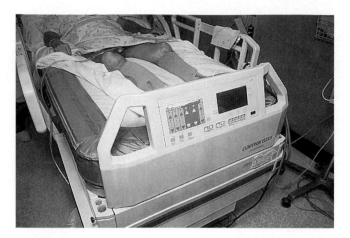

FIGURE 8-1
Air fluidized therapy to promote patient comfort and prevent development of pressure areas in the body.

pain. As skeletal destruction increases, deformities in the sternum and rib cage may develop, with some individuals losing stature (as much as 5 inches or more). Cord compression may result from vertebral collapse.

Diffuse osteoporosis with a negative calcium balance also occurs. As the diseased bones become demineralized, renal stones develop, especially if the patient is confined to bed rest. Hypercalcemia can also cause neurologic disturbances, gastrointestinal distress, altered musculoskeletal status, fluid and electrolyte imbalance, and altered cardiopulmonary function.

Renal disease may result not only from hypercalcemia and the development of renal calculi, but also from the toxic effect of Bence Jones proteins on the tubular epithelial cells of the kidneys.

COMPLICATIONS

- Impaired production of erythrocytes, leukocytes, and thrombocytes (with resultant anemia, bleeding tendencies, and increased danger of infection)
- Recurrent infections (from suppression of humoral immune response, probably by unknown factors secreted from malignant plasma cells)

DIAGNOSTIC STUDIES AND FINDINGS

Diagnostic test	Findings
Complete blood count	Moderate or severe anemia, 40% to 50% lymphocytes, approximately 3% plasma cells
Erythrocyte sedimentation rate	Elevated
Serum calcium	Elevated
Total protein	Elevated
Serum uric acid	Elevated

DIAGNOSTIC STUDIES AND FINDINGS—cont'd

Diagnostic test	Findings
Serum creatinine	Elevated
Urinalysis	Bence Jones protein, increased calcium
Bone marrow aspiration	Abnormal number of immature plasma cells
Serum electrophoresis	Elevated globulin spike
Skeletal x-rays	Several sharply circumscribed osteolytic lesions, particularly on skull, pelvis, and spine; vertebral compression fractures; demineralization

MEDICAL MANAGEMENT

Chemotherapy

Melphalan and prednisone at monthly intervals.

Vincristine, cyclophosphamide, doxorubicin, and prednisone.

Human leukocyte interferon and intermittent combinations of vindesine and prednisone.

Radiation therapy

Adjuvant local treatment to alleviate pain and reduce acute lesions.

Bone marrow transplantation

1 ASSESS

ASSESSMENT	OBSERVATIONS
Skeletal integrity	Backache or bone pain that worsens with movement; signs and symptoms of pathologic fracture
Sensory and motor function	Hypotonia, fatigue, muscle weakness, hyporeflexia of deep tendons; progressive central or radicular back pain; numbness, paresthesia, coldness; confusion, disorientation, drowsiness, lethargy, shortened attention span, inappropriate behavior, headache, stupor, coma
Renal function	Signs and symptoms of calculi; renal failure
Gastrointestinal function	Anorexia, nausea and vomiting, weight loss, constipation, vague abdominal pain
Fluid and electrolyte balance	Polyuria, polydipsia, dehydration, pruritus
Cardiopulmonary function	Chest pain, irregular pulse, bradycardia

→ > >

2   DIAGNOSE

NURSING DIAGNOSIS	SUBJECTIVE FINDINGS	OBJECTIVE FINDINGS
Pain related to bone fragility, pathologic fractures, and cord compression	Reports backache or bone pain, numbness, and tingling	Facial grimaces, shallow breathing, tachycardia; difficulty with movement; loss of feeling in extremities
Impaired physical mobility related to altered motor function secondary to pathologic fractures and cord compression	Reports difficulty walking, weakness, and easy fatigability	Hypotonia, hyporeflexia of deep tendons, muscle weakness
Altered patterns of urinary elimination related to calcium nephropathy, severe proteinuria, hyperuricemia, and hypercalcemia	Reports excessive thirst, itching, and pain in hips	Polyuria or decreased urine, renal calculi, imbalance between intake and output
Altered nutrition: less than body requirements related to hypercalcemia and response to treatment	Reports lack of appetite, nausea, and abdominal pain	Vomiting, weight loss, constipation
Altered cerebral tissue perfusion related to hypercalcemia	Reports confusion, drowsiness, and headaches	Disorientation, lethargy, reduced memory span, shortened attention span, inappropriate behavior, stupor, coma
Altered cardiopulmonary tissue perfusion related to hypercalcemia	Reports chest pain and rapid heart beat	Irregular pulse, bradycardia

3   PLAN

Patient goals

1. The patient will be comfortable.
2. The patient will be able to ambulate and carry out activities of daily living (ADLs).
3. The patient will have adequate urinary elimination.
4. The patient will have adequate nutrition.
5. The patient will be oriented and show appropriate behavior.
6. The patient will maintain adequate cardiopulmonary tissue perfusion.

4 IMPLEMENT

NURSING DIAGNOSIS	NURSING INTERVENTIONS	RATIONALE
Pain related to bone fragility, pathologic fractures, and cord compression	Position patient for comfort, and change the patient's position slowly.	To lessen pain and reduce trauma.
	Maintain patient in normal body alignment, using support as needed.	To prevent injury.
	Apply heat.	To reduce muscle spasm.
	Massage patient gently.	To reduce muscle spasm and swelling.
	Use firm mattress or specialty bed.	To support skeletal structure without pressure.
	Work with patient on ways to reduce pain, including analgesics and nonpharmacologic methods.	To give patient sense of control over pain management.
	Assess patient for evidence of pathologic fractures (pain on movement, swelling, and impaired movement).	To intervene early and prevent further damage.
	Assess patient for evidence of cord compression (progressive central or radicular back pain, numbness, paresthesia, and coldness) and for signs and symptoms specific to the level of compression.	To intervene early and prevent further damage.
Impaired physical mobility related to altered motor function secondary to pathologic fractures and cord compression	Assist with ambulation as patient's strength allows; mobilize patient as necessary using a walker, cane, or wheelchair.	To prevent injury.
	Provide range-of-motion exercises and assistance with turning.	To maintain mobility and prevent injury.
	Remove environmental barriers (chairs, tables, or rugs).	To prevent injury.
	Teach patient how to balance rest with activity.	To prevent fatigue.
	Provide trapeze over bed.	To enable patient to move himself in bed.
	Observe patient's gait, coordination, and stability.	To assess changes in musculoskeletal function.
Altered patterns of urinary elimination related to calcium nephropathy, severe proteinuria, hyperuricemia, and hypercalcemia	Provide adequate hydration (3,000 to 4,000 ml of fluid per 24 hours).	To prevent dehydration and urinary stasis.
	Monitor patient's complaints of frequency and urgency; report findings to physician.	To detect early evidence of inflammation or infection.
	Monitor intake and output (should be at least 1,500 ml per 24 hours).	To monitor renal function.

→ > >

NURSING DIAGNOSIS	NURSING INTERVENTIONS	RATIONALE
	Observe color of urine.	To detect bleeding or infection.
	Strain all urine.	To detect calculi.
	Encourage a diet low in calcium and phosphorus.	To prevent formation of calculi.
	Offer patient urine-acidifying juices.	To maintain normal urinary pH.
	Administer IV normal saline and other drugs as prescribed (may include plicamycin, corticosteroids, calcitonin, IV phosphate, and gallium).	To correct hypercalcemia.
Altered nutrition: less than body requirements related to hypercalcemia and response to treatment	Encourage diet high in protein and vitamins.	To enhance bone mineralization.
	Encourage decreased intake of calcium-rich foods.	To prevent formation of renal calculi.
	Encourage increased fluid intake, especially water.	To maintain adequate hydration.
	Refer patient to nutritionist.	To plan a diet that patient will eat.
	Encourage patient to ambulate.	To help prevent bone demineralization.
	Instruct patient not to take thiazide diuretics or vitamins A and D.	These drugs elevate the serum calcium level.
	Use oral hygiene, antiemetics, and nonpharmacologic interventions for management of nausea and vomiting.	To increase patient's appetite and decrease nausea and vomiting.
	Encourage use of fluids, fiber, and nonirritating laxatives.	To prevent and manage constipation.
	Use heat and mild analgesics.	To help control abdominal pain.
	Weigh patient daily.	To monitor nutritional status.
	Monitor blood studies, especially serum calcium and urinary calcium.	To monitor effectiveness of treatment.
Altered cerebral tissue perfusion related to hypercalcemia	Assess patient for orientation to time, place, and person; level of consciousness; attention span; and appropriateness of behavior.	To monitor cerebral function and detect problems early.
	Orient patient frequently to time, place, and person.	To decrease incidence and severity of confusion.
	Assist family and significant others in understanding patient's behavior.	To gain their assistance in supporting patient.

NURSING DIAGNOSIS	NURSING INTERVENTIONS	RATIONALE
	Give prescribed analgesics.	To decrease incidence and severity of headaches.
	Maintain a calm, supportive manner.	To prevent agitation.
Altered cardiopulmonary tissue perfusion related to hypercalcemia	Place patient in semi-Fowler's position.	To enhance cardiopulmonary function.
	Assist patient with ADLs and ambulation.	To prevent stress on cardiac function.
	Observe patient's skin color and temperature, level of consciousness, orientation, and mood.	To determine adequacy of circulation.
	Monitor pulse rate and rhythm.	To detect irregular pulse and bradycardia.
	Report patient's complaints of chest pain and palpitations to physician.	To detect dysfunction early.

5 EVALUATE

PATIENT OUTCOME	DATA INDICATING THAT OUTCOME IS REACHED
Patient is comfortable.	Patient has no complaints of bone or back pain.
Patient can ambulate and carry out ADLs.	Patient walks without difficulty or assistance; patient is coordinated, and his gait is steady
Urinary elimination is adequate.	Intake and output are balanced; patient does not complain of frequency or urgency; urine is clear and slightly acid; there is no evidence of calculi.
Nutrition is adequate.	Patient's weight is normal, and he does not complain of anorexia, nausea, or abdominal pain.
Patient is calm and oriented.	There is no evidence of confusion, disorientation, or inappropriate behavior; patient has adequate attention span and memory and does not complain of headaches.
Cardiopulmonary tissue perfusion is adequate.	Patient does not complain of chest pain or palpitations.

PATIENT TEACHING

1. Discuss the need for good body mechanics, mechanical support as needed, and avoiding environmental barriers (e.g., chairs, tables, or rugs).
2. Review general safety measures (see Patient Teaching Guide, page 209).
3. Plan with the patient ways to control pain, including nonpharmacologic means.
4. Teach the patient the importance of drinking adequate fluids and of controlling intake of high-calcium and alkaline foods and fluids; instruct the patient to focus on foods high in protein and vitamins.
5. Teach the patient and family how to monitor for signs and symptoms of inadequate renal, cerebral, or cardiopulmonary perfusion.

CHAPTER 9

Lymphomas

The malignant lymphomas are a heterogeneous group of cancers that arise from the lymphoreticular system. They include lymphosarcoma, reticulum cell sarcoma, Burkitt's lymphoma, T-cell cutaneous lymphoma, and Hodgkin's disease. Even though this group constitutes only the seventh most common type of cancer in the United States, it accounts for more years of life lost than do many of the more common cancers because of the relatively younger population affected.

These disorders are among the most curable of all cancers, and as knowledge about the pathogenesis and treatment of lymphomas advances, even higher cure rates should be seen.

Hodgkin's Disease

Hodgkin's disease is a cancer of the lymphatic system characterized by the abnormal proliferation of histiocytes called Reed-Sternberg cells.

Approximately 14% of all malignant lymphomas are Hodgkin's disease. In 1991 it was estimated that 7,400 new cases would occur and that 1,600 deaths would result. This disease shows a bimodal age-incidence distribution; that is, the incidence rises sharply after age 10, peaks in the late twenties, and then declines until age 45. After age 45, the incidence again increases steadily with age. Men are affected twice as often as women and boys five times more often than girls.

The clinical symptoms of Hodgkin's disease have suggested an infectious cause. The childhood social environment has been implicated as influencing the risk of the disease in young adulthood. The risk of acquiring the disease is associated with factors that diminish or delay exposure to infectious agents, such as higher social class, more education, small family size, and early birth order position.

The Epstein-Barr virus (EBV) is a possible causative agent, as suggested by the virus' ability to transform lymphocytes and by the presence of Reed-Sternberg–like cells in the lymphoid tissue of patients with infectious mononucleosis. Hodgkin's disease is also associated with some of the prodromal manifestations seen in acquired immunodeficiency syndrome (AIDS) when it appears in advanced stages with a higher incidence of bone marrow involvement. The risk of Hodgkin's disease is increased sevenfold for siblings of diagnosed patients, and other first-degree relatives have a threefold increase in risk, suggesting the important role of genetic factors in the etiology.

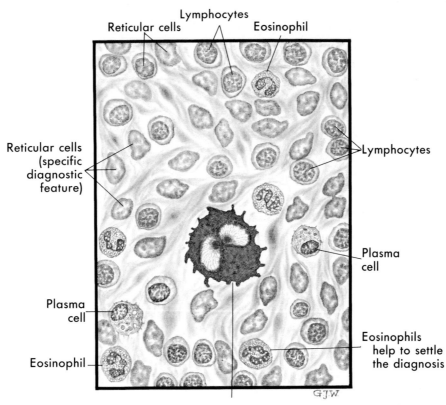

Reticular cells

Lymphocytes

Eosinophil

Reticular cells (specific diagnostic feature)

Lymphocytes

Plasma cell

Plasma cell

Eosinophils help to settle the diagnosis

Eosinophil

FIGURE 9-1
Reed-Sternberg giant cell in Hodgkin's disease. Giant cell is most often binucleated. Within nuclei are large "owl-eyed" nucleoli surrounded by a halo, often appearing as mirror images of each other.

PATHOPHYSIOLOGY

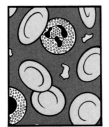

The Reed-Sternberg cell (Figure 9-1), which is present in Hodgkin's disease and not in other lymphomas, is believed to be derived from the monocyte-macrophage cell line. These cells have been shown to secrete the monokine interleukin-1, which causes proliferation of T lymphocytes and fibroblasts and acts as an endogenous pyrogen, common histologic features of Hodgkin's disease.

Abnormalities in cellular immunity have been demonstrated in batteries of skin tests. Lymphocyte depletion is seen in 40% to 50% of patients and is more common in advanced disease. These lymphocytes proliferate poorly when stimulated. Macrophages adhere poorly to foreign surfaces and have abnormal antigen processing.

The histologic pattern and anatomic distribution of Hodgkin's disease vary with age. The nodular sclerosis form of the disease predominates in young adults, and the mixed cellularity form is most common in the older age group. Twenty-five percent of elderly patients have only subdiaphragmatic disease at diagnosis, compared with fewer than 5% of young adult patients. More than half of the young patients have mediastinal involvement, compared with fewer than 25% of the elderly patients.

Hodgkin's disease initially affects one lymph node and then travels via lymphatic channels to nodes throughout the body; it may also appear in the liver and spleen, vertebrae, ureters, and bronchi. Staging of the disease is based on the microscopic appearance of the lymph nodes, the extent and severity of the disease, and the prognosis. Both clinical staging and pathologic staging are recommended. The clinical stage is determined by completing a thorough history and physical examination, blood counts and chemistries, chest x-ray, abdominal computed tomography (CT) scan, and bipedal lymphangiography. The pathologic stage is based on the clinical stage and information gained by the histologic review of tissue obtained by bone marrow biopsy or laparotomy or from other sites.

The stages of the Ann Arbor staging system (Figure 9-2) are described in the box on the next page.

The Rye classification system (Table 9-1) is used by pathologists and physicians to subclassify the histology of Hodgkin's disease into four groups.

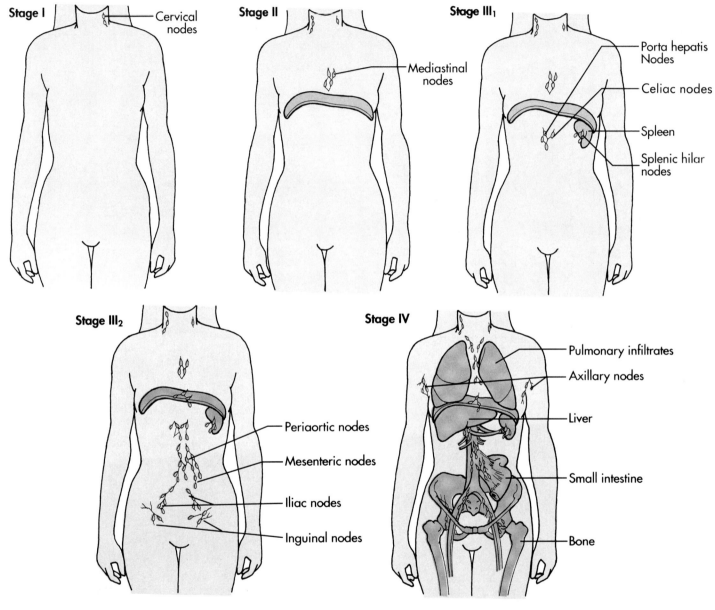

FIGURE 9-2
Nodal involvement by stage in Hodgkin's disease. (Based on modified Ann Arbor staging system.)

Table 9-1

HISTOPATHOLOGIC CLASSIFICATION OF HODGKIN'S DISEASE (RYE CLASSIFICATION)

Histologic subtype	Relative frequency
Lymphocyte predominant	5% to 10%
Nodular sclerosis	30% to 60%
Mixed cellularity	20% to 40%
Lymphocyte depleted	5% to 10%

(From the American Cancer Society.)[1]

ANN ARBOR STAGING SYSTEM FOR HODGKIN'S DISEASE

Stage I
Involvement of a single lymph node region or a single extranodal site

Stage II
Involvement of two or more lymph node regions on the same side of the diaphragm or localized involvement of an extranodal site and one or more lymph node regions on the same side of the diaphragm

Stage III
Involvement of lymph node regions on both sides of the diaphragm. May include a single extranodal site, the spleen, or both; now subdivided into lymphatic involvement of the upper abdomen in the spleen (splenic, celiac, and portal nodes) and the lower abdominal nodes in the periaortic, mesenteric, and iliac regions

Stage IV
Diffuse or disseminated disease of one or more extralymphatic organs or tissues with or without associated lymph node involvement; the extranodal site is identified as H (hepatic), L (lung), P (pleura), M (marrow), D (dermal), or O (osseous)

The patient's symptoms are also indicated in this system by "A" and "B." **A** refers to patients without certain general symptoms; **B** refers to those with certain general symptoms, including unexplained fever with oral temperatures above 38° C (100.4° F), night sweats, and unexplained weight loss of more than 10% of body weight during the previous 6 months.

The **lymphocyte predominant** histology accounts for 5% to 10% of patients. Abundant numbers of mature lymphocytes diffusely infiltrate the abnormal lymph nodes. The prognosis is excellent for patients with this subtype (i.e., a 5-year survival rate of 90%).

Nodular sclerosis accounts for 30% to 60% of cases. Interlacing bands of collagen that divide the cellular infiltrate into discrete islands produce the lymph node's nodular appearance. The prognosis is good, with a high 5-year survival rate. This subtype is seen most frequently in young adult women and at diagnosis is most often localized in the cervical nodes and mediastinum.

Mixed cellularity is the second most common subtype, accounting for about 33% of cases. The nodes contain a pleomorphic infiltrate of eosinophils, normal lymphocytes, and readily identifiable Reed-Sternberg cells. The 5-year survival of all stages is 50% to 60%.

The **lymphocyte depleted** subtype is the least common. The Reed-Sternberg cell predominates, and mature lymphocytes are virtually absent in affected lymph nodes. This pattern occurs primarily in older patients and is associated with B symptoms and an advanced stage at presentation. The 5-year survival rate is less than 50%.

CLINICAL MANIFESTATIONS

Young adults typically have painless lymphadenopathy, although associated symptoms of malaise,
fever, night sweats, pruritus, and weight loss
may be present. The enlarged lymph node usually is supradiaphragmatic (90% of cases) and
frequently is in the cervical region (60% to
80% of cases) (Figure 9-3.) Axillary or mediastinal lymphadenopathy is less common. Massive mediastinal lymph nodes may cause symptoms of coughing, wheezing, dyspnea, or superior vena cava syndrome. Subdiaphragmatic symptoms are uncommon in young patients but represent the only site of disease in 25% of older patients. Involvement of the retroperitoneal nodes,
liver, spleen, and bone marrow usually occurs
after the disease has become generalized. Mesenteric lymph nodes are rarely involved, although in advanced disease any organ can be
involved.

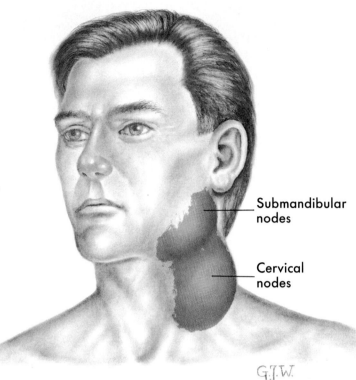

Submandibular
nodes

Cervical
nodes

FIGURE 9-3
Severe case of swollen lymph nodes in Hodgkin's disease.

DIAGNOSTIC STUDIES AND FINDINGS

Diagnostic test	Findings
Staging workup	
Lymph node biopsy of largest, most central node in an involved group, preferably cervical	Reed-Sternberg cells
Complete blood count	Mild normochromic-normocytic anemia, neutro-philic leukocytosis, lymphopenia, eosinophilia, hemolytic anemia (in advanced disease), ele-vated erythrocyte sedimentation rate
Blood chemistry	Elevated serum alkaline phosphatase, hypergam-maglobulinemia (in early disease); immunoglob-ulin levels may decline in advanced disease or during treatment; elevated serum copper and ceruloplasmin
Posteroanterior (PA) and lateral chest x-ray; chest computed tomography (CT) scan	Lung or pleural involvement
Bipedal lymphangiography	Abnormal nodes
Abdominal CT scan	Suspicious and enlarged nodes
Bone marrow biopsy (bilateral)	Abnormal cells
Laparotomy with splenectomy	Nodal and extranodal sites of disease

---

MEDICAL MANAGEMENT

Surgery

Therapeutic splenectomy.

Radiation therapy

External beam treatment.

Chemotherapy

Multiagent chemotherapy—MOPP (nitrogen mustard, vincristine, procarbazine, and prednisone).

ABVD (doxorubicin [Adriamycin], bleomycin, vinblastine, dacarbazine).

Single-agent chemotherapy.

SURGERY

The primary roles of surgery in Hodgkin's disease are to obtain biopsy specimens and to perform a staging laparotomy (see the box below) when needed. Therapeutic excision of enlarged nodes in early-stage disease is not done; removal of bulky masses after therapy usually reveals fibrosis.

Therapeutic splenectomy may be appropriate for treatment of an enlarged spleen, to increase tolerance to chemotherapy, or to reduce the size of the radiation field.

STAGING LAPAROTOMY

A staging laparotomy should be performed only when the information to be gained is deemed to affect both therapy and outcome. It should include *all* the following procedures:
1. Inspection
2. Splenectomy
3. Liver biopsies (wedge biopsy of left lobe, needle biopsies of right and left lobes)
4. Lymph node biopsies (splenic hilar, celiac, porta hepatis, mesenteric, periaortic, and iliac)
5. Placement of clips at biopsy site
6. Oophoropexy in women who want to avoid sterilization

RADIATION THERAPY

Radiation therapy (RT) is curative in most patients with stage I, stage II, and some cases of stage IIIA disease. Chemotherapy may be added to the RT protocol for patients with such adverse prognostic factors as B symptoms, bulky disease, and stage III disease.

Megavoltage RT is used to treat opposed fields in tumoricidal doses, with careful field simulation and verification and close follow-up of all patients.

The use of extended fields to include the adjacent, clinically negative nodal sites is essential for high cure rates. Total nodal irradiation sequentially treats a mantle field above the diaphragm. Subtotal nodal irradiation refers to a mantle field followed by irradiation to the periaortic nodes and splenic pedicle. Carefully constructed field shapes and blocks for shielding are used to protect the lungs, heart, spinal cord, larynx, kidneys, gonads, and iliac crests (Figure 9-4, page 150).

The tumoricidal dosage level is approximately 40 to 45 Gy, delivered at the rate of 10 Gy per week; this dosage may be reduced when combined with chemotherapy.

The use of an opposed field technique to treat deep-lying tissues, usually anterior and posterior, provides a homogenous dose distribution throughout the treatment area and decreases the chance of radiation damage to such structures as the heart and liver.

Consolidation RT involves lower doses given to areas of known disease in individuals with advanced stage IIIB or stage IV disease after a complete response to chemotherapy.

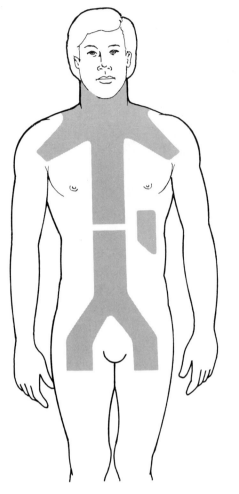

FIGURE 9-4
Radiation therapy ports used for total nodal irradiation.

CHEMOTHERAPEUTIC AGENTS USEFUL WITH LYMPHOMAS

Alkylating agents
Nitrogen mustard (mechlorethamine), chlorambucil, cyclophosphamide, carmustine (BCNU), lomustine (CCNU)
Vinca alkaloids
Vincristine (Oncovin), vinblastine
Antibiotics
Doxorubicin (Adriamycin), bleomycin
Other
Prednisone, procarbazine, methotrexate, dacarbazine (DTIC)

(From the American Cancer Society.)[1]

COMPLICATIONS

Radiation pneumonitis
Pericarditis
Hypothyroidism
Transverse myelitis

CHEMOTHERAPY

Multiagent chemotherapy of advanced Hodgkin's disease can produce a complete remission and a 5-year disease-free interval in most patients. Single-agent chemotherapy can produce complete and partial responses in 50% to 70% of patients, although the remissions last only a few months, and complete responses are unusual. Single agents are useful in palliating advanced disease in older patients or those who are heavily pre-

treated and, because of severe myelosuppression, cannot tolerate combined therapy (see the box above).

The MOPP regimen has resulted in a high complete response rate and a durable remission. Numerous other drugs have been added or substituted by researchers in an effort to reduce toxicity and improve results. For example, ABVD has a similar complete response rate and can salvage MOPP failures. ABVD is often considered a second-line regimen because of potential cardiac and pulmonary toxicity; however, recent research demonstrated no increased cardiopulmonary toxicity and less risk of secondary leukemia.

Certain groups of patients benefit from combinations of RT and chemotherapy: those showing localized disease with masses exceeding one third the diameter of the thoracic cavity (stage I or stage II disease with massive mediastinum); patients with stage IIIA disease with bulky sites; patients with stage IIIB or stage IV disease who achieve only a partial remission with chemotherapy who are converted to complete remission with added RT; and children in whom the use of combination chemotherapy will allow for reduced doses of RT, which spares bone growth.

COMPLICATIONS

Increased risk of secondary malignancies, particularly acute leukemia
Non-Hodgkin's lymphomas

NURSING CARE

See pages 153 to 157.

Non-Hodgkin's Lymphoma

Non-Hodgkin's lymphomas are cancers of the lymphatic system that commonly arise from a monoclonal population of B cells.

The American Cancer Society estimated that 37,200 new patients with non-Hodgkin's lymphoma would be diagnosed in 1991, 19,600 men and 17,600 women. It was estimated that 18,700 deaths would occur. Higher age-adjusted incidence rates have been attributed to increases among older people, with lesser increases in the 35 to 64 age group and relatively unchanged rates among young adults. The incidence of diffuse large-cell lymphoma is increasing among older people.

A viral cause has been implicated in such non-Hodgkin's lymphomas (NHLs) as Burkitt's lymphoma, Mediterranean lymphoma, and T-cell leukemia/lymphoma, which is associated with human T-cell leukemia/lymphoma virus I (HTLV-I). NHLs have been seen with increasing frequency in patients with AIDS and in people who are immunosuppressed following kidney and heart transplantation (particularly central nervous system NHL). There is also an increased risk of NHL in Wiskott-Aldrich syndrome, X-linked immunodeficiency, ataxia telangiectasia, and possibly Sjögren's syndrome.

PATHOPHYSIOLOGY

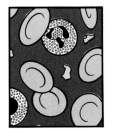

Cytogenetic abnormalities are seen in most non-Hodgkin's lymphomas. In Burkitt's lymphoma translocation between chromosome 8 and chromosome 14 often occurs, and other translocations have been observed.

NHLs are now characterized as cancers of the immune system. Subclasses of lymphoma manifest similarities in immunologic phenotype to stages in the normal differentiation of T and B lymphocytes.

Histologic classifications for NHLs include low grade (B-cell tumors), intermediate grade (B-cell and some T-cell lymphomas), high grade (immunoblastic lymphomas/predominantly B-cell; lymphoblastic/T-cell tumors; Burkitt's and non-Burkitt's small noncleaved cell tumors/predominantly B-cell), and miscellaneous histiocytic (mycosis fungoides and others). All of the low-grade NHLs and some of the intermediate-grade tumors with long natural histories have a good prognosis. Tumors with a poor prognosis include the rapidly progressive high-grade tumors, and some from the intermediate-grade group.

FOLLICULAR SMALL-CLEAVED CELL LYMPHOMA

Most common; patients usually manifest stage III or stage IV disease and have a high incidence of bone marrow involvement

Follicular mixed small-cleaved and large-cell lymphomas

Second most common group; marrow involvement is common, and most patients have stage III or stage IV disease at diagnosis

Diffuse large-cell lymphoma

Tends to appear frequently in extranodal as well as nodal sites; disseminates rapidly; involves such unusual areas as the CNS, bone, and GI tract

Immunoblastic lymphomas

The histologic features of the most common subgroups of NHLs are described in the box above.

The staging for NHL is the same as that for Hodgkin's lymphoma; however, because NHL frequently is disseminated at the time of diagnosis, surgical staging is not commonly done. The predictability of the spread of NHL is less certain than in Hodgkin's disease.

CLINICAL MANIFESTATIONS

The presenting symptom of NHL is an enlarged node or an abnormal chest x-ray (i.e., pleural effusion). The patient may also present with superior vena cava syndrome. Gastrointestinal involvement may manifest as jaundice, abdominal cramping, bloody diarrhea, or signs and symptoms of total colonic obstruction. Ascites may be evident. The patient may also have hydronephrosis as a result of ureteral obstruction by retroperitoneal masses. Cord compression may occur in the rare incidence of neurologic involvement. Later in the course of the disease, hemolytic or unexplained anemia may be detected.

Immunodeficiencies are more pronounced in diffuse disease and include marked impairment of recall, reduced serum IgA, and lymphopenia, resulting in infections.

DIAGNOSTIC STUDIES AND FINDINGS

Diagnostic test	Findings
Staging workup	
Surgical biopsy	Malignant cells
Bone marrow biopsy (bilateral)	Malignant cells
PA and lateral chest x-ray; computed tomography (CT) chest scan	Evidence of pleural effusion
Abdominal computed tomography (CT) scan	Involvement of upper retroperitoneal and mesenteric nodes, liver, and spleen
Bipedal lymphadenopathy	Borderline lymphadenopathy
Staging laparotomy (see box, page 149)	Increased incidence of hepatic, mesenteric, and GI involvement
Peritoneoscopy with directed biopsies	Liver involvement
Bone scans	Bone involvement

MEDICAL MANAGEMENT

Surgery

Resection of extranodal GI involvement; splenectomy.

Radiation therapy

External beam treatment.

Chemotherapy

COP (cyclophosphamide, vincristine, prednisone).

CHOP (cyclophosphamide, doxorubicin, vincristine, prednisone).

BACOP (bleomycin, doxorubicin, cyclophosphamide, vincristine, prednisone).

MACOP-B (methotrexate with leucovorin rescue, doxorubicin, cyclophosphamide, vincristine, prednisone, bleomycin).

m-BACOD (cyclophosphamide, doxorubicin, vincristine, bleomycin, dexamethasone, methotrexate with leucovorin rescue).

ProMACE-CytaBOM (cyclophosphamide, doxorubicin, etoposide, prednisone, cytarabine, bleomycin, vincristine, methotrexate with leucovorin rescue).

SURGERY

Resection of extranodal GI involvement with staging at the time of removal of the affected nodes lessens the likelihood of RT- or chemotherapy-related risk of perforation and/or bleeding. Splenectomy enables patients with hypersplenism to undergo more extensive chemotherapy.

RADIATION THERAPY

The goal of RT in NHL is to control disease within the confines of the clinically evident disease and not to irradiate adjacent areas. Low-grade lymphomas generally are highly responsive to irradiation, with local control rates exceeding 90%. Long-term follow-up of patients treated for stage I and stage II lymphomas indicates a

10-year survival and 50% freedom from relapse, particularly among younger patients. Total lymphoid irradiation given alone or in combination with chemotherapy, as well as whole-body irradiation, have been used to treat patients with stage III and stage IV disease, with a high remission rate.

Intermediate- and high-grade lymphomas appear almost equally in localized stage I and stage II disease and in disseminated stage III and stage IV disease; they also are more common in such extranodal sites as the GI tract, bone marrow, CNS, and skin. Current trials for these tumors combine chemotherapy with RT.

RT must be tailored to the site of origin of the localized NHL; for example, Waldeyer's ring is treated in patients with disease in the nasopharynx, tonsillar area, or base of the tongue; low-dose, whole-abdominal RT with shielding of the kidneys, followed by a boost to adjacent nodes, is used with GI involvement; radiation of the bone with local node treatment is used for primary bone lymphomas; and irradiation of the thyroid bed on both sides of the neck and the superior mediastinum is used for thyroid-localized NHL. Radiation is important in the treatment of primary CNS non-Hodgkin's lymphoma and is effective for palliating symptoms in individuals with advanced NHLs, such as obstruction of the superior vena cava, compression of the spinal cord, occlusion of the ureters, and painful tumor masses.

CHEMOTHERAPY

Chemotherapy is the primary treatment for disseminated NHL. The choice of agents is based on histology, disease stage, and such general patient information as age and performance status. The quality of life usually is good, with long periods of symptom-free survival.

Such combinations as COP, CHOP, BACOP, MACOP-B, m-BACOD, and ProMACE-CytaBOM have been used. Although these regimens have a high remission rate, the average remission lasts only 2 to 3 years. After successive relapses, the remissions induced with second courses of therapy generally are shorter. There is little evidence of curability for stage III and stage IV disease.

Research is focused on the use of progressive chemotherapy earlier in the course of the disease and/or biologic response modifiers in combination with chemotherapy or during maintenance. In addition, initial chemotherapy followed by RT for patients who have incomplete responses is being studied in patients with stage I and stage II disease.

Because increasing CNS involvement has been observed, especially with diffuse large-cell lymphomas and extensive marrow involvement, the cerebrospinal fluid (CSF) should be evaluated for lymphoma involvement. Patients should then be given either systemic agents at dosage levels known to penetrate the CSF or prophylactic intrathecal chemotherapy; this appears warranted in most cases of NHL among children.

1 ASSESS

ASSESSMENT	OBSERVATIONS
Skin	Painless swelling of lymph nodes
Comfort	Bone pain, nerve pain
Respiratory function	Coughing, wheezing, dyspnea
Immunologic function	Increased susceptibility to infection
Gastrointestinal function	Abdominal distention and discomfort, weight loss, anorexia
Energy level	Malaise
Psychosocial	Fear regarding impact of disease on fertility

→ > >

2 DIAGNOSE

NURSING DIAGNOSIS	SUBJECTIVE FINDINGS	OBJECTIVE FINDINGS
Impaired skin integrity related to swelling of lymph nodes and impaired function	Complains of pruritus and night sweats	Swollen lymph nodes
Pain related to disease progression to bones and nerves	Complains of bone pain, nerve pain, numbness, and tingling	Grimacing, limited movement, splinting
Ineffective breathing pattern related to disease progression to lungs and mediastinum	Complains of shortness of breath	Coughing, wheezing
High risk for infection related to impaired immunologic function	Complains of upper respiratory infections Complains of urinary tract infections Complains of painful itching, general malaise	Coughing, sneezing, nasal discharge Frequency, urgency, dysuria Herpes zoster
Altered nutrition: less than body requirements related to disease progression to gastrointestinal tract	Reports nausea, lack of appetite	Decreased intake, abdominal distention, weight loss
Fear related to possible infertility and altered body image	Expresses fear about changes in body and sexual function	Appears sad, withdrawn, angry, and depressed

3 PLAN

Patient goals

1. The patient will have normal skin integrity.
2. The patient will be comfortable.
3. The patient will have no difficulty breathing.
4. The patient will be free of infection.
5. The patient will have adequate nutrition.
6. The patient will be less fearful about the perceived and potential changes in body image and fertility.

4 IMPLEMENT

NURSING DIAGNOSIS	NURSING INTERVENTIONS	RATIONALE
Impaired skin integrity related to swelling of lymph nodes and impaired function	Bathe patient in cool water or apply cool, moist compresses.	To enhance comfort.

NURSING DIAGNOSIS	NURSING INTERVENTIONS	RATIONALE
	Apply calamine lotion, cornstarch, sodium bicarbonate, and medicated powder.	To relieve itching.
	Use a bed cradle and lightweight blankets and clothing.	To relieve pressure.
	Lubricate skin with baby oil, bath oil, body lotion, or petrolatum.	For comfort.
	Maintain adequate humidity and cool room.	To decrease itching.
	Avoid adhesive, alkaline soap, and local heat.	To avoid irritating skin.
Pain related to disease progression to bones and nerves	Position patient comfortably, change position gradually, and handle patient gently.	To prevent trauma (for bone pain).
	Support affected body part.	To prevent pressure.
	Encourage adequate rest.	To reduce incidence of pain related to activity.
	Give analgesics as ordered; provide pain relief measures based on patient's choice.	To decrease pain.
	Provide safety measures (assistive devices for ambulation, pads for elbows and feet).	To prevent trauma related to numbness and tingling.
Ineffective breathing pattern related to disease progression to lungs and mediastinum	Place patient in sitting position.	To increase chest expansion.
	Remove constrictive clothing.	To relieve pressure on chest.
	Encourage deep breathing.	To enhance alveolar expansion.
	Administer oxygen as needed.	To ensure tissue oxygenation.
	Keep emergency equipment at hand.	To relieve airway obstruction if needed.
	Inspect chest for respiratory rate and rhythm and symmetric expansion.	To monitor changes from baseline values.
	Auscultate lungs for abnormal breath sounds, aeration, rales, and rhonchi.	To detect development of infection or progression of disease.
	Observe for hoarseness, coughing, stridor, pain, and change in skin color (cyanosis).	To detect complications.
	Monitor blood studies	To detect abnormal gas exchange.
High risk for infection related to impaired immunologic function	Have the patient turn, cough, and deep breathe at regular intervals.	To prevent respiratory tract infection.

→ 〉 〉

NURSING DIAGNOSIS	NURSING INTERVENTIONS	RATIONALE
	Encourage fluids and balanced diet.	To maintain general well-being.
	Maintain reverse isolation.	To protect patient from microorganisms.
	Observe patient for nasal discharge, sore throat, anorexia, pain on urination, and increases in temperature, pulse, and respirations.	These indicate infection.
	Administer antibiotics as ordered.	To treat infection.
	Assess patient's skin for development of herpes zoster, and notify physician of need for appropriate medication.	To detect infection early and treat appropriately.
Altered nutrition: less than body requirements related to disease progression to gastrointestinal tract	Provide small meals of high-calorie, high-protein foods and fluids.	To increase nutritional intake.
	Assist with oral care, general hygiene, and environmental control (temperature, appearance, odors).	To enhance appetite.
	Identify food preferences, and provide them as often as possible.	To promote adequate nutritional intake.
	Place patient in a sitting position after meals.	To decrease feeling of fullness.
Fear related to possible infertility and altered body image	Assess appetite, weight loss, sleep patterns, and activity level.	Depression may be manifested by changes in these areas.
	Assess quality of support system.	To determine whether someone is available and helpful to patient.
	Monitor changes in communication with others.	Withdrawal or silence may indicate anger or depression.
	Listen and accept patient's fears and anger.	To foster constructive expression of negative feelings and fears.
	Encourage patient to discuss specific fears with other patients, a support group, or a sexual counselor.	Talking with someone who has had these experiences can validate fears and stimulate problem-solving, such as sperm banking.

5 EVALUATE

PATIENT OUTCOME	DATA INDICATING THAT OUTCOME IS REACHED
Skin is intact.	There is no evidence of irritation or pruritus.

PATIENT OUTCOME	DATA INDICATING THAT OUTCOME IS REACHED
Patient is comfortable.	Patient has no bone or nerve pain.
Patient's breathing is normal.	Patient has no dyspnea, coughing, or wheezing.
Patient has no infection.	There is no evidence of respiratory, urinary, or skin infection; temperature is within normal limits.
Nutrition is adequate.	Patient's weight is normal; patient has no anorexia, nausea, or abdominal distention.
Progress has been made in eliminating fear.	Patient discusses plans for sperm banking or other methods of retaining ability to conceive and plans realistically for possible changes in body image.

PATIENT TEACHING

1. Explain the need to avoid scratching and to correctly care for skin to reduce susceptibility to infection and mechanical skin damage.
2. Teach correct maintenance of body alignment, use of body mechanics and ambulatory aids, and the early symptoms of vertebral compression and paralysis to report to the physician or nurse.
3. Teach ways to relieve pain without the use of medications as often as possible; bone, nerve, and abdominal pain is chronic and increases with the pressure of disseminated disease.
4. Emphasize the importance of respiratory therapy to prevent or decrease the severity of symptoms of mediastinal lymph node enlargement, involvement of lung parenchyma, and invasion of pleura.
5. Teach the need for adequate rest and exercise and a balanced diet.
6. Help the patient make use of coping methods after exploring these with the patient and family.

Cutaneous T-cell Lymphoma

Cutaneous T-cell lymphoma represents a spectrum of diseases with preferential involvement of the skin by malignant lymphocytes with T-cell membrane characteristics.

Cutaneous T-cell lymphoma (CTCL), commonly called mycosis fungoides, begins superficially, with skin lesions ranging in appearance from eczema to parapsoriasis, and progresses to involve lymph nodes and visceral organs. The malignant cells in both this disorder and Sézary syndrome are lymphocytes; the specific lymphocyte involved is the T-cell lymphocyte. The characteristic histopathologic feature of the disease is marked infiltration of the epidermis by malignant lymphocytes.

Each year 400 to 1,000 new cases of CTCL are diagnosed in the United States. The disease is found in equal numbers of whites and blacks, but it is more

ALIBERT-BAZIN CLASSIFICATION OF SKIN LESIONS IN CTCL

Premycotic

Nonspecific skin eruptions resembling eczema, atopic dermatitis, or psoriasis; the lesions may precede or be accompanied by pruritus, may wax and wane, may change in character, and may disappear, only to reappear in the same place or in another area; exfoliation may occur; the lesions usually are present for about 6 years before a diagnosis of CTCL finally is made

Plaque

Irregular thickening of the skin, with raised plaques that may be accompanied by palpable lymph nodes; hyperkeratosis of the palms and soles may develop, causing painful fissures; scalp involvement can cause alopecia; leonine facies and eversion of the eyelids may develop

Tumor

Manifested by nodular growths that may ulcerate; tumors may arise on previously uninvolved skin

common in men than in women. The average age of onset is 52 years. It is believed that environment and heredity may be contributing factors; for example, those affected often are employed in manufacturing (petroleum, rubber, metal, machinery, and printing materials) or have a long-standing history of skin diseases or allergies.

The Alibert-Bazin system categorizes the skin involvement in CTCL into three stages (see the box above). Each stage can last from months to years, with gradual advancement from one stage to the next. The amount of skin involved at each stage may vary from 10% to the entire body.

Those whose disease is confined to the skin usually live about 9 years; those with organ dissemination survive less than 4 years. The most common sites of extracutaneous disease are the lymph nodes, liver, spleen, and lungs. The other major cause of morbidity is infec-

tion, most commonly caused by *Staphylococcus aureus* and *Pseudomonas aeruginosa*.

Treatment is aimed at palliation, with a variety of topical therapies used, including nitrogen mustard and BCNU. Electron beam radiation therapy, which penetrates only the skin, has provided good response of long duration. Radiosensitive areas such as the eyes and fingernails are protected with lead shields. In recent years, PUVA (psoralen and ultraviolet light A) has been used with some success in malignant infiltrates located in the epidermis and superficial dermis. Treatment consists of oral 8-methoxypsoralen (methoxsalen) followed in 2 hours by exposure to ultraviolet radiation. Methoxsalen is a phototoxic compound that is activated by ultraviolet light and, once activated, effects cell death by inhibiting DNA synthesis and cell division. PUVA is relatively expensive and has a principal long-term complication of second nonmelanoma cutaneous malignancies. In addition, when maintenance therapy is discontinued, the patient tends to relapse promptly.

Systemic chemotherapy generally is indicated when the skin disease has become resistant to all cutaneous therapies, when visceral extension is suspected or confirmed, or when other treatments have failed to control the disease. Single agents used include methotrexate, cyclophosphamide, and chlorambucil, vinca alkaloids and VP-16, and bleomycin and doxorubicin. Overall responses have been of short duration. Combination therapy may include MOPP, CHOP, CVP, and others.

The most frequently used combined modalities include RT plus chemotherapy and topical nitrogen mustard plus systemic chemotherapy. Biologic response modifiers are a promising treatment for CTCL. These include alpha-interferon, interleukin-2, and monoclonal antibodies.

Several retinoids have shown beneficial effects in CTCL and probably are best used in conjunction with PUVA or combined chemotherapy.

Leukapheresis, which can result in both a reduction in circulating blood cells and a regression of cutaneous lesions, provides temporary benefit for a small group of patients with the high leukemic counts associated with the Sézary syndrome. Extracorporeal photopheresis, the exposure of the circulating leukocytes to long-wave ultraviolet radiation in the presence of psoralen, is also promising.

NURSING CARE OF THE PATIENT WITH CTCL

NURSING DIAGNOSIS	NURSING INTERVENTIONS	RATIONALE
Impaired skin integrity related to infiltration of the epidermis by malignant lymphocytes	Monitor vital signs; skin temperature, color, and moisture; presence and character of ulcerations.	To detect and treat infection at an early stage.
	Apply topical chemotherapeutic drugs as prescribed; observe for hyperpigmentation and delayed hypersensitivity reaction.	To determine therapeutic effect of treatment and prevent adverse effects.
	Treat radiation-induced pruritus with cornstarch, baby powder, bland emollients, and antipruritic drugs.	To relieve itching.
	Treat moist desquamation with gentle cleansing (plain water; saline; combination of saline and hydrogen peroxide; or combination of saline, hydrogen peroxide, and water).	To promote healing and comfort.
	Use diet manipulation, food timing, and rectal or oral antiemetics as needed.	To control nausea and vomiting induced by phototoxic compounds used in ultraviolet light therapy.
Body image disturbance related to visible lesions	Encourage patient to discuss sexual concerns as needed.	To provide information and dispel misconceptions.
	Discuss with patient how to deal with co-workers and others.	To prevent patient from isolating himself from work and social settings.
	Suggest ways to apply hypoallergenic makeup to exposed lesions.	To enhance self-image.
	Provide information, dispel misconceptions, and provide support and encouragement.	To help patient feel accepted by himself and others.

CHAPTER 10

Therapeutic Interventions

BLOOD TRANSFUSIONS

Infusion of blood may be lifesaving for the patient with a blood disorder, whose blood loss may be caused by the disease itself, for example, thrombocytopenia or disseminated intravascular clotting; surgical intervention; bone marrow suppression during chemotherapy or radiation therapy; or trauma.

The transfusion immediately increases the body's ability to receive oxygen and transmit it to the cells, thereby avoiding severe and sometimes irreversible tissue damage.

Blood component therapy, which is the transfusion of a specific part of the blood rather than whole blood, conserves precious resources, allows for treatment of specific problems such as thrombocytopenia and anemia, and is the best method for patients who require numerous transfusions of a specific blood component. Frequently used blood components include packed red blood cells to treat anemia.

Packed RBCs are produced by centrifuging a unit of whole blood, forcing the RBCs (which are heavier than plasma) to the bottom of the container. After the plasma is removed, the percentage by volume of packed RBCs (hematocrit) increases. Whole blood has a hematocrit of about 40%; a unit of RBCs has a hemato-

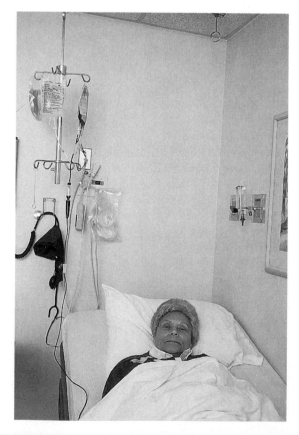

FIGURE 10-1
Woman receiving blood transfusion.

CAUTIONS FOR THE USE OF BLOOD

1. Blood to be transfused must be checked by at least two care providers to prevent infusion of mismatched blood, which causes a severe hemolytic reaction characterized by chills and fever, tachycardia, nausea and vomiting, hematuria or oliguria, headache, backache, dyspnea, cyanosis and chest pain. If such a reaction occurs, the transfusion should be discontinued immediately, the remaining blood and a sample of the patient's blood sent to the laboratory for repeat type and cross-match, and intravenous fluids, oxygen, and such drugs as vasopressor agents, epinephrine, sedatives, and mannitol administered.
2. Contaminated blood can cause a bacterial reaction; thus the nurse must observe the patient for fever, chills, lumbar pain, headache, malaise, bloody vomitus, diarrhea, or red shock (skin warm, dry, and pink): if these occur, the transfusion should be discontinued immediately, the remaining blood and a sample of the patient's blood send to the laboratory for repeat type and cross-match, and intravenous fluids, cooling measures, and medications such as vasopressors, steroids, broad-spectrum antibiotics, analgesics, and antiemetics administered.
3. Allergic reactions can occur, although their cause is unknown; the signs and symptoms vary from mild edema and hives to bronchial wheezing or anaphylaxis; if a mild reaction occurs, the nurse should slow the rate of transfusion; if the reaction is severe, the nurse should stop the transfusion, administer intravenous fluids, give medications such as a bronchodilator or epinephrine, and provide oxygen therapy.
4. Too rapid an infusion or too great a quantity of blood can result in circulatory overload, particularly if the patient has concurrent renal or cardiac disease. The signs and symptoms include cough; dyspnea; tachycardia; hemoptysis; frothy, pink-tinged sputum; and distended neck veins. If these occur, the nurse should slow the rate of transfusion, notify the physician, give digitalis as ordered to enhance cardiac output, prepare for venisection or rotating tourniquets, and monitor vital signs.

crit of about 70% to 80%. RBCs can be refrigerated up to 35 days.

The use of granulocyte concentrates is controversial and expensive and carries the possibility of numerous recipient complications. However, this therapy may be of value to the neutropenic patient with a diagnosed infection that is unresponsive to antibiotic therapy. Granulocytes are obtained by filtration or by differential centrifugation of donor blood.

Platelet transfusions are used to treat patients with thrombocytopenia or active bleeding disorders such as disseminated intravascular clotting. Platelet concentrates are prepared from whole blood by a series of differential centrifugations. Initially centrifugation is a soft spin (a slow spin for a short time). Platelets remain suspended in the plasma while the heavier RBCs and WBCs settle to the bottom. The plasma is then transferred to another bag and respun at a faster speed, which separates the excess plasma from the platelet concentrate.

Platelet concentrate is best preserved at room temperature in a plastic container with gentle agitation to prevent clumping or aggregating. Correct storage guarantees the shelf-life of platelet concentrate for 3 to 5 days. Refrigerated platelet concentrate lasts only 2 days.

BONE MARROW TRANSPLANTATION

Until recently most bone marrow transplants have involved donors of two types, an identical twin (syngeneic transplant) or an HLA-matched, mixed lymphocyte culture (MLC)-compatible sibling (allogeneic transplant). A syngeneic (identical twin) transplant is ideal, because the donor is matched with the recipient at all genetic loci.

A transplant using bone marrow from anyone other than an identical twin or the patient himself is called an allogeneic transplant. In most allogeneic bone marrow transplants, a sibling who matches at HLA-A, HLA-B, HLA-C, and HLA-D loci is the donor. The HLA loci are on a small region of chromosome 6, and these loci usually are inherited as a unit, known as a haplotype. Each parent has two haplotypes, and a child inherits one haplotype from each parent. A 25% probability exists that two siblings will be HLA identical.

An unrelated HLA-identical donor may also be used when no related donor is available. There is a 1 in 25,000 chance that two unrelated individuals will be HLA identical. A number of centers worldwide perform unrelated transplants, and the International Bone

Table 10-1

TYPES OF BONE MARROW TRANSPLANTS

Type	Advantages	Disadvantages
Autologous	Low risk of graft versus host disease Availability of donor Fewer treatment-related side effects and complications	Greater risk of relapse
Syngeneic	Low risk of graft versus host disease Fewer treatment-related side effects and complications	Greater risk of relapse Few donors available
Allogeneic	Less risk of relapse Greater availability of donors (compared with syngeneic type)	Greater risk of graft versus host disease Increased number and severity of treatments, related side effects, and complications

From Freedman et al.[19]

Marrow Registry is available to try to match donors and recipients. Initial reports on the use of unrelated donors are available; however, results have been poor, and further research is needed.

A partially matched donor, such as a sibling, parent, or uncle, may be selected when no HLA-identical sibling is available. Preliminary reports on the use of partially matched donors are encouraging, but further investigation is needed.

Another form of bone marrow transplantation (BMT), the autologous graft, involves the use of the patient's own bone marrow. As with identical twins, no clinically significant graft-versus-host disease (GVHD) will occur. However, with autologous grafts, tumor cells may be present in the marrow harvested during remission; therefore attempts to purge the marrow of occult tumor cells before cryopreservation (freezing of the marrow) are being studied. Autologous bone marrow transplantation currently is under investigation as a treatment for a variety of malignancies.

Advantages and disadvantages of the three types of BMT are compared in Table 10-1.

INDICATIONS

Allogeneic bone marrow transplantation is the treatment of choice for patients with aplastic anemia who are under 50 years of age and who have an HLA-identical donor. It is also a treatment for severe immunodeficiency disorders, acute leukemias, myelodysplastic syndromes, chronic myelogenous leukemia, multiple myeloma, and hematopoietic defects.

Autologous bone marrow transplantation is being used with increasing success to treat acute leukemia, multiple myeloma, lymphoma, both Hodgkin's and non-Hodgkin's disease, and responsive solid tumors, including neuroblastomas, cancers of the breast and testes, and small cell lung cancer.

HARVEST

With both allogeneic and autologous transplants, marrow is harvested in the operating room with the donor under general or spinal anesthesia. About 100 aspirations are obtained from the posterior iliac crest (if necessary the anterior iliac crest may also be used) (Figure 10-2). Because children require a smaller amount of marrow, fewer aspirations are necessary than for an adult. A small amount of bone marrow (20 ml) is collected with each aspiration and placed in a tissue culture medium containing heparin. This solution is filtered through a stainless steel screen to remove bone chips, fat globules, and clots. The marrow is filtered initially through a large-screen filter and again through a smaller screen filter. The marrow is then transferred to a blood transfusion bag. The amount of bone marrow aspirated depends on several factors: the donor's weight, the concentration of cells in the donated marrow, and the processing procedure used before the marrow is transfused. If no special processing is done, the amount of marrow obtained is approximately 10 to 15 ml/kg of the recipient's body weight. Some of the cells are destroyed when the marrow is processed, leaving fewer cells for infusion. In a typical adult, a unit of 500 to 750 ml of blood and bone marrow contains 10 billion to 20 billion nucleated marrow cells.

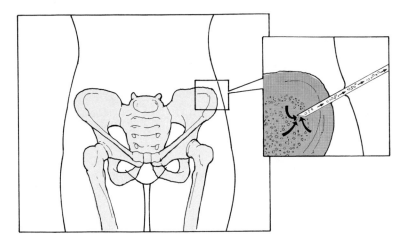

FIGURE 10-2
Bone marrow harvest.

ADMINISTRATION OF MARROW

After harvesting, the marrow is administered intravenously through a central venous access device (such as a Hickman or Cook catheter) or frozen in liquid nitrogen. If the marrow is to be purged either with a chemotherapeutic agent (e.g., 4-HC-4 hydroperoxycyclophosphamide) or a monoclonal antibody, this is done before cryopreservation. Purging eliminates any occult tumor cells in the marrow. Cell volume and viability are also evaluated before cryopreservation.

In the stem cell disorders, bone marrow transplantation is used to replace defective or missing hematopoietic stem cells with healthy ones. In the treatment of hematogenously spread malignant diseases, transplantation is done after chemotherapy to replace defective stem cells with healthy ones. In the treatment of solid tumors, transplantation is done after high-dose chemotherapy has eradicated the marrow. The high-dose chemotherapy destroys normal bone marrow, and transplantation is done to repopulate or rescue the patient's own hematopoietic system.

COMPLICATIONS: GRAFT-VERSUS-HOST DISEASE

Graft-versus-host disease (GVHD) is a major cause of mortality following allogeneic transplantation, with an incidence as high as 45%. GVHD results when the mature lymphocytes in the marrow (graft) recognize the recipient (host) as foreign. Since most patients are HLA-A, HLA-B, and HLA-D/DR identical to their donors, minor antigenic differences are thought to cause

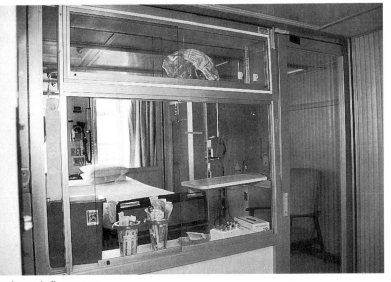

Laminar air flow room.

GVHD. In any mismatched transplants, the probability of GVHD developing increases with the degree of mismatch. A number of factors increase the probability of GVHD, as shown in the box below.

FACTORS INCREASING THE PROBABILITY OF GVHD

Recipient over 30 years of age
Advanced disease
Donor of the opposite sex
High degree of mismatch
Diagnosis other than acute lymphocytic leukemia
From Gale et al, 1987.[22]

Clinical Presentation

In GVHD, the lymphocyte in the graft attacks the patient's skin, liver, and gastrointestinal tract. With acute GVHD, peak onset occurs 30 to 50 days after transplantation, although the disorder may start as early as day 10 and last up to day 100. The median duration of onset is 25 days. Patients may manifest symptoms in one or all three systems. Skin GVHD usually starts as a fine maculopapular rash on the trunk, palms, soles, and ears; this may progress to generalized erythroderma with desquamation of the skin. The major complaints associated with gastrointestinal involvement are abdominal pain, nausea, vomiting, and diarrhea. The diarrhea usually is watery and may amount to as much as several liters in a 24-hour period. GVHD involving the liver is characterized by an increase in liver enzymes and alkaline phosphatase. Patients may complain of pain in the right upper quadrant, and hepatomegaly may develop.

Chronic GVHD has an onset of 100 days after transplantation, although in rare cases it has been diagnosed at 1 year afterward. The disease occurs as an extension of acute GVHD (progressive-type onset), subsequent to a period of resolution of acute GVHD (quiescent onset), or without preceding acute GVHD (de novo onset). The signs and symptoms of chronic GVHD in the skin are itching and burning, particularly on the palms and soles; patchy hyperpigmentation that may appear mottled; erythema; rough, flaky bronze-colored hyperpigmentation; and possibly contractures.

The incidence of chronic GVHD affecting the liver may be as high as 90%. Symptoms may include increases in alkaline phosphatase, serum glutamate oxaloacetate transaminase (SGOT), and bilirubin.

Other manifestations of chronic GVHD include involvement of the oral mucosa and ocular lining, esophageal abnormalities, vaginal problems, and immunodeficiencies.

Diagnosis and Treatment

The diagnosis usually is made by biopsy of the skin or gastrointestinal tract. GVHD may be treated with cyclosporin A, prednisone, methotrexate, monoclonal antibodies, and antithymocyte globulin. Investigational agents include thalidomide and xomazyme. These agents may be used individually or in combination, and a number of studies are attempting to determine the best combination for treatment and prophylaxis.

The diagnostic tests for chronic GVHD include skin and oral mucosa biopsies, liver and pulmonary function tests, the Schirmer tear test, and autoimmune blood tests (Table 10-2). Therapy for chronic GVHD includes immunosuppressive agents and antibiotics to prevent infection. Immunosuppressive agents include predni-

Table 10-2

DIAGNOSTIC STUDIES AND FINDINGS IN GRAFT-VERSUS-HOST DISEASE

Diagnostic test	Findings	
	Acute GVHD	**Chronic GVHD**
Biopsy of skin, gut, or oral mucosa	Infiltration of T cells into skin or gastrointestinal tract	Infiltration of lymphocytes and T cells into skin and oral mucosa
Liver function test	Elevated bilirubin, alkaline phosphatase, and SGOT	Elevated bilirubin, alkaline phosphatase, and SGOT
Pulmonary function test	Decreased diffusion capacity and lung capacity	Decreased diffusion capacity and lung capacity
Schirmer tear test	Dry eyes with increased risk of corneal abrasions and ulcerations	Dry eyes with increased risk of corneal abrasions and ulcerations
Autoimmune blood test	Not applicable	Positive test result; patient may have patchy dispigmentation and lichen planus–like papules on the skin and may have salivary changes similar to those in Sjögren's syndrome

Table 10-3

SEVERITY OF ACUTE GRAFT-VERSUS-HOST DISEASE

Stages of GVHD according to organ system

Skin	*Liver*	*Gastrointestinal*
Stage	Stage	Stage
+1 Maculopapular eruption involving less than 25% of the body surface	+1 Moderate increase in SGOT (150 to 170 IU) and bilirubin (2 to 3 mg/dl)	Diarrhea, nausea, and vomiting are also grade +1 through +4 in severity. The severity of GI involvement was assigned to the most severe of the three involvements noted. It is difficult to quantitate most of these manifestations, except diarrhea.
+2 Maculopapular eruption involving 25% to 50% of the body surface	+2 Rise in bilirubin (3 to 5.9 mg/dl) with or without an increase in SGOT	
+3 Generalized erythroderma	+3 Rise in bilirubin (6 to 14.9 mg/dl) with or without an increase in SGOT	+1 500 ml of stool/day
+4 Generalized erythroderma with bulbous formation and often with desquamation	+4 Rise in bilirubin (15 mg/dl) with or without an increase in SGOT (increases in SGOT are temporarily related to either onset or worsening of the skin rash)	+2 1,000 ml of stool/day
		+3 1,500 ml of stool/day
		+4 2,000 ml of stool/day

Adapted from Thompson et al.[60]

Table 10-4

CLINICAL GRADING OF GRAFT-VERSUS-HOST DISEASE

Grade	Degree of organ involvement
I	+1 to +2 skin rash; no gut involvement; no liver involvement; no decrease in clinical performance
II	+1 to +3 skin rash; +1 gut involvement or +1 liver involvement (or both); mild decrease in clinical performance.
III	+2 to +3 skin rash; +2 to +3 gut involvement or +2 to +3 liver involvement, or both; marked decrease in clinical performance
IV	Similar to grade III with +2 to +4 organ involvement and extreme decrease in clinical performance

From Thomas ED: Reprinted by permission of the *New England Journal of Medicine* 292:896, 1975.

sone, procarbazine, cyclophosphamide, and azathioprine. It has been reported that thalidomide may be useful in the treatment of chronic GVHD. The antibiotic most commonly used to prevent infection is trimethoprim-sulfamethoxazole (Bactrim), and acyclovir is given for prophylaxis against recrudescence of the herpes virus.

Tables 10-3 and 10-4 present two systems for clinical staging of GVHD. In about 40% of patients, acute GVHD is mild and limited to the skin. As many as 15% to 20% of allograft recipients have severe multiorgan disease, which may be fatal.

CONDITIONING REGIMEN

The purposes of conditioning are to eliminate defective stem cells; to provide immunosuppression, thereby minimizing the possibility of rejection; and to eliminate any residual malignant cells.

The conditioning regimen used before bone marrow transplantation depends on the disease being treated. Conditioning regimens include high-dose chemotherapy with or without radiotherapy (see box on page 164).

The patient, family, donor, and significant others are provided with instructions about the procedure, its course, and complications.

Radiation

Typical side effects of total body irradiation (TBI) include nausea and vomiting, which may be severe; diarrhea; erythema of the skin; and parotitis. These side effects usually are of short duration when moderate fractionated radiotherapy is used. Except for erythema of the skin, these side effects usually resolve within 7 days.

Cyclophosphamide

Cyclophosphamide may cause hemorrhagic cystitis. This may be counteracted by inserting a three-way Foley catheter and providing continuous saline irrigation at the rate of 1 L/hour. The Foley catheter remains in place for 24 hours after the last dose of cyclophosphamide. Removal of the catheter is delayed because of the prolonged half-life of cyclophosphamide (21 hours). Uric acid is released as cells are destroyed, resulting in deposition of uric acid crystals in the kidneys. This can be decreased by providing an alkaline environment. Maintaining a urine pH above 6.5 reduces the potential for uric acid nephropathy. Allopurinol may be used to prevent the formation of uric acid from cell byproducts. Cardiotoxicity is another problem with cyclophosphamide, yet it is found in fewer than 5% of the patients receiving this drug.

Busulfan

Because busulfan is available only in 2 mg tablets, the patient must swallow a significant number of pills for each dose. The tablets should not be swallowed all at once, since this increases the risk of emesis. The patient should be instructed to take five to eight of the tablets at a time. The dose should be taken over a period no longer than 30 minutes.

The toxicities associated with busulfan include severe pancytopenia, potential pulmonary toxicity, severe nausea and vomiting (at high doses), and skin alterations such as ulcerations and erythema of the palms, soles, axillae, and groin. Busulfan also has been reported to lower the seizure threshold, and grand mal seizures have been reported. The toxicities most often seen in transplant recipients are nausea, vomiting, and skin alterations. Appropriate skin care measures should be instituted to prevent infection in the affected areas.

Etoposide (VP-16)

Fever and chills usually are noted within a few hours of starting etoposide. Acetaminophen is given to control the fever, and if the chills progress to rigors, meperidine (25-50 mg IV) may be used to diminish the shaking. Metabolic changes include acidosis, which may be

---

PREPARATIVE SCHEDULES FOR BONE MARROW TRANSPLANT

The days before transplant are indicated by negative numbers, with day 0 being the day of transplant.

An allogeneic conditioning regimen:

Wednesday	Day −8	Admission
Thursday	Day −7	Cyclophosphamide, Foley catheter, continuous bladder irrigation
Friday	Day −6	Cyclophosphamide, Foley catheter with continuous bladder irrigation
Saturday	Day −5	Removal of Foley catheter; rest
Sunday	Day −4	Rest
Monday	Day −3	TBI, fractionated bid
Tuesday	Day −2	TBI (as above)
Wednesday	Day −1	TBI (as above)
Thursday	Day 0	Marrow infusion

An autologous conditioning regimen:

Wednesday	Day −8	Admission
Thursday	Day −7	Busulfan PO
Friday	Day −6	Busulfan PO
Saturday	Day −5	Busulfan PO
Sunday	Day −4	Busulfan PO
Monday	Day −3	Etoposide (VP-16) IV
Tuesday	Day −2	Rest
Wednesday	Day −1	Rest
Thursday	Day 0	Marrow infusion

noted by a decreasing carbon dioxide level within 24 hours after administration. Significant mucositis is noted within 5 to 7 days after completion of the therapy. Significant skin toxicity is also seen within 1 week of completion of therapy and may last for 3 weeks. Hypotension, dysrhythmias, hepatic toxicity, and neurotoxicity have also been reported with use of this drug in high doses.

ADMINISTRATION

The goal of BMT is to restore defective or missing stem cells. For autologous marrow, blood bags containing approximately 50 ml of cryopreserved marrow are thawed quickly, one at a time, in a basin of warm water at approximately 37.7° C (100° F). The contents of the bag are removed with a 50-ml syringe and a 16-gauge needle and then administered rapidly through a central line (double-lumen Cook or Hickman catheter). A solution of 0.9% normal saline is infused during the procedure. Before the infusion the patient usually is given diphenhydramine (50 mg), acetaminophen (650 mg), and hydrocortisone (50 mg). Because the patient may react to the preservative dimethylsulfoxide (DMSO) used in the marrow bags, epinephrine, diphenhydramine, and hydrocortisone are kept at the bedside. The patient may experience fever, chills, rash, chest pain, bradycardia, heart block, and nausea and vomiting. Major hemolytic reactions, along with elevated serum creatinine, have also been reported.

For a syngeneic or allogeneic donation, a standard-type blood bag containing fresh bone marrow just obtained from the donor and appropriately filtered is transported from the operating room. After the recipient is given diphenhydramine (50 mg) and acetaminophen (650 mg), the donated marrow is administered (over a period of no more than 4 hours) through a Hickman catheter without a filter. Patients receiving the marrow may have some chest pain, shortness of breath, or flushing, but these symptoms usually subside with appropriate intervention. The usual interventions for any side effects of marrow infusion are steroids, oxygen, and nitroglycerin tablets.

UNIVERSITY OF CALIFORNIA–SAN FRANCISCO SKIN CARE PROGRAM

1. Wash affected areas tid with water, no soap.
2. Apply Aquaphor cream tid to erythematous areas without skin breakdown.
3. For skin breakdown other than on the scrotum or in the pubic area, use Burow's soaks (one capful of solution in 1 quart of water) for 20 minutes, followed by application of Silvadene cream. (**Silvadene cream should not be used if the patient is allergic to sulfa.**) Wrap the affected areas with Kerlix. Repeat the procedure tid until all areas have healed.
4. For skin breakdown on the scrotum and in the pubic area, apply soda bicarbonate soaks to decrease the irritation; then apply Aquaphor or nystatin cream to affected areas.

MEDICAL MANAGEMENT

GENERAL MANAGEMENT

Physical therapy: Activate referral on admission; daily exercise program.

Vital signs: Check q 4 h or more frequently as necessary.

Diet: Regular diet as tolerated; calorie count when unable to eat; obtain orders for hyperalimentation (hyperalimentation usually lasts for at least 3 weeks).

IV therapy: To maintain hydration and renal perfusion.

Pain management: Intermittent use of narcotics for pain control, followed by continuous infusion via patient-controlled analgesia as needed.

Antiemetic therapy: Used to decrease nausea from conditioning regimen and results of alteration in gastrointestinal tract from chemotherapy: metoclopramide, lorazepam, diphenhydramine, dexamethasone, ondansetron.

Skin care management: To decrease effects of toxicity from combination chemotherapy and/or radiation therapy (see the box above): Aquaphor, Burow's solution, Silvadene (for those not allergic to sulfa).

MEDICAL MANAGEMENT—cont'd

Treatment for rigors: Meperidine, 25-50 mg IV, to control rigors from preparative regimen or reaction to blood products and/or antifungal agents.

PROPHYLACTIC DRUG THERAPY

Antibiotics: Usually given for prophylaxis after right atrial catheter is placed; trimethoprim-sulfamethoxazole (Bactrim) is given to prevent *Pneumocystis carinii* pneumonia; often started when absolute neutrophil count drops below 500/mm^3.

Antiviral drugs: Acyclovir to prevent recrudescence of herpes virus.

Antifungal drugs: To prevent fungal infections (e.g., fluconazole, amphotericin).

CONDITIONING REGIMEN

Chemotherapy: Usually given for 2-6 days, depending on protocol.

TBI: Dosage varies from 800 to 1,200 rad (e.g., 1,200 rad given in fractionated doses of 200 rad two times per day).

DRUG THERAPY—CONDITIONING REGIMEN

Cyclophosphamide: Usually given for 2-4 days.
Busulfan: Usually given over 4 days at dosing interval of q 6 h.
Etoposide (VP-16):   Can be given over 2-4 days or as a single large dose.
Methotrexate: 12 mg intrathecally for leukemic patients or those with lymphoma; for CNS prophylaxis.

DRUG THERAPY—GVHD PROPHYLAXIS (ALLOGENEIC TRANSPLANT ONLY)

Cyclosporin A; prednisone; methotrexate; gamma globulin: given on a regular basis to provide antibodies that were ablated during preparative regimen; antipyretics: for fever.

NURSING ASSESSMENT FOR THE BONE MARROW TRANSPLANT PATIENT

ASSESSMENT	OBSERVATIONS
Volume status	Anxiety; tachycardia; cool, moist skin; cyanotic lips and nail beds; if edema worsens, confusion and stupor appear; dyspnea and air hunger are accompanied by a productive cough and frothy, blood-tinged sputum; rales and rhonchi are also heard on examination
Pulmonary	Dyspnea; rapid, shallow respirations; shortness of breath; chest pain; cyanosis; increased heart rate; diaphoresis
Reaction to white cells in marrow	Chills, fever, rash, urticaria, chest pain, malaise, hypotension, shortness of breath

ASSESSMENT	OBSERVATIONS
Renal	Grossly red urine and Hemastix-positive urine (normal for 24 hours after transplant)
Bacterial contamination of marrow	Hypotension, fever, rigors, diaphoresis, shaking chills, shortness of breath
Engraftment	Hematologic recovery, increasing neutrophil count within 10-14 days after marrow infusion; granulocytes, platelets, and erythrocytes within normal limits (normal time period, 21-160 days)
Rejection/failure to engraft	Marrow function does not return; obligatory 7 to 10 days for marrow recovery or to engraft after a period of recovery
Infection	Fever, chills, rigors, redness, swelling of any site, skin rash, wound drainage, cough, dyspnea, sore throat, mucositis, headache, dysuria, frequency, urgency, diarrhea, hypotension, positive blood cultures, spontaneous bacterial peritonitis, change in mental status
Anemia	Decreased RBCs, decreased Hct ($<$25%), decreased Hb ($<$8.2), excessive fatigue, dyspnea on exertion, shortness of breath, pallor, tachycardia, palpitations
Stomatitis	Oral soreness, pain, burning or tingling in mouth, thick secretions, inability to swallow, erythema, ulceration, pseudomembrane formation, taste changes, oozing from oral membranes
Thrombocytopenia	Petechiae, purpura, bleeding from any body orifice or site of catheter, epistaxis, hemoptysis, hematemesis, hematuria, hematochezia, change in mental status (e.g., headache, confusion, lethargy, nausea, change in pupil size, seizures)
Nutritional status	Anorexia, weight loss ($>$2 kg/wk), decreased albumin ($<$3.5), nausea, vomiting, diarrhea, fluid imbalance
GVHD	Mild maculopapular rash, generalized erythroderma that may progress to desquamation, increase in serum bilirubin, increase in SGOT or alkaline phosphatase, abdominal cramping, diarrhea (green and watery), hematochezia
Venoocclusive disease (VOD)	Sudden weight gain, increasing abdominal girth, right upper quadrant pain, jaundice, hepatomegaly, ascites, encephalopathy; elevated SGOT, alkaline phosphatase, and bilirubin; coagulation abnormalities (PT, PTT, fibrinogen)
Interstitial pneumonitis	Dry cough, dyspnea, nasal flaring, tachypnea (40-60 beats/min), rales; diffuse pulmonary infiltrates on chest x-ray; hypoxemia at room air (Pao_2 $<$70 mm Hg)
Cardiac toxicity	Dyspnea on exertion, orthopnea, weakness, fatigue, peripheral edema, chest pain, syncope, dysrhythmias, pericardial effusion, and tachypnea; changes noted on ECG and echocardiogram
Renal insufficiency	Decreased urine output; marked increase in body weight ($>$2 kg); peripheral edema; postural changes in BP ($<$20 mm Hg); thirst; complaints of dizziness; flat, distended neck veins; changes in specific gravity ($<$1.005) and urine electrolytes
Psychosocial status	Fear, anger, depression, anxiety, remorse, acting out, inappropriate behavior

→ › ›

NURSING CARE OF THE BONE MARROW TRANSPLANT PATIENT

NURSING DIAGNOSIS

Altered nutrition: less than body requirements related to nausea and vomiting, indigestion, and loss of appetite from chemotherapy.

NURSING INTERVENTIONS AND RATIONALE

1. Administer antiemetic drug before treatment and at frequent intervals afterward as ordered to relieve nausea and anxiety related to nausea, and monitor patient response.
2. Consider using behavioral relaxation techniques to reduce the onset and duration of nausea.
3. Instruct patient to avoid quick movements while nauseated. Quick movements can trigger the gag reflex and increase nausea.
4. Encourage patient to eat slowly and chew thoroughly to aid digestion.
5. Instruct patient to avoid lying flat for at least 1 hour after eating to aid digestion.
6. Encourage patient to drink liquids (clear, cool beverages or soups) slowly through a straw before, not during, meals to maintain adequate fluid intake.
7. Provide carbonated beverages, dry crackers or toast, tart foods (e.g., lemons or sour pickles), ice pops, and gelatin desserts to curb nausea.
8. Suggest high-protein, high-calorie diet and small, frequent meals to ensure adequate nutrient intake and curb nausea.
9. Maintain optimum nutritional status; check weight daily; monitor calorie counts; arrange dietary consultation; administer TPN as ordered to maintain adequate nutritional intake.
10. Monitor serum electrolytes daily, and check urine for glucose, ketones, and protein to identify electrolyte accumulations.

NURSING DIAGNOSIS

Pain related to parotitis.

NURSING INTERVENTIONS AND RATIONALE

1. Encourage increased fluid intake to provide adequate hydration and to compensate for lack of saliva.
2. Encourage frequent oral hygiene to eliminate bad taste in patient's mouth.
3. If xerostomia is present, suggest hard candies, sugarless gum, or a commercial product such as Xero-Lube or Orabase to increase salivary secretion.
4. Administer medications as ordered to alleviate pain, and monitor patient response; narcotic analgesics may be required.
5. Tell patient to avoid using irritants such as alcohol or tobacco to prevent further discomfort.

NURSING DIAGNOSIS

Hyperthermia related to total body irradiation.

NURSING INTERVENTIONS AND RATIONALE

1. Maintain adequate hydration to compensate for dryness of mucosa caused by irradiation.
2. Administer antipyretics as ordered, and monitor patient response.
3. Alleviate patient's concern by informing him that fever usually disappears 4 to 6 days after TBI.
4. Monitor temperature every 2 to 4 hours to detect persistent or resolving hyperthermia.
5. Monitor intake and output and daily weights to ensure optimal fluid balance and prevent dehydration.
6. Adjust environmental temperature to patient's comfort (e.g., remove excess clothing and bedding). Body heat is lost through convection and evaporation of sweat.
7. Administer acetaminophen rather than aspirin to children, since aspirin has been implicated in Reye's syndrome in children.

NURSING DIAGNOSIS

Diarrhea related to effects of total body irradiation on gastrointestinal mucosa.

NURSING INTERVENTIONS AND RATIONALE

1. Administer antidiarrheal agents as ordered to prevent and control diarrhea, and monitor patient response.
2. Maintain adequate fluid intake to prevent dehydration.
3. Suggest a bland, low-residue diet high in potassium to provide adequate potassium from food that can be digested easily (irradiation can increase transit time in the colon).
4. Instruct patient in meticulous perianal skin care; tell him to use sitz baths after each bowel movement and to apply a soothing lubricant to the perianal area to prevent infection and alleviate pain and discomfort.

NURSING DIAGNOSIS

High risk for impaired skin integrity related to erythema of skin from irradiation.

NURSING INTERVENTIONS AND RATIONALE

1. Instruct patient to keep skin clean and dry before irradiation. Use mild soap such as Dove or Dial for bathing, rinse skin well, and pat dry, because irradiation dries and irritates the skin at the level of the dermis and epidermis.
2. Instruct patient to avoid using perfumed powders or lotions and extremes of temperature to skin (e.g.,

hot or cold baths, ice packs, and heating pads) to prevent further skin irritation.
3. Use lubricated cream (Aquaphor, Nutriderm) tid after irradiation to increase patient's comfort and minimize itching.

NURSING DIAGNOSIS

Altered bladder tissue perfusion (hemorrhagic cystitis) related to local effects of cyclophosphamide.

NURSING INTERVENTIONS AND RATIONALE

1. Begin IV hydration 4 h before cyclophosphamide administration, and continue for 24 h after therapy as ordered (IV fluids should be administered 1½ to 2 times maintenance rates) as a cleansing measure, because cyclophosphamide metabolites can destroy the uroepithelial lining of the bladder.
2. Perform continuous bladder irrigation using a three-way Foley catheter if ordered (not needed if patient can void qh) to eliminate toxic products of cyclophosphamide that irritate the bladder lining.
3. Monitor urine for blood q 4 h to identify destruction of bladder lining.
4. Maintain accurate intake and output records to detect altered fluid status.

NURSING DIAGNOSIS

Altered renal tissue perfusion related to potential toxicity from chemotherapy.

NURSING INTERVENTIONS AND RATIONALE

1. Maintain adequate hydration, check urine output hourly, and administer furosemide (Lasix) as ordered to prevent interference with renal function and damage to renal tubules that sometimes occurs with chemotherapy. Monitor patient response.
2. Check urine pH q 4 h; maintain at or above 7, and monitor BUN/creatinine to determine adequacy of renal function.
3. Administer allopurinol as ordered, and monitor patient response. Allopurinol may increase the incidence and degree of bone marrow suppression by prolonging the half-life of cyclophosphamide, which may cause further insult to the kidneys.

NURSING DIAGNOSIS

Decreased cardiac output (potential) related to cardiotoxicity from chemotherapy.

NURSING INTERVENTIONS AND RATIONALE

1. Check results of ECG to detect alterations indicating damage to myocardial muscle or the presence of a cardiomyopathy (ECG is obtained daily while patient is being treated with high-dose cyclophosphamide).

2. Monitor patient's level of consciousness, changes in baseline vital signs, and ECG. Changes in clinical status may indicate decreased cardiac output.
3. Monitor heart rate and rhythm to identify dysrhythmias.

NURSING DIAGNOSIS

High risk for infection related to leukopenia.

NURSING INTERVENTIONS AND RATIONALE

1. Maintain protective environment to reduce the risk of infection (reverse isolation protocols vary among centers).
2. Monitor WBC and absolute granulocyte count daily to detect evidence of infection induced by prolonged leukopenia.
3. Monitor vital signs q 4 h, and check skin and mucous membranes; inspect all body orifices daily for redness, swelling, and pain, and inspect insertion site of venous access device for redness, swelling, pain, and drainage, to detect infection early.
4. Auscultate lungs q 8 h for increased or decreased breath sounds, rhonchi, and rales to determine adequacy of gas exchange and detect presence of possible infection.
5. Maintain meticulous mouth care to prevent infection and eliminate bad taste in patient's mouth.
6. Use strict aseptic technique when changing dressings and in IV preparation and administration to prevent infection.
7. Avoid bladder catheterization, except when necessary; avoid administering enemas and suppositories and taking rectal temperatures to prevent introduction of bacteria.
8. Encourage patient to use deodorant rather than antiperspirant to avoid blocking axillary sweat glands, which may promote infection.
9. Obtain surveillance cultures of throat, urine, stool, skin, or other areas as ordered to detect colonization before infection spreads.
10. Do not allow fresh-cut flowers or plants in patient's room, and eliminate stagnant water to prevent colonization of bacteria.
11. Limit the number of visitors, and screen them for infection, recent vaccinations (e.g., oral polio vaccine is shed in the stool), or exposure to communicable diseases (especially children) to protect patient from exposure to communicable diseases.
12. Provide mask for patient when he leaves his room (isolation protocol varies) to protect him from infection.
13. Administer antibiotics on schedule per physician's orders to control proliferation of infection. Monitor patient response.
14. Patient's CMV status should be determined before

transfusions. If the patient is CMV negative, administer only CMV-negative blood to prevent serious illness that can be caused by the virus, especially in organ transplant patients.

NURSING DIAGNOSIS

Alteration in protection related to decreased function of hemopoietic system (platelets).

NURSING INTERVENTIONS AND RATIONALE

1. Monitor platelet count regularly (the risk of bleeding is high when platelet count is <10,000 cells/mm^3) to prevent increased risk of bleeding caused by prolonged thrombocytopenia.
2. Monitor skin and mucous membranes for increased tendency to bruise, petechiae, bleeding gums, and epistaxis; test stool, urine, and emesis for occult blood to detect bleeding early.
3. Look for any changes in patient's vital signs, behavior, or pupil size to detect intracranial hemorrhage.
4. After invasive procedures such as bone marrow aspiration and biopsy, monitor site frequently to detect any oozing of blood.
5. Do not take rectal temperatures or administer rectal suppositories and enemas, to avoid irritating the rectal tissue and to decrease the risk of bleeding.
6. Encourage adequate fluid intake and use of stool softener to prevent constipation and straining, which may increase the risk of bleeding.
7. Place a sign indicating bleeding precautions over patient's bed to alert others to the potential for bleeding.
8. Administer medroxyprogesterone acetate as ordered to control menses, and monitor patient's response.
9. Apply topical agents (e.g., topical thrombin, ε-aminocaproic acid, topical cocaine, tranexamic acid, or Gelfoam) to bleeding sites per physician's order to control bleeding. Monitor patient response.
10. Administer irradiated platelet transfusions rapidly as ordered (families are encouraged to find donors for blood products), and monitor platelet count 1 h after transfusion to prevent further bleeding.

NURSING DIAGNOSIS

Activity intolerance related to anemia, nutritional status, disruption of sleep, anxiety, or depression.

NURSING INTERVENTIONS AND RATIONALE

1. Administer irradiated RBC transfusions as ordered to counteract fatigue and decreased activity tolerance caused by BMT process. Monitor patient response.
2. Check Hb levels and Hct values regularly to assess the need for more blood.

3. Maintain optimum nutritional status to improve strength and minimize fatigue.
4. Arrange nursing care so that patient has uninterrupted periods of rest and sleep, especially during the night, to relieve fatigue.
5. Encourage patient to discuss his feelings and concerns to alleviate or minimize anxiety or depression, which may contribute to persistent fatigue.
6. Encourage a progressive activity program as tolerated to prevent adverse effects of bed rest and increase activity.

NURSING DIAGNOSIS

Altered oral mucous membrane related to conditioning regimen or infection.

NURSING INTERVENTIONS AND RATIONALE

1. Implement nursing care related to stomatitis, based on assessment using grading system developed by Capizzi (see the box on the next page), to care for patient's mucositis/stomatitis.

NURSING DIAGNOSIS

Altered protection related to graft-versus-host disease (occurs only in allogeneic BMT).

NURSING INTERVENTIONS AND RATIONALE

1. Assess skin integrity each shift; assess level of pain and pruritus, and administer analgesics and antihistamines as needed, because donor T cells destroy host in areas of skin, gastrointestinal tract, and liver. Monitor patient response.
2. Provide meticulous skin care, including daily bath with povidone-iodine and normal saline or other antibacterial solution. Oatmeal or baking soda baths may be indicated for pruritus to prevent infection and to help healing.
3. Apply creams or lotions (Aquaphor or A&D Ointment with mineral oil) on intact skin to minimize breakdown of healthy skin and to promote healing of affected skin.
4. Apply mixture of silver sulfadiazine and nystatin on open areas of skin (other creams and ointments such as fluocinonide, hydrocortisone, and petroleum gauze may be used) to promote healing of affected skin.
5. Explain need to prevent scratching. Use mittens if necessary on infant or child. Use KenAire, Mediscus, or other flotation-type bed for patient with extensive skin involvement to prevent further irritation of skin.
6. Use bed cradle to prevent linens from touching skin, to alleviate pressure.
7. Assist patient frequently with active and passive

ORAL CARE FOR STOMATITIS

For grade 1 or grade 2 stomatitis

1. Perform oral hygiene regimen every 2 hours while patient is awake and every 6 hours during night as follows:
   a. Use normal saline mouthwash if crusts are absent (1 teaspoon of salt in 1 L of sterile water may be used). If crusts and debris are present, use sodium bicarbonate solution (1 teaspoon in 8 ounces of water). Perform mouth care every 2 hours while patient is awake. Alternate bicarbonate solution with normal saline. Rinse with normal saline after bicarbonate.
   b. Floss gently with unwaxed dental floss every 24 hours if platelet count is above 50,000/mm^3.
   c. Brush after each meal and before sleep, using a soft toothbrush and nonabrasive toothpaste such as Colgate.
   d. Remove dentures or partial plates; replace only for meals.
   e. Apply lip lubricant (e.g., Vaseline, Blistex, or K-Y Jelly) four times a day and as needed.
2. Measures for oral care include routine culture of mouth for bacteria, fungus, and virus. If these are present, use the following:
   a. For bacteria: Peridex, 15 ml bid.
   b. For fungus: nystatin, 15 ml qid; clotrimazole troche, 1 tablet 5 times a day; ketoconazole, 200 mg bid.
   c. For virus: acyclovir, 200 mg tablet 5 times a day, or 5 mg/kg IV q 8 h.
3. Suggestions for control of mouth pain:
   a. Initiate low-dose narcotics on a prn schedule; if necessary, proceed to continuous infusion (morphine, 2-4 mg q 2-4 h prn). If required more than q 2 h, switch to continuous infusion. If patient has problems with morphine, use Dilaudid, 0.5-1.5 mg q 2-4 h prn. If required more than q 2 h, change to continuous infusion. Patient-controlled analgesia may also be used at this time.
4. Implement dietary measures, including the following:
   a. Instruct patient to avoid abrasive foods such as toast, apples, and celery.
   b. Encourage intake of pureed, bland foods.
   c. Instruct patient to avoid tart or acid foods such as pickles or tomatoes.
   d. Instruct patient to avoid spices and vinegar.
   e. Instruct patient to avoid alcohol.
   f. Arrange for dietary consultation.
5. Discourage smoking.
6. Recommend use of artificial saliva for xerostomia. No comparative research on various agents is available.

For grade 3 or grade 4 stomatitis

1. Obtain sample from suspicious area and culture for bacteria, fungus, and virus per physician's order.
2. Institute oral hygiene regimen:
   a. Alternate antifungal or antibacterial suspension with warm saline mouthwash q 2 h while patient is awake and q 4 h during night.
   b. Do not floss.
   c. Brush gently with toothettes or cotton-tipped applicators.
   d. Remove dentures or bridge; do not replace for meals.
   e. Apply lip lubricant q 2 h.
3. In addition to local measures indicated for grades 1 and 2 stomatitis, systemic analgesics may be indicated, especially before eating.
4. Liquid diet may be indicated. If not, use pureed diet. See other measures as indicated in no. 3 for grade 1 and grade 2 stomatitis.
5. Discourage smoking.

---

range-of-motion exercises to prevent adverse effects of bed rest.

8. Note character and quantity of stool; test stool for occult blood to monitor blood loss.
9. Administer antidiarrheal agents as ordered (usually not helpful in controlling diarrhea with GVHD) to control diarrhea. Monitor patient response.
10. Provide meticulous perianal skin care to prevent infection.
11. Permit nothing by mouth as ordered to allow bowel to rest.
12. Reinstate oral feedings with isosmotic, low-fat, lactose-free beverages as ordered; increase diet as tolerated to provide adequate nutrients. Monitor patient response.
13. Monitor closely for dehydration, electrolyte imbalance, and weight change to monitor hydration and nutrition.

14. Ausculate bowel sounds q 8 h to monitor for development of ileus.
15. Check bilirubin and SGOT levels regularly to monitor for development of acute liver disease.
16. Measure abdominal girth twice a day to evaluate for ascites, hepatomegaly, or splenomegaly.
17. Position patient on left side to decrease pressure on liver.
18. Administer drugs to decrease the effects of GVHD (e.g., steroids, cyclosporin A, methotrexate, and antithymocyte globulin) as ordered according to protocol, and monitor patient response.

NURSING DIAGNOSIS

Altered protection related to venoocclusive disease stemming from fibrous obliteration of small hepatic venules.

NURSING INTERVENTIONS AND RATIONALE

1. Assess and monitor for sudden weight gain, right upper quadrant pain, ascites, jaundice, and disorientation, and measure abdominal girth twice a day at the level of the umbilicus with patient supine to detect fibrotic obliteration of hepatic venules and alterations in hepatic function sometimes created by chemotherapy and irradiation.
2. Restrict sodium intake as ordered, and administer all intravenous medication in minimum volume of fluid to prevent fluid retention.
3. Monitor urine sodium levels and BP daily for orthostatic changes and to assess for fluid accumulation.
4. Monitor patient closely for toxic side effects of medication, which can be caused by impaired liver function.
5. Monitor liver function tests frequently to assess and monitor liver function.

NURSING DIAGNOSIS

Body image disturbance related to alopecia, weight loss, and sterility.

NURSING INTERVENTIONS AND RATIONALE

1. Encourage patient and significant others to express their feelings and concerns, and help them explore perceived meaning of loss, to facilitate recognition of body image changes.
2. Help minimize anxiety and promote adjustment of patient and significant others by informing them that alopecia and weight loss are temporary.
3. Help patient find ways to improve appearance (use of clothing, scarves, hats, or hairpieces) to enhance healthy self-image.
4. Convey an attitude of acceptance and understanding to enhance patient's feelings of self-worth.

5. Emphasize that negative reactions to altered body image are normal and expected, to minimize or alleviate patient's concern and anxiety.
6. Refer patient to community resources, organizations, and peer support group information. Shared experiences and methods of improving self-image may promote a positive body image and an improved sense of self.

NURSING DIAGNOSIS

Fear related to uncertain outcome of treatment, threat of death, isolation, and treatment protocols.

NURSING INTERVENTIONS AND RATIONALE

1. Encourage patient and significant others to express feelings and concerns and to ask questions, to facilitate recognition of fear and uncertainty.
2. Help patient decrease feelings of isolation through use of radio, television, tape recorder, or video cassette recorder.
3. Reinforce and restate information given to patient and significant others, to promote understanding of procedures and treatments.
4. Encourage patient and significant others to discuss hopes for positive outcome, to promote positive thinking, which generates energy and decreases feelings of fear and loneliness.
5. Consult other health care providers in planning a comprehensive approach to patient's care, to ensure that patient's needs are met and questions answered.

PATIENT TEACHING

Preparation for discharge includes teaching the following:

1. Teach the patient daily care for the central venous access device to maintain the patency of the catheter and prevent infection and bleeding.
   a. Cleanse area around catheter regularly and follow with povidone-iodine; cover with a gauze square and apply plastic dressing or paper tape.
   b. Monitor for signs of redness, pain, or swelling at catheter exit site.
   c. Heparinize line daily, according to the specific instructions given by your nurse.
   d. Contact your doctor if you experience chills, fever, or rigors (shaking chills after you flush the catheter).
2. Explain diet needed for optimum nutritional status (ideally the patient should be able to tolerate 1,000 calories a day to be discharged). All fresh fruits and vegetables should be thoroughly washed. Do not eat from salad bars or eat any raw food in restaurants. Make sure all your food is cooked and served

at the appropriate temperature. Try to drink at least 2 quarts of fluid a day.

3. Teach the patient measures for preventing infection. Precautions are more rigid during the first 3 months after bone marrow transplantation and are relaxed as the year progresses.
   a. Monitor your temperature daily for the first month after discharge. Take your temperature in the late afternoon; it usually is highest at this time. If your temperature is over 38.5° C (101° F) call your doctor. Do not take medication to lower your temperature without first checking with your physician.
   b. Wear a face mask when you are out in crowds.
   c. Avoid contact with anyone who has had a cold or the flu or who has been exposed to such diseases as measles, mumps, or chickenpox.
   d. Avoid contact with young children who attend school. If you have young children and they are exposed to someone who has been ill, try to decrease your close contact for at least 24 hours.
   e. Make sure to wash your hands well before eating, after using the toilet, and after contact with anyone who might have a cold.
   f. Avoid crowds for the first 3 months; go grocery shopping and to theaters and restaurants during off peak hours.
   g. Avoid uncooked or rare meat for the first 3 months.
   h. Children who have had a bone marrow transplant should not attend school for 1 year.
   i. Do not swim in a private or public pool for 1 year after a bone marrow transplantation.

4. Teach the patient about contact with pets.
   a. Avoid contact with pets for the first 3 months after transplantation. Do not clean litter boxes or come in contact with animal feces.
   b. If you have an indoor/outdoor cat, do not allow the cat in your bedroom for the first 3 months. Cats carry organisms and may transmit diseases obtained while outdoors.

5. Instruct the patient about contact with plants and flowers.
   a. Do not garden for at least 3 months after transplantation.
   b. Do not cut fresh flowers or change their water; the water has bacteria that may cause infection.
   c. Try to decrease your contact with dirt and dust for at least 3 months after transplantation.

6. Instruct the patient in the importance of strict dental hygiene.
   a. See your dentist regularly.
   b. Brush your teeth at least twice a day.
   c. Continue your mouth care for the first month after discharge from the hospital.
   d. Floss your teeth daily if your platelet count is above 50,000/mm^3.
   e. Do not use toothpicks.
   f. Use a soft-bristled toothbrush. If your platelet count is below 20,000/mm^3, use a toothette instead of a toothbrush.
   g. Do not have elective dental work done during periods of thrombocytopenia, since it increases the risk of bleeding. Platelets must be above 50,000/mm^3 before any dental work can be done.
   h. Do not use aspirin or products containing aspirin.
   i. If bleeding in your mouth occurs, control it with iced saline mouth rinses.

7. Provide the patient with information about immunizations.
   a. Do not have immunizations without your physician's approval.
   b. Avoid coming in contact with individuals who have recently been immunized with live viruses (e.g., measles, mumps, rubella, and oral polio).

8. Discuss sexuality with the patient.
   a. You may resume your normal sexual function when your platelets are above 50,000/mm^3 and your energy level is sufficient.
   b. Avoid anal intercourse for at least 3 months after transplantation.

9. Discuss with patient necessary changes in activities of daily living.
   a. Take prophylactic antibiotics as prescribed.
   b. Take your temperature daily, and notify the physician of any elevation 2° above baseline.
   c. Eliminate sharp objects in your environment (e.g., shave with an electric razor rather than a hand razor).
   d. Wear shoes or slippers at all times—no bare feet while walking.
   e. Do not use any beverages containing alcohol.
   f. Avoid blowing your nose or sneezing forcefully.
   g. Avoid bruising or bumping yourself.
   h. If epistaxis occurs, stay in a sitting position and apply ice to constrict small blood vessels. Applying pressure to your nose may control bleeding.

10. Teach the patient to call the doctor if:
    a. His temperature is over 38.5° C (101° F).
    b. He notices any rash, change in the color or consistency of his stool, change in the color of his urine, nausea or vomiting, pain, dryness of the mouth, difficulty swallowing, or change in skin color.
    c. He has a cough or shortness of breath.
    d. He notices any physical change that concerns him.

SPLENECTOMY

Although it serves various important functions, the spleen can be surgically removed from adults without harm. Hypersplenism, the destruction of excessive numbers of blood cells by the spleen, is a major reason for its surgical removal. Another frequent indication is splenic rupture with severe hemorrhage, often caused by trauma. Other therapeutic indications include auto-immune anemia or thrombocytopenia refractory to systemic therapy, or persistent symptomatic splenomegaly. The procedure is relatively simple unless the spleen is greatly enlarged or surrounded by adhesions.

Long-term effects of splenectomy are not entirely beneficial, however, and may include leukocytosis, decreased levels of serum iron, and slight decreases in immune function.

RADIATION THERAPY

Radiation therapy is a major modality in the treatment of cancer. It involves using high-energy ionizing radiation to treat malignancies. It is estimated that 60% of individuals with cancer receive radiation at some point during the course of their disease. Radiation is used at all phases of the cancer trajectory. As a primary therapy, radiation is used with curative intent in early-stage Hodgkin's disease, skin cancers, and head and neck and gynecologic malignancies. Radiation is used as an adjuvant treatment in small cell lung cancer and head and neck cancer; after definitive chemotherapy in small cell cancer; and after surgery with head and neck malignancies. In the palliative phase of treatment, radiation alleviates pain from bony metastases, controls bleeding from extensive gynecologic malignancies, and relieves obstruction and compression from advanced lung cancer and brain and spinal cord lesions.

Radiation is one of the oldest treatments for cancer. From the discovery of x-rays by Roentgen in 1895, radioactivity by Becquerel in 1896, and radium by the Curies in 1898, attempts have been made to use radiation to treat cancer. Early efforts were hampered by lack of equipment and an inadequate understanding of radiobiology. Treatment units could deliver significant radiation doses to the skin but lacked the energy to treat tumors below the skin's surface without causing unacceptable side effects. Skin cancers and other superficial lesions could be treated, but it was not until high-energy cobalt and linear accelerators (Figure 10-3) were developed in the 1950s that tumors well below the skin's surface could be treated. Linear accelerators deliver the maximum radiation below the skin's surface and are known as skin sparing.

CELLULAR RESPONSE TO RADIATION

Physical: Phase of excitation and ionization; the energy imparted by the radiation disrupts molecules by ejecting electrons from orbit

Physicochemical: Powerful oxidizing and reducing agents are formed within the cells

Chemical: Chemical reactions occur within the cell, producing changes in DNA

Biologic: Cellular death occurs as cells divide; single- and double-stranded breaks in chromosomes occur, rendering cells incapable of proliferation

---

Along with the development of sophisticated equipment, the sciences of radiation biology and physics emerged. Understanding the effect of radiation on normal and tumor cells and the properties of ionizing radiation was essential to the safe, effective use of radiation in individuals with cancer.

The types of radiation commonly used in treatment include electromagnetic radiation with x-rays and gamma rays. X-rays are photons generated within a machine; gamma rays are photons emitted from a radioactive source. Particulate radiation uses electrons, protons, and, less commonly, neutrons and pi mesons produced within a machine. Radiation is measured in units known as the rad (radiation absorbed dose) or the Gray, which is equal to 100 rad.

The target organ in the cell for radiation damage is the DNA. Cellular death from radiation is mitotically linked in that the cell can function but cannot survive division. The rate at which normal and cancer cells react to radiation is determined by their mitotic rate. Normal cells with high mitotic rates (e.g., hair follicles, gastrointestinal mucosa, and bone marrow cells) and cancers such as lymphomas, leukemias, and seminomas respond quickly to treatment. These are radiosensitive tumors. Cells with slower rates (e.g., muscles, nerves, and vessels) and tumors such as rhabdomyosarcomas are radioresistant, requiring a higher radiation dose and a longer response time.

The cellular response to radiation occurs in several phases (see box above).

Normal cells are better able to recover from the damage caused by radiation than are cancer cells. Because malignant cells lack the capacity for repair, more cancer cells than normal cells are damaged by radiation. However, normal cells do have a maximum dose of radiation that they can tolerate before irreversible damage occurs. Simulation and treatment planning are designed to minimize the radiation dose to normal structures (Figures 10-4 and 10-5). Radiation tolerance varies widely, from sensitive organs (e.g., the gonads

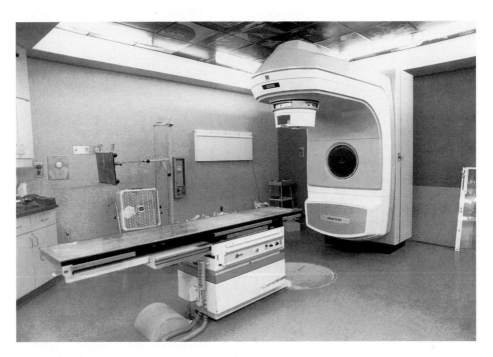

FIGURE 10-3
Linear accelerator. Used for the treatment of patients with a wide variey of cancers.

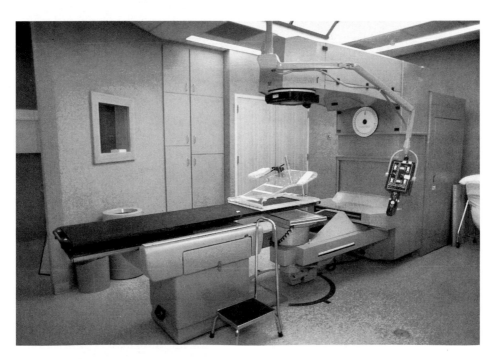

FIGURE 10-4
Simulator. Used to take treatment planning films and to set up treatment fields.

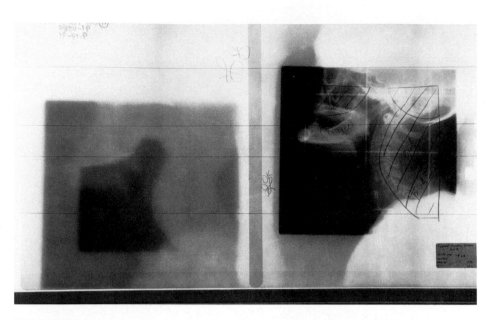

FIGURE 10-5
Treatment planning for radiation therapy. The film on the left is a port film of a patient with head and neck cancer. The film on the right is a simulation film showing the treatment field with blocks.

and small intestine) to tolerant tissue (e.g., the uterus and bladder). Spinal cord tolerance, at 4,500 rad, is a dose-limiting factor, since overdose to the spinal cord causes cord necrosis and results in functional loss. Meticulous planning and recording of spinal cord dose are essential.

EFFECTS OF RADIATION

Radiation effects may be categorized as acute (during treatment to 6 months), subacute (after 6 months), and chronic (with variable time to expression). The effects are seen sooner in cell lines with a high mitotic index (the skin, mucous membranes, and hair follicles) and later in cell lines that divide more slowly (the vascular system and muscles). Early side effects are believed to be reparable, whereas late effects are more often permanent.

Radiation produces most of its effects in the area being treated; however, general effects such as fatigue and anorexia do occur. Fatigue is a commonly reported problem that has been shown to increase during the course of treatment. Research suggests a weekly pattern to the fatigue, with patients feeling better on some days than others. Fatigue is expected to occur by the third or fourth week of treatment. The patient should be encouraged to chart a pattern of fatigue and to plan activities accordingly, with rest planned before activities.

Megavoltage radiation therapy with skin-sparing

techniques has resulted in less severe skin reactions than in the past. However, patients continue to express a fear of being burned. Transient erythema may appear as early as the first treatment, but it is usually during the second or third week of therapy that a lasting reaction appears. A dry desquamation may develop, with peeling of the skin. The cells may become darker before they peel off because of radiation effects on melanocytes. Patients complain of dryness and itching. Areas of wet desquamation may occur in areas subjected to higher doses or pressure (e.g., skin folds, perineum, axilla, collar area, and areas under the breast). This is a result of the destruction of all cells of the basal layer, exposing the dermis, which creates small but painful oozing areas. Permanent skin changes may result from dermal fibrosis and atrophy. The skin may feel hard, look shiny, and become darker than surrounding tissue. Telangiectasia (a dilation of capillaries related to late vascular effects and increased pressure of blood flowing through superficial vessels) results in spidery purple-red vessels visible in the treated area. This area may always react differently to sun exposure and should be protected (see Patient Teaching Guide).

Acute pulmonary effects of chest radiation therapy include increased cough, which may become more productive with the release of material that has been trapped in blocked alveoli as a result of lung cancer. As the mucosa dries during treatment, the cough becomes nonproductive and may require cough suppressant therapy if it becomes persistent and debilitating. Patients also report dyspnea, which is difficult to manage and heightens the patient's anxiety. The primary acute effect is pneumonitis, with symptoms such as dyspnea, cough, fever, and night sweats appearing within 3 to 6 weeks after radiation therapy is begun, although pneumonitis often may be asymptomatic. The late effect is fibrosis in the treated area. This usually is asymptomatic, although extensive fibrosis with very high doses of radiation therapy may cause infection, fever, chills, dyspnea, clubbing, and abscesses.

Gastrointestinal effects reflect the area being irradiated. Irradiation of the small and large intestine causes vomiting, anorexia, diarrhea, and gastric distention. Gastric emptying is delayed, returning to normal 1 to 2 weeks after treatment ends. Patients receiving radiation therapy to the gastrointestinal tract may complain of nausea, vomiting, and diarrhea.

Radiosensitive cells, those most likely to be adversely affected by radiation, include relatively undifferentiated and rapidly dividing cells such as those of the gonads, the mucosa of the gastrointestinal tract, and lymphoid tissue. The most radioresistant cells are those originating from the connective tissue. At the cellular level the degree of sensitivity is related to the degree of cellular differentiation, rate of mitosis, and mitotic potential. The degrees of vascularity and oxygenation are also important in determining tissue responsiveness.

The toxic effects of radiation therapy depend on the site of irradiation, the volume of tissue irradiated, the total dosage delivered, and the time frame within which it is administered. Although newer technology has allowed tumors to be treated more precisely, surrounding or underlying healthy tissue will still be damaged.

The dose of radiation that can be delivered to any tumor is limited by the radiation tolerance of the adjacent normal tissues. A method of allowing for recovery of normal tissue is the fractionation of treatment, or dividing the total dosage of radiation into several equal daily doses (five days a week). This allows the following processes to occur: repair of sublethal tissue damage, repopulation of clonogenic cells, reassortment of cells in the cell cycle, and reoxygenation of hypoxic cells. The best results are achieved with predetermined doses given five times a week for 4 to 6 weeks (depending on the type of tumor).

Before initiating therapy, the radiation oncologist localizes the treatment field with a simulator, which reproduces the geometric factors of actual therapy. Computed tomography (CT) scanning that defines both the tumor-bearing volume and critical normal structures is also used. The information obtained is used, with computer assistance, to devise an individualized treatment plan (see photographs).

Using chemotherapy with radiation requires careful monitoring of peripheral blood counts and observation for combined modality disorders such as dysuria (cyclophosphamide) and enhanced mucositis (methotrexate, bleomycin). Actinomycin D and doxorubicin produce a recall phenomenon in which skin reactions appear in previously irradiated tissues when the drug is given as late as 1 year after the patient's radiation therapy. When radiation therapy is combined with other treatment modalities, acute and chronic reactions may be exacerbated. The nurse caring for these individuals must coordinate assessments and interventions to provide continuity of care.

PATIENT TEACHING

Teaching patients receiving radiation involves explaining the complex treatment in terms they can understand, predicting anticipated acute and long-term effects, and providing information about symptom management. With these tools, patients can undergo treatment with minimal disruption of their activities. Symptom management is a critical aspect of the care of the individual receiving radiation therapy.

1 ASSESS

ASSESSMENT	OBSERVATIONS
Gastrointestinal tract	Nausea and vomiting, anorexia, taste changes, esophagitis, sore throat, xerostomia, mucositis, tooth decay, diarrhea, perianal irritation
Genitourinary	Bladder irritation, vaginal discharge, amenorrhea, impotence, sterility
Dermatologic	Hair loss, dry desquamation, moist desquamation
Central nervous system	Headache, irritability, confusion, restlessness
Neuromuscular system	Fatigue, transient myelitis
Cardiopulmonary	Pneumonitis, pericarditis, myocarditis
Hematologic	Leukopenia, thrombocytopenia

2 DIAGNOSE

NURSING DIAGNOSIS	SUBJECTIVE FINDINGS	OBJECTIVE FINDINGS
Fluid volume deficit related to nausea and vomiting	Complains of nausea	Vomiting
Altered nutrition: less than body requirements related to gastrointestinal irritation and increased body requirements	Complains of anorexia, taste changes, sore throat	Esophagitis, xerostomia, mucositis
Diarrhea related to gastrointestinal irritation	Complains of urgency to defecate, perianal irritation	Frequent loose, liquid, or semiliquid stools
Altered oral mucous membranes related to treatment-induced irritation	Complains of sore throat, dry mouth	Mucositis, xerostomia
Altered patterns of urinary elimination related to bladder irritation	Complains of urgency, burning during urination	Frequency, hematuria

NURSING DIAGNOSIS	SUBJECTIVE FINDINGS	OBJECTIVE FINDINGS
Sexual dysfunction related to treatment-induced changes in hormonal status and local effects of radiation	Complains of impotence; discomfort during sexual activity	Vaginal discharge, amenorrhea, sterility, vaginal dryness
Impaired skin integrity related to treatment-induced changes	Complains of dry, itchy feeling	Hair loss, dry desquamation (reddened area, dry in appearance), moist desquamation (blistering, sloughing)
Pain (headache) related to increased intracranial pressure	Complains of headache	Grimacing, holding head in hands, pupillary changes, increased blood pressure
Impaired physical mobility related to fatigue and myelitis	Complains of fatigue, painful sensations	Weakness, guarding of extremities, Lhermitte's sign
Altered cardiopulmonary tissue perfusion related to pneumonitis, pericarditis, myocarditis, anemia, and bleeding	Complains of chest pain	Cough, dyspnea, friction rub, electrocardiogram (ECG) changes, dysrhythmias, anemia, thrombocytopenia

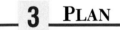

3   PLAN

Patient goals

1. The patient will maintain adequate hydration and nutrition.
2. The patient will maintain normal fecal and urinary elimination patterns.
3. The patient will have healthy oral mucous membranes.
4. Sexual function will be normal.
5. The patient will have healthy skin.
6. The patient will have no pain.
7. The patient will ambulate without difficulty.
8. The patient will have adequate oxygenation, as evidenced by normal cardiopulmonary function.

4　IMPLEMENT

NURSING DIAGNOSIS	NURSING INTERVENTIONS	RATIONALE
Fluid volume deficit related to nausea and vomiting	Administer antiemetic as needed before treatment of areas known to cause nausea and vomiting.	To control incidence of nausea and vomiting.
	Plan rest periods before and after meals.	To enhance patient's appetite.
	Provide small, bland feedings and increased fluids.	To maintain nutrition and hydration.
	Offer frequent mouth care.	To promote comfort and appetite.
	Provide clean environment with fresh air and no odors.	To decrease noxious stimuli.
	Administer intravenous therapy as ordered.	To maintain hydration.
	Monitor intake and output, daily weight, and electrolytes.	To determine need for further intervention.
Altered nutrition: less than body requirements related to gastrointestinal irritation and increased body requirements	Encourage patient to eat high-calorie, high-protein diet.	For maximum nutrition.
	Offer small, frequent feedings.	To increase intake.
	Do not rush meals.	To increase intake.
	Keep room free of odors and clutter.	To reduce noxious stimuli.
	Provide meticulous mouth care.	To increase comfort and appetite.
	Use enteral feeding tube or total parenteral nutrition if necessary.	To maintain nutritional balance.
	Monitor weight daily.	To detect nutritional imbalance.
	Encourage clear liquids, low-residue diet, and antacids.	To increase comfort.
Diarrhea related to gastrointestinal irritation	Offer antidiarrheal agents per physician's order.	To control intestinal irritability.
	Maintain good perineal care.	To prevent pain, infection, and fear of eating caused by painful bowel movement.
	Test stools for occult blood.	To identify intestinal bleeding.
	Record number and consistency of stools.	To monitor effect of therapy.
	Observe for dehydration and electrolyte imbalances.	To determine need for further intervention.

NURSING DIAGNOSIS	NURSING INTERVENTIONS	RATIONALE
Altered oral mucous membranes related to treatment-induced irritation	Encourage good oral hygiene with use of dental floss or Water Pik unless thrombocytopenia is present.	To prevent infection and assist in healing.
	Discourage foods that are spicy, hot, dry, or thick.	They increase discomfort.
	Offer topical relief of pain—viscous lidocaine.	To promote comfort and nutrition.
	Apply water-soluble lubricant (K-Y Jelly) to lips.	To maintain moisture.
	Offer sugar-free popsicles.	To increase comfort and hydration.
	Offer artificial saliva.	To moisten mucosa.
	Encourage increased fluid intake with meals.	To maintain hydration.
	Use mouth irrigations (e.g., salt and bicarbonate with water).	For oral hygiene.
	Encourage use of sugarless lemon drops or mints.	To promote feeling of freshness and to stimulate saliva.
	Discourage smoking, alcohol, or ginger ale.	They irritate mucosa.
	Assess mouth for dryness, lesions, bleeding, discharge, and tooth decay.	To determine need for specific interventions.
	Consult dentist before treatment for dental problems, including fluoride therapy.	To prevent further irritation and infection and to prevent radiation caries.
Altered patterns of urinary elimination related to bladder irritation	Force fluids.	To maintain renal and bladder hydration.
	Encourage patient to empty bladder completely.	To avoid distention.
	Administer urinary antiseptics as prescribed.	To reduce inflammation.
	Observe for signs of infection (e.g., burning, cloudy urine, hematuria, and fever).	To determine the need for antibiotics and other interventions.

→ 〉 〉 〉

NURSING DIAGNOSIS	NURSING INTERVENTIONS	RATIONALE
Sexual dysfunction related to treatment-induced changes in hormonal status and local effects of radiation	*For sterility:* Help patient explore alternatives (e.g., sperm banking) if an option and hormonal therapy.	To counteract sterility.
	Refer patient to sexual counselor as necessary.	To treat impotence.
	For vaginal discharge: Encourage patient to douche as needed and to perform thorough perineal care.	To maintain hygiene.
	Observe for redness, tenderness, discharge, or drainage.	These may indicate need for further intervention.
	For vaginal dryness: Observe for skin integrity and lubrication of mucosa; offer lubricants and vaginal dilator.	To maintain integrity of mucosa, facilitate comfort during intercourse, and prevent vaginal fibrosis.
Impaired skin integrity related to treatment-induced changes	*For alopecia:* Help patient plan for wig with soft underside to minimize skin irritation; use only for special occasions.	To avoid scalp damage.
	Have patient wear scarf or turban.	For daily protection of scalp.
	Have patient gently wash and comb hair.	To avoid further hair loss.
	Tell patient that hair loss secondary to whole brain radiation for primary brain tumors is permanent.	To avoid false hope about regrowth.
	For dermatitis: Observe irradiated area daily.	To monitor for inflammation or other reactions.
	Apply baby oil or ointment as prescribed: lanolin or Aquaphor.	To maintain moisture.

NURSING DIAGNOSIS	NURSING INTERVENTIONS	RATIONALE
	Keep reddened area dry and aerated.	To avoid infection.
	Use cornstarch, A & D ointment, hydrocortisone ointment, aloe vera.	To relieve dryness and itching.
	For moist desquamation: Provide saline soaks, moisture-permeable dressings, topical vitamins, steroids, or antibiotic ointments; expose area to air.	To enhance healing.
	Do not use adhesive tape.	It irritates the skin.
	Help patient with bathing.	To maintain markings.
	Have patient avoid excessive heat, sunlight, soap, and tight, restrictive clothing.	They further irritate damaged skin.
	Provide special skin care to tissue folds (e.g., buttocks, perineum, groin, and axilla).	They are subject to increased pressure and damage.
	Do not apply deodorant or aftershave lotion to treated area.	They may irritate the skin.
Pain (headache) related to increased intracranial pressure	Assess presence and characteristics of headache.	To monitor need for intervention.
	Administer medications (e.g., steroids, analgesics) as prescribed.	To relieve pain.
	Offer patient other pain relief measures if desired.	To encourage patient involvement in pain management.
	Monitor pupillary response and changes in vital signs, irritability, confusion, and restlessness.	These indicate increasing intracranial pressure.

NURSING DIAGNOSIS	NURSING INTERVENTIONS	RATIONALE
Impaired physical mobility related to fatigue and myelitis	Plan frequent rest periods.	To avoid fatigue.
	Assist patient with ambulation and remove environmental barriers.	To avoid injury.
	Assess reflexes, tactile sensation, and movement in extremities; report abnormal findings.	To detect complications.
	Observe for Lhermitte's sign (sensation of electric shock running down back and over extremities).	This indicates transient myelitis.
Altered cardiopulmonary tissue perfusion related to pneumonitis, pericarditis, myocarditis, anemia, and bleeding	Auscultate lungs, and report signs of pleural rub.	To detect respiratory problems early.
	Observe for cough, dyspnea, and pain on inspiration.	These indicate respiratory dysfunction.
	Treat with antibiotics and steroids as prescribed.	To reduce irritation and prevent infection.
	Auscultate heart, and report signs of friction rub, dysrhythmia, or hypertension.	To detect complications.
	Observe for chest pain and weakness.	These indicate cardiac dysfunction.
	Monitor ECG reports.	To monitor cardiac function.
	Administer drugs as prescribed.	To counteract dysrhythmias.
	Encourage adequate rest; alternate rest and activity periods.	To avoid stress on respiratory system.
	Observe patient for dyspnea and increased weakness.	These are signs of further anemia.
	Administer oxygen therapy as needed.	To increase oxygenation of tissues.
	Monitor hemoglobin and hematocrit.	To determine effect of therapy on bone marrow.
	Administer transfusions as ordered.	To increase circulating red blood cells.

5 EVALUATE

PATIENT OUTCOME	DATA INDICATING THAT OUTCOME IS REACHED
Patient has adequate hydration.	Patient has no nausea or vomiting, intake and output are balanced, and electrolytes are within normal limits.
Patient's nutrition is adequate.	Patient has no complaints of anorexia or unusual taste sensations and can eat and swallow without pain; weight is normal.
Patient has normal bowel elimination.	Patient has no diarrhea.
Patient's oral mucous membranes are healthy.	Mucous membranes, lips, tongue, and gingiva are moist and normal in color; the teeth are clean and saliva is adequate; patient can swallow and has a normal voice.
Patient has normal urinary elimination.	Patient has no complaints of urinary distress, and intake and output are balanced.
Patient's sexual function is normal.	Patient has a satisfactory libido and has made plans for dealing with possible sterility; there is no vaginal discharge (women) or erectile ability has been maintained (men).
Patient's skin is healthy and intact.	Patient has no complaints of itching, and there is no evidence of rash, blistering, or redness.
Patient has no pain.	Patient has no complaint of headache.
Patient has normal physical mobility.	Patient can ambulate without assistance.
Patient has adequate cardiopulmonary tissue perfusion.	Patient has no complaints of chest pain, cough, or dyspnea, and CBC is within normal limits.

PATIENT TEACHING

1. Discuss the need for skin care such as maintenance of dye markings, avoiding soap and other ointments, and avoiding sunbathing or heat applications (see Patient Teaching Guide).
2. Emphasize the need to avoid injury to the skin (see Patient Teaching Guide).
3. Explain the maintenance of adequate nutrition and hydration (see Patient Teaching Guide).
4. Explain the patient's "radioactive state," if present, and precautions to be taken.
5. Discuss how to manage fatigue and maintain mobility.

CHEMOTHERAPY

Chemotherapy is still considered a relatively new form of cancer treatment, the first patient having been treated with nitrogen mustard in 1942. Chemical agents are especially important in the treatment of systemic disease. Researchers strive to discover drugs that kill cancer cells without extensively damaging normal tissues. In addition, combinations of chemotherapeutic agents, as well as chemotherapy combined with other treatments, have increased the number of cures, remissions, and palliative outcomes.

Chemotherapeutic agents are highly toxic, attacking all rapidly dividing cells, both normal and malignant. Thus the contraindications for and precautions in the use of the various agents reflect the patient's pretreatment condition, stage of disease, response to therapy, and allergies or sensitivities. The nurse involved in administering the drugs and monitoring the patient's responses must have a comprehensive baseline assessment for evaluating the patient's condition and ability to tolerate the therapy. Many health care providers monitor the patient's functional status in a systematic manner, using such instruments as the Karnofsky Performance Scale (Table 10-5). Preset values guide the health care provider in determining the patient's tolerance of the therapy, as well as the need to delay or discontinue treatment.

ROUTES OF ADMINISTRATION

Depending on the drug's pharmacodynamics, chemotherapy may be administered by a variety of routes: oral, intravenous, central venous catheter, venous access via an implantable access device, intraarterial, intraperitoneal, intrapleural, or intrathecal via the Ommaya reservoir. The intramuscular and subcutaneous routes are used less frequently than other routes.

In recent years venous access has become increasingly important because of the ease of access to the venous system for drug delivery, increased patient comfort, and the addition of external or internal pump systems for more continuous infusion of drugs (Figure 10-6) (see Patient Teaching Guide). Although most central venous lines have similarities, the nurse should become familiar with the variations; for example, a Broviac line has a smaller inner lumen than a Hickman catheter. Injection caps, repair kits, and surgical insertion techniques also vary with the brand, as do the materials the catheters are made of. Most central venous lines (except the Groshong catheter) should be flushed with 2 to 5 ml of normal saline before medication is administered. After the medication has been instilled, the

Table 10-5 ⟍⟍⟍

KARNOFSKY PERFORMANCE SCALE

Activity status	%	Description
Normal activity	100	Normal, with no complaints or evidence of disease
	90	Able to carry on normal activity but with minor signs or symptoms of disease present
	80	Normal activity but requiring effort; signs and symptoms of disease more prominent
Self-care	70	Able to care for self but unable to work or carry on other normal activities
	60	Able to care for most needs but requires occasional assistance
	50	Considerable assistance required, along with frequent medical care; some self-care still possible
Incapacitated	40	Disabled and requiring special care and assistance
	30	Severely disabled; hospitalization required but death from disease not imminent
	20	Extremely ill; supportive treatment, hospitalized care required
	10	Imminent death
	0	Dead

nurse or patient should flush again with saline and then a heparin solution. When not in use, the catheter should be flushed regularly with a heparin solution to maintain patency. There is increasing evidence that the catheter does not have to be flushed daily; nursing research continues in this area. Unlike other central lines, the Groshong catheter has a rounded tip and a valve that prevents venous blood from entering the catheter and also blocks out air if the line is left uncapped. This catheter should be flushed with normal saline after use; no heparinization is required. The Groshong is a more transparent and flexible catheter and should not be clamped when uncapped. When caring for a patient who has a central line, the nurse should don a mask and sterile gloves, hold the catheter away from the patient's body, and clean the site and 3 inches

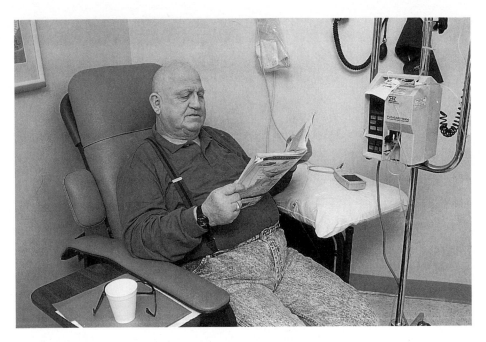

FIGURE 10-6
Chemotherapy.

GENERAL PRINCIPLES THAT GUIDE THE USE OF CANCER CHEMOTHERAPEUTIC AGENTS

1. Combination chemotherapy, when carefully designed, has been consistently superior to single-agent therapy.
2. Complete remission is the minimum requirement to achieve cure and even significantly prolonged survival.
3. The best chance for a significant response is with the first attempt; thus the type of treatment should be the approach with maximum effectiveness.
4. Drugs should be used in the highest possible doses to attain maximum tumor-cell kill.
5. Drug dosage reduction to minimize toxicity is itself the most toxic side effect of chemotherapy.
6. Adjuvant chemotherapy is now well established in the treatment of breast cancer and holds promise for other types of cancer.
7. The development of analogs of existing drugs has made it possible to at least partly modify those drugs' toxicity while preserving their antitumor activity (e.g., carboplatin and iproplatin are second-generation platinum compounds that are less nephrotoxic than cisplatin).
8. Various therapeutic maneuvers are used to lessen toxicity (e.g., doxorubicin is much less toxic when given by 96-hour infusion than when given as a bolus).
9. "Neoadjuvant," or induction, chemotherapy is the initial use of drugs to reduce a tumor's bulk and lower its stage, making it amenable to cure with local therapy (e.g., as in osteogenic sarcoma).
10. Chemoprevention of cancer is becoming a reality (e.g., 13-cis-retinoic acid has been shown to produce marked regression of leukoplakia, a premalignant lesion in the oral cavity).

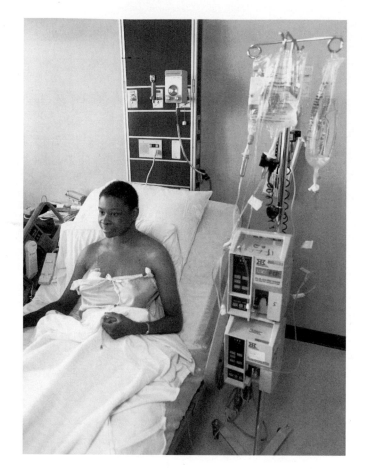

FIGURE 10-7
Hickman-Brovlac catheter. This patient has a Hickman-Brovlac catheter for venous access. Note the catheter's lift over the right breast, with a protective dressing and tape to prevent dislodgment. The patient is receiving multiple intravenous infusions via the catheter.

up the catheter with povidone-iodine. It is also important to observe the site for redness, tenderness, drainage, or swelling, each of which requires further assessment and intervention.

Unlike central venous lines, which provide external access, the implanted venous infusion device remains completely under the patient's skin, which serves as a defense against infection. Vascular access ports (Figure 10-7) such as the Infuse-A-Port and the Port-A-Cath consist of a resealable silicone rubber septum, a housing or body of molded plastic and silicone rubber or stainless steel, and an attached silicone rubber catheter or a separate catheter and locking ring. The port is implanted subcutaneously with the indwelling catheter positioned in a vein, artery, peritoneum, pericardial cavity, or pleural cavity. The advantages of the port include repeated access to blood vessels or a body cavity with minimal trauma and distress for the patient; the ability to inject bolus or continuous infusions of drugs, blood, nutritional products, or other fluids; access to blood samples; and promotion of the patient's normal body image and ability to conduct activities of daily living. The system is flushed weekly or monthly, depending on whether the catheter is in an artery or a vein.

The implantable pump (Figure 10-8) provides a refillable reservoir; a permanent, nonreplaceable power source; few moving parts; a variable infusion rate; and a double septum for continuous and bolus drug delivery. The pump is approved for use with floxuridine (FUDR), methotrexate, heparin, morphine, and some aminoglycosides.

The Ommaya reservoir (Figure 10-9) is a mushroom-shaped device made of silicone rubber and con-

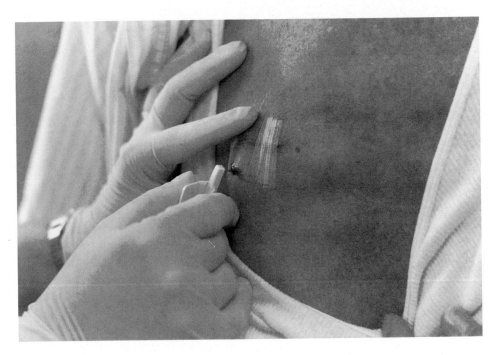

FIGURE 10-8
Implanted pump. The nurse is accessing the patient's implanted pump for the purpose of infusing a chemotherapeutic agent. The needle is taped to the skin surface for the duration of the infusion and then removed.

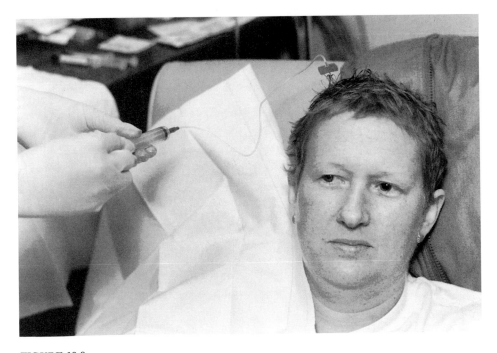

FIGURE 10-9
Ommaya reservoir. This patient is receiving chemotherapy via the Ommaya reservoir, which is implanted within the scalp. The drug is delivered directly into the cerebrospinal fluid.

nected to a catheter in the lateral ventricle. The hollow dome, a reservoir with an internal volume of 1.25 ml, is made of specially thickened self-sealing silicone rubber that allows for at least 200 separate needle punctures. The dome also functions as a pump when compressed through the skin with a fingertip. The Ommaya reservoir is used to deliver drugs directly into the cerebrospinal fluid (CSF), to obtain CSF specimens, and to measure CSF pressure, thus eliminating the need for repeated lumbar punctures. In addition, drug distribution is better when the drug is delivered into the ventricles.

Intraperitoneal chemotherapy is used to treat minimal residual disease, with the goal of enhancing local tumor control while decreasing systemic exposure to drug toxicity. The peritoneal cavity acts as a tumor refuge, since it is separated from the bloodstream by a cellular enclosure similar to the blood-brain barrier. Direct administration of chemotherapeutic drugs ensures greater exposure of malignant cells to the drugs. The slower peritoneal clearance or absorption leads to greater pharmacologic advantage. In addition, the drug is partly detoxified and metabolized by the liver before entering the systemic circulation, thus reducing the number and severity of systemic toxicities. Cisplatin currently is the drug of choice for intraperitoneal infusion, although interferon-alpha, methotrexate, fluorouracil (5FU), doxorubicin, and other agents are being studied.

The Tenckhoff peritoneal dialysis catheter most often is used for intraperitoneal chemotherapy, with the intraperitoneal end surgically placed in the abdominal cavity. The distal end of the catheter and the abdominal exit site are cared for meticulously to prevent infection. The nurse must help the patient in the management of abdominal fullness or pressure, which results from drastic fluid changes in the abdominal cavity. Effective interventions include having the patient wear loose-fitting clothing and change position every 15 minutes, and maintaining the bed in semi-Fowler's position during the infusion. If the patient experiences severe dyspnea during the procedure, the nurse may need to withdraw the fluid early. If leakage occurs around the catheter site, the placement of the catheter should be checked. Complications include bacterial peritonitis and infection at the exit site.

CLINICAL TRIALS

Many cancer chemotherapeutic agents currently are under study. Patients often are asked to participate in clinical trials of single agents or combinations of drugs.

It is important for the nurse to understand the phases of drug testing to teach the patient about clinical trials and to ensure the patient's informed consent if he or she agrees to participate (see Patient Teaching Guide).

OTHER ISSUES RELATED TO CHEMOTHERAPY

Although chemotherapy often is of great value to the patient with cancer, it may also create chemotherapy-related malignancies. The class of drugs most commonly associated with long-term damage to normal cells is the alkylating agents, which include busulfan (Myleran), chlorambucil (Leukeran), cyclophosphamide (Cytoxan), and melphalan (Alkeran). The most frequently reported second cancer is acute nonlymphocytic leukemia (ANL), which has a short latency period (2 to 5 years after treatment). Most patients die within 6 months of diagnosis. Patients at greatest risk for second malignancies are those treated for Hodgkin's lymphoma, non-Hodgkin's lymphoma, multiple myeloma, ovarian cancer, breast cancer, gastrointestinal cancers, lung cancer, and testicular cancer.

Another interesting phenomenon is multidrug resistance, which is seen in cancers that are (1) highly responsive to chemotherapy and frequently curable but that show a drug-resistant relapse (e.g., diffuse lymphomas and testicular cancers); (2) initially highly responsive to cytoreductive therapy but eventually relapse or progress (e.g., disseminated breast cancer, ovarian cancer, and small cell lung cancer); or (3) refractory at initial diagnosis; that is, de novo resistance (e.g., colon cancer and disseminated malignant melanoma). If satisfactory tumor-cell kill is achieved only at the cost of unacceptable patient toxicity, then for all practical purposes the tumor is resistant.

The nurse who administers cancer chemotherapeutic drugs must be concerned about and careful with not only the patient but also herself. It has been proved that unsafe handling of these drugs may heighten the nurse's reproductive risks as well as endanger the environment. The Occupational Safety and Health Administration (OSHA) offers recommendations for safe handling of antineoplastic drugs, which can be obtained from the U.S. Department of Labor. Nurses preparing and administering chemotherapy must be familiar with these guidelines and see that they are implemented for the protection of all who come into contact with these drugs. The guidelines address avoiding exposure via inhalation, absorption through the skin, and ingestion. There are also recommendations for protective equipment, safe disposal, and monitoring of biologic safety cabinets and personnel health.

1 ASSESS

ASSESSMENT	OBSERVATIONS
Gastrointestinal	Nausea and vomiting, diarrhea, constipation, stomatitis, esophagitis, anorexia
Dermatologic	Alopecia, dermatitis, changes in skin color, hyperpigmentation of nail beds, rash, jaundice, pruritus, extravasation
Hematologic	Fatigue and dyspnea (anemia), petechiae, ecchymoses, frank bleeding (thrombocytopenia), fever, chills, hypotension (leukopenia)
Reproductive	Sterility, amenorrhea, decreased libido
Urinary	Hemorrhagic cystitis, as evidenced by hematuria, burning during urination, and backache; nephrotoxicity, as evidenced by renal failure or decrease or absence of urinary output
Neurologic	Ototoxicity, as evidenced by vertigo, tinnitus, and loss of hearing; peripheral neuropathies, as evidenced by muscular weakness, paresthesia, absence of deep tendon reflexes
Musculoskeletal	Myalgia, muscle weakness, osteoporosis, gout
Respiratory	Pulmonary fibrosis, as evidenced by dyspnea, chest pain, or cyanosis
Cardiac	Congestive heart failure, as evidenced by exertional dyspnea, cough, rales, and ECG changes
Psychosocial	Fear, depression, anger, anxiety

2 DIAGNOSE

NURSING DIAGNOSIS	SUBJECTIVE FINDINGS	OBJECTIVE FINDINGS
Fluid volume deficit related to nausea and vomiting	Complains of nausea	Vomiting
Constipation related to impaired intestinal motility	Complains of fullness, inability to defecate	Absence of bowel movements
Diarrhea related to intestinal irritation	Complains of urgency to defecate	Frequent loose, liquid, or semiliquid stools
Altered oral mucous membranes related to poor oral hygiene, pre-existing dental disorders, or drug-induced irritation	Complains of pain in mouth, difficulty swallowing, unusual taste sensations	Redness, ulcers or lesions, dry or cracked lips, coated tongue, thick saliva, edematous gums, plaque or debris around teeth, deep, raspy voice

→ > >

NURSING DIAGNOSIS	SUBJECTIVE FINDINGS	OBJECTIVE FINDINGS
Altered nutrition: less than body requirements related to gastrointestinal irritation and increased body requirements	Complains of anorexia, unusual taste sensations	Stomatitis, esophagitis
Impaired skin integrity related to drug-induced changes, extravasation	Complains of itching	Alopecia, dermatitis/rash, changes in skin color (e.g., jaundice), hyperpigmentation of skin and nail beds
Impaired gas exchange related to anemia, pulmonary fibrosis, cardiotoxicity	Complains of fatigue, chest pain	Pallor, exertional dyspnea, cough, fever, ECG changes
Altered peripheral tissue perfusion related to bleeding	Complains of weakness	Tachycardia, hyperpnea, hypotension, petechiae, ecchymoses, melena, hematuria, frank bleeding
Potential for infection related to leukopenia, bone marrow suppression	Complains of fever	Chills; hypotension; damp, warm, red skin; odor; leukocytosis or leukopenia
Sexual dysfunction related to drug-induced changes in hormonal status	Complains of decreased libido	Sterility, amenorrhea
Altered patterns of urinary elimination related to drug-induced nephrotoxicity	Complains of burning during urination, urgency, backache	Frequency, decreased urination, hematuria
Sensory/perceptual alterations (auditory, tactile) related to drug-induced neurotoxicity	Complains of vertigo, dizziness, loss of hearing, numbness and tingling, weakness	Appears not to hear speaker; asks speaker to repeat words; muscle weakness; loss of deep tendon reflexes
Impaired physical mobility related to drug-induced gout, osteoporosis, myelotoxicity	Complains of weakness, muscle pain	Muscle weakness, difficulty ambulating
Altered cardiopulmonary tissue perfusion related to pneumonitis, pericarditis, myocarditis, anemia, and bleeding	Complains of chest pain	Exertional dyspnea, cough, rales, ECG changes

NURSING DIAGNOSIS	SUBJECTIVE FINDINGS	OBJECTIVE FINDINGS
Ineffective individual coping related to stress of dealing with chemotherapy	Expresses fear, anger, sadness	Appears afraid, angry, anxious, withdrawn

3 PLAN

Patient goals

1. The patient will maintain adequate hydration and nutrition.
2. The patient will maintain normal fecal and urinary elimination patterns.
3. The patient will have healthy oral mucous membranes and skin.
4. The patient will have adequate oxygenation, as evidenced by normal cardiopulmonary function and warm, pink skin.
5. The patient will have no evidence of infection.
6. Sexual function will be normal.
7. The patient will demonstrate normal sensory/perceptual function with regard to hearing, touch, and sensation.
8. The patient will ambulate without difficulty.
9. The patient will be able to cope with the stress of chemotherapy.

4 IMPLEMENT

NURSING DIAGNOSIS	NURSING INTERVENTIONS	RATIONALE
Fluid volume deficit related to nausea and vomiting	Administer antiemetic (prochlorperazine, thiethylperazine, trimethobenzamide, metoclopramide, intravenous dexamethasone, or ondansetron prophylactically before chemotherapy and on regular schedule after therapy per physician order.	To decrease incidence of nausea and vomiting.
	Withhold food and fluids for 4 to 6 hours before treatment.	To decrease gastric irritation.
	Provide small feedings and increase fluids.	To maintain nutrition and hydration.
	Provide frequent mouth care.	To promote patient's comfort.
	Provide clean environment with fresh air and no odors.	To reduce noxious stimuli.
	Monitor intake and output, weight, and electrolytes.	To avoid dehydration.
	Administer intravenous therapy as ordered.	To maintain fluid and electrolyte balance.
	Use relaxation techniques, guided imagery, self-hypnosis, and distraction as indicated.	To reduce nausea.

NURSING DIAGNOSIS	NURSING INTERVENTIONS	RATIONALE
Constipation related to impaired intestinal motility	Offer fluids and foods high in fiber and bulk; offer stool softeners or laxatives.	To stimulate motility.
	Avoid enemas.	They may traumatize the intestinal mucosa.
	Use warmth, such as a heating pad.	To relieve discomfort caused by abdominal distention.
Diarrhea related to intestinal irritation	Offer clear liquids.	To prevent dehydration.
	Offer antidiarrheal agent, such as Kaopectate or diphenoxylate (Lomotil), per physician's order.	To control amount and frequency of diarrhea.
	Maintain good perineal care.	To avoid irritation and discomfort.
	Test stools for occult blood.	To identify evidence of blood.
	Record number and consistency of stools.	To monitor need for further intervention.
	Observe for dehydration and electrolyte imbalance.	To detect complications early.
Altered oral mucous membranes related to poor oral hygiene, preexisting dental disorders, or drug-induced irritation	Avoid alcohol and tobacco.	They irritate mucous membranes.
	Encourage good oral hygiene.	To promote comfort and prevent infection.
	Discourage spicy and hot foods.	To avoid irritation or pain.
	Offer topical agents for relief of pain (lidocaine or dyclonine) per physician's order.	To soothe irritated mucous membranes.
	Apply water-soluble lubricant (K-Y Jelly) to lips.	To maintain moisture.
	Offer popsicles.	For hydration and comfort.
	Use oral assessment guide to monitor changes in voice and ability to swallow, as well as condition of lips, tongue, mucous membranes, gingiva, teeth, and saliva.	To evaluate response to interventions.
	Avoid foods that are difficult to chew, such as apples, and highly acidic beverages such as citrus juices.	To avoid irritation.
	Administer nystatin oral suspension or suppository or clotrimazole (Mycelex) troche per physician's order.	To combat infection.

NURSING DIAGNOSIS	NURSING INTERVENTIONS	RATIONALE
	Have patient postpone dental work if possible; have patient brush teeth gently and use toothettes.	To avoid further trauma.
Altered nutrition: less than body requirements related to gastrointestinal irritation and increased body requirements	Offer bland or pureed foods.	To facilitate swallowing.
	Have patient avoid spicy foods, alcohol, and tobacco.	To decrease irritation.
	Offer antacids.	To counteract gastric acid.
	Identify food preferences.	To increase patient's interest in eating.
	Offer small, frequent feedings.	To avoid distention.
	Do not rush meals.	So patient will increase intake.
	Keep room free of odors and clutter.	To reduce noxious stimuli.
	Provide meticulous mouth care.	To enhance appetite.
	Use enteral feeding tube or total parenteral nutrition if necessary.	To maintain nutritional balance.
	Weigh daily.	To monitor nutritional status.
Impaired skin integrity related to drug-induced changes, extravasation	*For alopecia:* Help patient plan for wig, scarf, or hat before hair loss.	To enhance patient's self-image.
	Offer tourniquet or ice cap preventive therapy based on policy and diagnosis.	To decrease hair loss.
	Have patient wash and comb remaining hair gently.	To decrease hair loss.
	Reassure patient that hair will grow back after therapy.	To lessen patient's anxiety regarding hair loss.
	For dermatitis: Use cornstarch, Alpha Keri, calamine lotion, or other agent.	To relieve itching.
	Warn against overexposure to sun.	To avoid further irritation.
	Keep skin clean and dry.	To avoid infection.
	For changes in color of skin or nail beds: Assure patient that discoloration will fade with time.	To lessen patient's anxiety regarding discoloration.

NURSING DIAGNOSIS	NURSING INTERVENTIONS	RATIONALE
	Use nail polish according to patient's wishes.	To mask discoloration.
	For jaundice: Monitor hepatic enzymes.	To determine liver function.
	Assess skin and sclera daily.	For evidence of increase or decrease in discoloration.
	For extravasation: Observe for early signs, which include pain or burning sensation at or above IV site, blanching, redness, swelling, slowing of infusion, absence of blood return.	To detect problem before tissue damage occurs.
	Stop infusion; aspirate remaining drug from needle, inject antidote, and apply topical ointment, heat, or cold as dictated by protocol.	To prevent tissue damage.
Impaired gas exchange related to anemia, pulmonary fibrosis, cardiotoxicity	Monitor respiratory function with pulmonary function tests.	To detect changes in status.
	Note limitation of lifetime dosage of bleomycin.	To prevent irreversible toxicity.
	Help with pulmonary function studies.	To detect changes in status.
	Provide oxygen therapy, sedative, cough suppressants, and steroids as prescribed.	For symptom management.
	Have patient change position slowly, and encourage adequate rest.	To conserve energy.
	Observe patient for dyspnea and increased weakness.	As evidence of further dysfunction.
	Monitor hemoglobin and hematocrit.	To determine effect of therapy.
	Administer transfusions as ordered.	To increase red blood cell count.
	Monitor heart rate, blood pressure, and ECG.	To detect cardiac dysfunction.
Altered peripheral tissue perfusion related to bleeding	Protect patient from injury (e.g., use precautions when shaving with razor blade, do not permit cluttered environment, and do not administer rectal suppositories).	To avoid trauma.
	Have patient avoid using aspirin and aspirin products.	They increase clotting time.

NURSING DIAGNOSIS	NURSING INTERVENTIONS	RATIONALE
	Avoid giving injections; if they are necessary, apply pressure at site for 3 to 5 minutes afterward.	To prevent bleeding.
	Use toothettes for oral care.	To avoid trauma to mucosa.
	Monitor skin (petechiae, ecchymoses), urine, and platelet count.	For evidence of bleeding.
	Evaluate neurologic status.	To identify intracranial bleeding.
	Have nasal packing available.	In case bleeding occurs.
	Administer platelet transfusions as necessary.	To control bleeding.
	Monitor vital signs.	To detect bleeding early.
	Support patient in ambulation.	To prevent injury related to weakness.
Potential for infection related to leukopenia, bone marrow suppression	Warn patient to avoid crowds and people with colds, flu, or cold sores.	To prevent exposure to infection.
	Use sterile technique whenever needed.	To prevent infection.
	Initiate reverse isolation as indicated.	To protect patient from pathogens.
	Monitor temperature and leukocyte count; observe skin temperature, color, and odor.	To detect signs of infection.
	Encourage careful hygiene.	To prevent infection.
	Discourage fresh-cut flowers.	They may carry microorganisms.
	Avoid using indwelling catheters or performing rectal procedures or examinations.	To prevent infection.
	Administer antibiotics as prescribed.	To treat infection.
	Provide analgesics as ordered.	To reduce fever.
	Encourage fluids.	To prevent dehydration.
Sexual dysfunction related to drug-induced changes in hormonal status	Help patient explore alternatives for sterility (e.g., sperm banking, hormonal therapy during treatment, and postponement of conception and childbearing). Refer to sexual counselor as needed.	To provide support regarding possible changes in sexuality.

NURSING DIAGNOSIS	NURSING INTERVENTIONS	RATIONALE
Altered patterns of urinary elimination related to drug-induced nephrotoxicity	Force fluids.	To maintain renal blood flow.
	Monitor blood urea nitrogen, serum creatinine, creatinine clearance, and electrolytes.	They indicate renal function.
	Monitor intake and output; check for edema.	To detect renal dysfunction.
	Administer diuretics as ordered.	To enhance renal excretion.
	Encourage foods high in potassium.	To prevent diuretic-related hypokalemia.
	Administer normal saline and mannitol before cisplatin therapy per physician's order.	To maintain fluid and electrolyte balance.
	Administer allopurinol as prescribed with high fluid intake.	To prevent uric acid accumulation in kidneys.
	Encourage patient to empty bladder frequently, especially at night.	To avoid stasis, inflammation, and infection.
	Provide adequate hydration.	To maintain renal function.
Sensory/perceptual alterations (auditory, tactile) related to drug-induced neurotoxicity	Monitor hearing with baseline and periodic audiograms.	To detect hearing loss early.
	Speak clearly and in normal tone of voice.	To enhance communication.
	Assess patient for numbness and tingling in extremities.	To detect development of paresthesias.
	Prohibit smoking and have patient observe placement of feet and hands.	To encourage safety.
Impaired physical mobility related to drug-induced gout, osteoporosis, myelotoxicity	Monitor calcium level.	To determine bone status.
	Provide safety measures.	To prevent injury.
	Be alert for complaint of pain over bony area; if patient has such a complaint, maintain bed rest until x-rays are taken for fracture.	To detect bone disease.
	Use assistive devices for ambulation.	To enhance tolerance of activity.
	Encourage range-of-motion exercises.	To maintain mobility.
	Position patient in proper anatomic alignment.	To avoid stretching, pressure, or fracture.

NURSING DIAGNOSIS	NURSING INTERVENTIONS	RATIONALE
Altered cardiopulmonary tissue perfusion related to pneumonitis, pericarditis, myocarditis, anemia, and bleeding	Auscultate lungs, and report signs of pleural rub.	To detect respiratory problems early.
	Observe for cough, dyspnea, and pain on inspiration.	These indicate respiratory dysfunction.
	Treat with antibiotics and steroids as prescribed.	To reduce irritation and prevent infection.
	Auscultate heart, and report signs of friction rub, dysrhythmia, or hypertension.	To detect complications.
	Observe for chest pain and weakness.	These indicate cardiac dysfunction.
	Monitor ECG reports.	To monitor cardiac function.
	Administer drugs as prescribed.	To counteract dysrhythmias.
	Encourage adequate rest; alternate rest and activity periods.	To avoid stress on respiratory system.
	Observe patient for dyspnea and increased weakness.	These are signs of further anemia.
	Administer oxygen therapy as needed.	To increase oxygenation of tissues.
	Monitor hemoglobin and hematocrit.	To determine effectiveness of therapy.
	Administer transfusions as ordered.	To increase circulating red blood cells.
Ineffective individual coping related to stress of dealing with chemotherapy	Assess patient's coping behavior, and determine its effectiveness.	To detect need for new coping strategies.
	Reassure patient that mood changes are temporary and dose related.	To reduce anxiety regarding mood changes.
	Allow independence in self-care.	To maintain patient's self-esteem and promote effective coping.
	Maintain supportive, nonjudgmental attitude.	To foster patient coping.
	Encourage use of resources, such as support groups.	To assist patient in coping.
	Encourage patient to express fears.	To identify problem-solving strategies.

5   EVALUATE

PATIENT OUTCOME	DATA INDICATING THAT OUTCOME IS REACHED
Patient has adequate hydration.	Patient has no nausea or vomiting, intake and output are balanced, patient's weight is normal, and electrolytes are within normal limits.
Patient has normal bowel elimination.	Patient has no constipation, diarrhea, or distention.
Patient's oral mucous membranes are healthy.	Mucous membranes, lips, tongue, and gingiva are moist and normal in color; patient's teeth are clean, and saliva is adequate; patient can swallow and speaks in a normal voice.
Patient's nutrition is adequate.	Patient has no complaints of anorexia or unusual taste sensations; patient can eat and swallow without pain, and weight is normal.
Patient has healthy, intact skin.	Patient has no complaints of itching, and there is no evidence of rash or changes in pigmentation; patient has hair on head.
Patient has adequate gas exchange and peripheral tissue perfusion.	Patient has no complaints of fatigue or weakness, and skin is warm and pink; respirations, pulse, blood pressure, and ECG are normal; there are no signs or symptoms of bleeding or cardiac dysfunction.
Patient has no infection.	Patient's temperature and WBC are normal; skin is cool and dry.
Patient has normal sexual function.	Patient has satisfactory libido and has made plans for dealing with possible sterility.
Patient has normal urinary elimination.	Patient has no complaints of urinary distress, and intake and output are balanced.
Patient has normal hearing and sense of touch.	Patient can hear speaker and is aware of sensations on body.
Patient has normal physical mobility.	Patient can ambulate without assistance.
Patient can cope with stress of therapy.	Patient discusses fears, anger, and sadness but focuses on problem solving.

PATIENT TEACHING

1. Encourage the patient to maintain adequate nutrition and hydration.
2. Emphasize the need for self-care to control nausea, vomiting, constipation, diarrhea, urinary distress, oral irritation, and itching, which may include appropriate use of medications (see Patient Teaching Guide).
3. Discuss the warning signs of bleeding that should be reported to the physician, as well as safety measures (see Patient Teaching Guide).
4. Emphasize the need to take temperature, use good hand-washing techniques, identify and report signs of infection, and avoid exposure to infected individuals (see Patient Teaching Guide).

NUTRITIONAL SUPPORT

Patients with cancer must deal not only with the metabolic effects of the disease on their nutritional status but also with the effects of treatment. In addition, being unable to eat or having difficulty eating may affect the patient psychologically, since eating is not only a basic human need but often a source of social interaction. Patients with cancer who have anorexia, nausea and vomiting, stomatitis, changes in taste, and difficulty swallowing face the challenge of eating when they least want or are able to do so, yet have the greatest need for good nutrition. Numerous research studies have shown that poor nutritional status adversely affects the patient's ability to tolerate both cancer and its treatment.

The body of an individual with cancer responds to the increased demand for glucose, which is required by both normal and cancer cells, by increasing the rate of gluconeogenesis. This is the synthesis of glucose by the liver and renal cortex from noncarbohydrate sources such as lactate and amino acids. When protein is broken down to provide amino acids for gluconeogenesis, muscle wasting is the result. Progressive muscle wasting, called cachexia, gives the patient a characteristic appearance of emaciation.

Fat metabolization is also adversely affected in individuals with cancer. Fat stored in the form of fatty acids is mobilized from adipose tissue and released into the bloodstream for use as fuel. This process, which is controlled by the inhibitory effects of insulin, is compromised in people with cancer, so that body stores of fat are depleted as the disease progresses.

People with cancer also have deficiencies in such vitamins as A, thiamine, and C. Iron deficiency may also occur. Fluid and electrolyte imbalances include hypercalcemia, hyperuricemia, hyperphosphatemia, and hyperkalemia. These alterations result from either the direct or indirect effects of tumors, such as paraneoplastic syndromes (see Chapter 4).

Poor nutrition also adversely affects immunocompetence, by decreasing the size of the lymphoid tissues, including the spleen, lymph nodes, and thymus. The resulting decreased function of B- and T-cell lymphocytes, directly correlated with the degree of malnutrition, produces delayed hypersensitivity response.

Local effects of cancer, such as tumors that adversely affect chewing, swallowing, and peristalsis, can alter the patient's nutritional status. Obstruction, pain, and distention affect the patient's ability to digest and metabolize food.

As discussed earlier, treatment modalities may also compromise the patient's nutritional status. Thus the nurse must assess the patient's nutritional status frequently to obtain a baseline measure and to identify the need for aggressive intervention. Clinical observation, including identification of concurrent health problems (diabetes, hypertension, malabsorption), psychosocial factors (home environment, methods of food preparation, the patient's body image), and physical assessment provide the data needed to monitor the patient's nutritional status. Examining the hair, teeth, gums, and general muscle tone can facilitate detection of early signs of nutritional deficiencies.

Dietary evaluation is also useful and includes a 24-hour food diary, a complete dietary history with food allergies and preferences, direct observation of dietary intake, and evaluation of nutrient composition. Biochemical measurements include such laboratory values as serum albumin, serum transferrin, total lymphocyte count, and urine urea nitrogen. Anthropometric measurements include the patient's midarm muscle circumference (MAMC), triceps skin fold thickness (SFT), subscapular skin fold thickness (SST), and weight for height.

Nutritional interventions for the person with cancer have been shown to decrease the morbidity and mortality of cancer by preventing weight loss, increasing response to therapy, minimizing the side effects of treatment, and improving the quality of life. The type of nutritional support the patient requires is based on functional abilities and limitations, severity of the nutritional deficiency, potential for complications, duration of therapy, cost, and psychologic effect.

Nutritional support may include oral, enteral, and parenteral nutritional management. The oral route is preferred, because it is more natural and least invasive. Oral nutritional support may range from adding sauces and gravies to foods to more complex interventions such as dietary supplements. The patient with anorexia may benefit from frequent small meals and snacks. Foods high in protein and calories are recommended, such as cheese, fish, poultry, milkshakes, peanut butter on crackers, and prepackaged puddings.

If the patient has stomatitis or taste alterations, a high-calorie bland diet may be helpful. The patient should avoid seasoning and liquids with high acidity such as orange and lemon juices. Measures such as using a topical analgesic, good mouth care, and avoiding commercial mouthwashes reduce oral discomfort. Cold foods such as popsicles and ice cream have a numbing effect, which patients tolerate better than warm or hot foods.

Psychosocial support is also critical. Both the patient and family should be encouraged to try a variety of strategies and to be supportive of one another, since this is a difficult and challenging problem. Sometimes eating at the table with family and friends in an attractive sociable environment can enhance the patient's appetite. Using small plates, eating more often, and decreasing exposure to strong food odors may also be helpful. Antiemetics and artificial saliva can be used to control the symptoms of gastrointestinal irritation.

High-calorie, high-protein supplements such as Isocal, Polycose, and Vivonex may be helpful to the patient; however, they are not well tolerated by patients with lactose intolerance.

The enteral route via a feeding tube may be needed by patients who are anorectic, hypermetabolic, or unconscious, as well as those who have a mechanical impairment. Parenteral feeding is indicated only for patients with totally nonfunctioning gastrointestinal tracts, who require bowel rest, or who cannot tolerate enteral nutritional support.

Patients with functioning gastrointestinal tracts who cannot ingest adequate nutrients to meet their metabolic demands should be considered for enteral feeding. These include patients with anorexia; cachexia; cancers of the head or neck, esophagus, and stomach; central nervous system disease that impairs swallowing; and intractable diarrhea.

Tube feedings may be administered by the nasogastric, nasoduodenal, nasojejunal, esophagostomy, gastrostomy, and jejunostomy routes (Figure 10-10). The most common routes involve passage of a small, flexible feeding tube through the nose into the stomach or intestine. Feeding ostomies, such as the gastrostomy, usually require surgical percutaneous insertion and are preferred for long-term nutritional support. The cervical esophagostomy is a surgically created, skin-lined canal extending from the border of the neck to the area below the cervical esophagus; the feeding tube is passed through this opening to the stomach for each feeding and then removed.

Aspiration may occur more often with gastric feedings, because only the gastroesophageal sphincter is functioning to prevent gastric reflux, whereas the intestinal feedings use both the gastroesophageal and pyloric sphincters to prevent reflux. When feedings are improperly selected or administered, nausea, diarrhea, and cramps can occur.

The volume and concentration of the nutrient provided by tube feeding should meet the needs of the individual and should be compatible with the size and location of the tube and the patient's tolerance of formula strength and rate of administration. Feedings may be delivered by bolus or gravity, as well as by enteral pump. The position of the tube and gastric residual should be checked frequently. The patient should be monitored for the development of dumping syndrome, aspiration, weight loss, or diarrhea, each of which requires evaluation of the formula and infusion rate for changes.

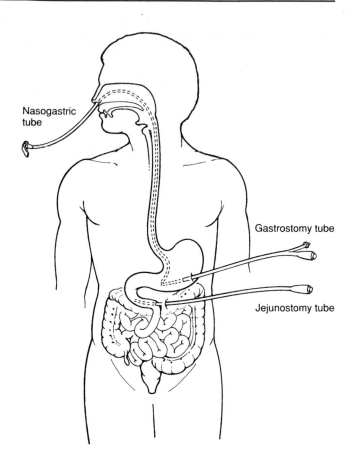

FIGURE 10-10
Three routes for tube feeding. (From Otto.[45])

The patient may also complain of thirst, taste deprivation, and inability to satisfy the appetite, as well as a sense of altered body image. The patient may be permitted to chew gum or suck on hard candies, drink fluids, and eat soft, bland foods. Referral to a support group may help the patient accept the changes in the social and aesthetic aspects of eating.

Complications of tube feedings may be mechanical (nasal irritation and erosion, esophagitis or pharyngitis, tube dislocation or occlusion), gastrointestinal (abdominal distention, nausea and vomiting, constipation, or diarrhea), respiratory (aspiration pneumonia), or metabolic (hyperglycemia, hypokalemia, hyperkalemia, hypernatremia, and dehydration). The nurse and patient should monitor the feedings to identify problems early and intervene before serious alterations occur. Since many patients now receive enteral feedings in the home, a caregiver and the patient should be taught general care of the patient and the tube to ensure safe and effective therapy.

Parenteral nutrition, also called hyperalimentation, supplies all of the essential nutrients by intravenous infusion. Total parenteral nutrition (TPN) supplies all of the daily requirements for protein and calories directly into the patient's bloodstream; it is indicated for patients with cancer of the gastrointestinal tract, other obstructions, radiation enteritis, and intractable diarrhea, to name but a few conditions.

Total parenteral nutrition is delivered via peripheral veins, most often those of the arm or the external jugular vein. Limitations of peripheral infusion include provision of limited calories, vein irritation, and limited usefulness for long-term therapy. Use of a central line into a major vein such as the superior vena cava provides for a large amount of calories and protein, high dextrose and amino acid concentrations, and usefulness for long-term therapy. Central lines used for total parenteral nutrition include ports, triple lumen catheters, and Broviac, Hickman, and Groshong catheters. When central infusion is used, the solution must be tapered by rate and concentration to discontinue therapy without inducing profound hypoglycemia.

Total parenteral nutrition contains glucose, amino acids, and fats to provide both immediate and long-term energy. Patients receiving total parenteral nutrition usually have a multilumen central venous catheter inserted to serve as access for administering medications and drawing blood.

Total parenteral nutrition may be given continuously or by cycling; cycling at night is used most often for patients receiving TPN at home. Cycling enables the patient to be mobile during the day but does require the ability to tolerate a high-volume load. Programmable pumps are used to prevent or minimize hypoglycemia and hyperglycemia. Ambulatory patients benefit from using the portable pump, which is worn in a backpack-type carrying bag.

The nurse should assess the patient's life-style, home environment, family and support systems, body image, and perceptions about total parenteral nutrition to plan for optimum acceptance of and adaptation to the therapy. Daily monitoring of vital signs, weight, and laboratory values enables the nurse to determine the need for adjusting the formula or rate of administration before the patient's discharge. Follow-up visits in the home are important and ensure the patient's compliance with and tolerance of TPN.

The nurse's role in nutritional support is a critical one that involves comprehensive assessment, monitoring, and patient education to maintain the individual with cancer in optimum nutritional status.

P AIN MANAGEMENT

Patients with cancer and other blood disorders may have pain at any point during the course of their disease and its treatment. In fact, of the 4 million people

---

DATA TO INCLUDE IN PAIN HISTORY

Onset of the pain (when it started)
Precipitating factors (what triggers the pain)
Alleviating factors (what lessens the pain)
Location of the pain
Associated signs and symptoms
Medications taken by the patient and the extent to which they provide relief
Quality and intensity of the pain
Patient's view of the pain
Actions that have helped or not helped to relieve the pain

---

throughout the world who die from cancer each year, 70% experience pain as a primary symptom. Unfortunately, many people believe that pain is an early symptom of disease and do not seek diagnosis until pain occurs. Pain is almost without exception a late symptom of cancer and indicates tumor obstruction, pressure on nerves, invasion of bone, phantom sensation, peripheral neuropathy, postherpetic neuralgia, mucositis, and/or incisional irritation.

It is estimated that 85% of patients with pain can be managed effectively with appropriate therapy. The American Cancer Society, the American Pain Society, the World Health Organization, and the Oncology Nursing Society, as well as many other organizations, consider pain control to be a major issue in the management of a person with cancer and other blood disorders. If not relieved, pain contributes to nausea, vomiting, anorexia, and insomnia. Anxiety, fear, and depression contribute to this pain and interfere with the patient's ability to cope with it.

One of many challenges facing the nurse who cares for the patient with pain is the assessment of the pain. The nurse must accept the definition of pain as whatever the person experiencing the pain says it is, existing wherever the person says it does.[39] This is frustrating to many nurses and physicians, who may doubt the presence and nature of the patient's pain when there are no physiologic parameters by which to measure it. Because there are no direct measures of pain, the nurse must gather data from the patient for use in diagnosing the pain, describing its characteristics, and deciding on the appropriate interventions.

In addition, the nurse should use observational skills to assess the patient's appearance, motor behavior, affective behavior, verbal behavior, brainstem automatic responses (e.g., increase in heart rate, respirations, and blood pressure), spinal cord reflex responses, and nonverbal pain clues. The psychosocial dimensions of the pain must also be explored. These include personality factors, cultural factors, religious factors, the patient's interpretation of pain, the patient's prior experience with pain, and the physical environment in which the patient is experiencing the pain.

Chemical means of pain management include the use of narcotics and nonnarcotics. Nonnarcotic analgesics of value in the treatment of cancer pain are acetaminophen, aspirin, and nonsteroidal antiinflammatory drugs such as ibuprofen, indomethacin, and naproxen. One potential drawback of aspirin is its antiplatelet effect, which can create problems in the myelosuppressed patient. Acetaminophen may be a problem in patients with impaired liver function. Both aspirin and the nonsteroidal antiinflammatory drugs are generally well tolerated but have the potential to cause gastrointestinal ulceration, renal toxic effects, and inhibition of platelet aggregation. If a nonnarcotic does not have a therapeutic effect initially, then the dosage should be increased before another type of drug is tried. When a ceiling is reached with a nonnarcotic, a moderately potent narcotic such as oxycodone or codeine can be added.

Narcotics (opioids) used in the management of pain include morphine (the prototype), hydromorphone, and methadone. Sustained-release morphine in an oral form, such as MS Contin or Roxanol SR, has been found to be of particular value in the management of the terminally ill person with pain. Administering narcotics via intravenous drips, intrathecally, and epidurally enhances the analgesic effect of the opioids. Avoiding the peaks and valleys of pain relief with bolus injections has provided a more constant analgesic effect for patients. The need for around-the-clock dosage has been noted, so that fixed dosage schedules with adequate doses for pain relief provide more constant blood levels and predictable pain relief. Some patients have breakthrough pain that requires additional doses, but the fixed dosage schedule should be maintained. Side effects of the narcotics that require monitoring and intervention by the nurse include constipation, vomiting, and respiratory and central nervous system depression.

Another category of drugs that may be used for pain management is the narcotic agonist/antagonists such as nalbuphine (Nubain), butorphanol (Stadol), pentazocine (Talwin), and buprenorphine (Buprenex). Analgesic potentiators include the phenothiazine derivatives such as promethazine (Phenergan), prochlorperazine (Compazine), and chlorpromazine (Thorazine); hydroxyzine (Vistaril); diazepam (Valium); lorazepam (Ativan); and diphenhydramine (Benadryl). Also used are stimulants such as cocaine, methylphenidate (Ritalin), dextroamphetamine, and caffeine; tricyclic antidepressants such as amitriptyline (Elavil), imipramine (Tofranil), and doxepin (Sinequan); and butyrophenones such as dro-

---

GENERAL GUIDELINES FOR THE USE OF PAIN RELIEF MEASURES

1. Use a variety of pain relief measures.
2. Use pain relief measures before the patient's pain becomes severe.
3. Include pain relief measures that the patient believes will be helpful.
4. Determine the patient's ability or willingness to participate actively in the use of pain relief measures.
5. Rely on patient behavior that indicates pain severity rather than relying on known physical stimuli.
6. Encourage the patient to try a pain relief measure at least two times before abandoning it as ineffective.
7. Have an open mind as to what may relieve the patient's pain, including nonpharmacologic measures.
8. Keep trying to relieve the pain; do not become discouraged and stop working with the patient.

---

peridol (Inapsine) and haloperidol (Haldol).

Patient self-control methods include distraction, massage, relaxation, biofeedback, hypnosis, and imagery (see Patient Teaching Guide). Many patients respond positively to the opportunity for self-care in the management of their pain and perceive that such self-control measures enhance the effectiveness of other prescribed pain interventions.

In each instance the nurse must develop the technical skill needed to initiate and monitor the therapy and to teach the patient and family how to use and maintain the system. Each of these technologies has expanded the options for the patient with pain and increased the degree of self-control.

Other interventions for pain include (1) anesthetic procedures such as nerve blocks, trigger point injections, and the use of nitrous oxide; (2) neuroaugmentive therapies such as counterirritation, rubbing, TENS, and percutaneous nerve stimulation; (3) neuroablative procedures such as cordotomy; and (4) physiatric supportive measures such as using a prosthesis, physical therapy, and occupational therapy.

The nurse's unique contributions to pain management are acting as key link between the patient and the health care team, the amount of time spent with the patient, the ability to assess the patient's response to the pain and its management, and the role of patient and

COMPONENTS OF PAIN TECHNOLOGY

1. External pumps for the intravenous, epidural, and intrathecal administration of narcotic analgesics
2. Implantable pumps for the intravenous, epidural, and intrathecal administration of narcotic analgesics
3. Patient-controlled analgesia (PCA), particularly for the management of acute pain such as postoperative pain (Figure 10-11)
4. Transcutaneous electrical nerve stimulation (TENS)
5. Continuous subcutaneous infusion (CSCI) with an ambulatory infusion pump

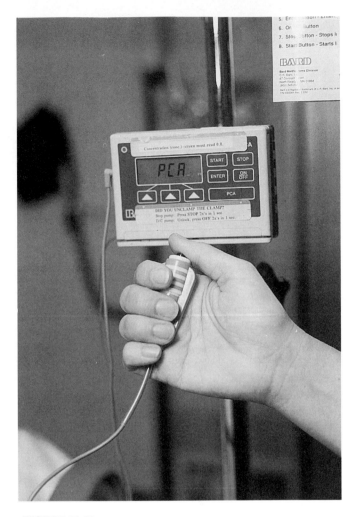

FIGURE 10-11
PCA pump.

family. In addition, the nurse has the ability to articulate a concise pain assessment, use equianalgesic charts for dosage guidelines, and anticipate and address patient, family, and health care provider misconceptions about pain management. For example, many patients and their families have opioid phobia, the irrational and undocumented fear that even appropriate use of narcotics causes addiction. This fear of addiction among both health care providers and the public seems to be a major reason for the undertreatment of pain. The nurse must understand and be able to articulate the differences between addiction, tolerance, and physical dependence in order to use pain management strategies appropriately and to enable patients and their families to accept the therapeutic value of drugs such as the narcotics.

CHAPTER 11

Patient Teaching Guides

Patient education has always been an important part of the nursing process. In today's hospitals, teaching patients about their disease and its treatment poses a great challenge as diagnostic and treatment methods become increasingly complex. Hospitalized patients often are confronted by an array of threatening-looking equipment, and many procedures are based on technology that is unfamiliar to the general public. Compounding these problems is the shortened hospital stay for most patients.

Written materials can help patients understand their treatments and what they must do to manage at home. This chapter provides handouts that can be photocopied and given to patients or their caregivers to take home and use for self-care. Specific materials that explain anticoagulant therapy and genetic counseling are among those used by nurses who care for patients with hematologic disorders. Some of the guides list step-by-step instructions for certain procedures.

More than one guide may be needed for a particular patient. For example, a patient undergoing chemotherapy will need to know how to deal with loss of appetite, how to prevent infection and bleeding, and how to manage pain without drugs. Guides that explain preventive measures such as dealing with stress and quitting smoking are also included.

Mosby's
Clinical Nursing
Series

General Safety Precautions

More deaths in the United States are caused by accidents than most people realize. In fact, accidents are the leading cause of death for children in this country. Yet about 90% of all accidents are preventable. Most households would reduce their annual need for emergency medical treatment, if they would simply observe general safety precautions in a few key areas of their life-style.

Take time to check your own surroundings for potential hazards, and reduce or eliminate them. Below are some general guidelines for preventing common accidents. These guidelines encompass motor vehicles, sports and recreation, electrical and mechanical equipment, preventing falls, poisonings and ingestions, fire, and swimming pools. Use this as a checklist to evaluate your safety standards.

Motor vehicles

Naturally all automobiles should be maintained in good mechanical condition. Seat belts should be worn at all times; never start the car until everyone has buckled up. You'll be surprised at how little time it takes for your friends and family to start buckling up automatically whenever they ride with you! Look carefully in front and in back of the car before accelerating and make sure all car doors are locked when a child travels in your car. Young children should never be left alone in a car, and heavy or sharp objects should not be placed on the same seat with a child. Small children should ride in a car seat appropriate for their age.

Sports and recreation

Many accidents in sports and recreation could be prevented by keeping equipment in good condition and proper working order.

We live in a rushed age. We often go directly from work to recreation or sports programs. Still, train yourself always to stop by the locker room first: always wear appropriate clothing and shoes (if needed) for the activity. You'll prevent a lot of injuries over the years by simply taking a few minutes before you play. Once involved in the sport or activity of your choice, do not attempt activities beyond your physical endurance. Injuring yourself will simply put you further back on the fitness scale.

Finally, keep all firearms and ammunition locked up.

Electrical and mechanical equipment

Only devices approved by Underwriters' Laboratories should be installed, and they should be inspected periodically. Dry your hands before touching appliances, and keep radios, fans, portable heaters, and hair dryers out of the bathroom. Discourage children from playing with or being in an area where appliances or power tools (e.g., washing machine, clothes dryer, saw, or lawn mower) are being used. Disconnect appliances after using them and before attempting minor repairs. Avoid overloading electrical circuits.

Keep garden equipment and machinery in a restricted area. As soon as each child in your household is old enough, teach him or her how to use the equipment properly.

Preventing falls

You might be surprised at the number of broken bones that are a result of falls in or around the house each year. These are not only painful, time-consuming, and expensive to fix—they can also be pretty embarrassing! Here are a few quick tips for saving bones, medical bills, and face:

Keep stairs well-lighted and free of clutter; provide sturdy railings. Anchor small rugs securely, and use rubber mats in the bathtub and shower. Use only sturdy ladders for climbing.

Poisonings and ingestions

Poisonings and ingestions are the most common type of household accident among children and the elderly, but they can happen to anyone. Below are a few general guidelines.

When cleaning, never mix bleaches with ammonia, vinegar, and other household cleaners. Label all medications clearly, and childproof your home by placing medications out of reach of children. But, just in case, keep emergency medical numbers clear, up-to-date, and easy to find.

Fire

Figure out an adequate fire escape plan, and routinely conduct home fire drills. Teach each child the escape routes as soon as he or she is old enough.

Keep a pressure-type hand fire extinguisher on each floor of your household. Instruct all family members who are old enough in its use. In addition, teach children about the danger of smoke inhalation. Use such slogans as "Stop, drop, and roll" to help children remember not to run if flames are on their clothing or bodies.

Fit fireplaces with snug fireplace screens. Store gasoline and other flammable fluids in tightly covered containers that are clearly labeled, and keep them away from heat and sparks. Dispose of paint- and oil-soaked cloth quickly.

Buy flame-retardant sleepwear, and mark the children's rooms so that they are obvious to firefighters.

Swimming pools

Completely enclose your pool with a fence that complies with local regulations. The gate should be self-closing and have a lock. It's a good idea to indicate water depth with numbers on the edge of the pool so that all swimmers can gauge how close they can go to the deep end. Place a safety float line where the bottom slope begins to deepen.

Install at least one ladder at each end of the pool. Ladders should have handrails on both sides, and the diameter of the rails should be small enough for a child to grasp.

Install underwater lighting as well as outdoor lights if the pool is used at night. A ground fault circuit interrupter should be installed on the pool circuit to cut off electrical power and thus prevent electrocutions in case of electrical fault.

Instruct everyone who uses your pool in such safety rules as not swimming alone and not running around the pool or pushing others. Do not use radios or other electrical appliances near the pool.

Use nonslip materials on ladders, deck, and diving boards. Finally, keep essential rescue devices and first-aid equipment close to the pool.

Emergency precautions

The first step in any effort to prepare for emergencies is to record emergency telephone numbers in an obvious and easily accessible place. Keep a well-stocked first-aid kit immediately available for emergencies.

Obtain instruction in the principles of first aid, and see that these are also taught to all family members as soon as they are old enough. Professional instruction can be obtained through an official Red Cross first-aid course or an adult education program.

Wherever they get their training in these important issues, be sure that everyone knows the first-aid procedures for burns; electrical shock; poisoning; cardiopulmonary arrest; cuts, scrapes, and punctures; drowning; and fractures.

Teach any children in your household safety precautions for bicycles, answering the telephone or door, keeping strangers outside the home, and crossing the street.

Finally, be sure you know the location of gas, water, and electrical switches and how to turn them off in an emergency.

Miscellaneous

Take advantage of preventive health care by obtaining recommended immunizations and by having regular physical examinations. Seek immediate treatment of all diseases and health problems. Finally, to maintain good health in general, balance work, rest, and exercise in daily living.

Therapeutic Exercise: Focus on Walking

What exactly is meant by "therapeutic exercise"?

Therapeutic exercise is the motion of the body or its parts to achieve symptom-free movement and function. It is used to develop and retrain deficient muscles; to restore as much normal movement as possible to prevent deformity; to stimulate the functions of various organs and body systems; to build strength and endurance; and to promote relaxation.

Various theories and methods have been proposed to improve health through exercise and movement. Decreased physical activity, which may be the result of illness or treatment, can lead to anxiety, depression, weakness, fatigue, and nausea. Regular, moderate exercise can prevent these feelings and help a person feel energetic.

Aerobic exercise (the sustained rhythmic activity of large muscle groups, which entails using large amounts of oxygen) increases heart rate, stroke volume, respiratory rate, and relaxation of blood vessels. Cardiovascular fitness and increased stamina are the goals. Body fat is also reduced. Aerobic exercises include running, jogging, brisk walking, swimming, aquadynamics, and aerobic dance.

Always check with your doctor before beginning any exercise program and for help in choosing the type of exercise that is best for you. Whatever type you choose, the goal should be to maintain a regular, moderate exercise program to enhance physical and emotional health. The exercise should involve large muscle groups in dynamic movement for about 20 minutes 3 or more days a week. The exertion should be within limits appropriate to your physical status and needs. At the end of exercise you should feel replenished rather than bored, burned out, or excessively fatigued.

What makes walking a good form of regular exercise?

Walking allows for psychomotor expression without the hazards of contact sports and is adaptable to a wide range of weather or geographic conditions, schedules, personalities, and body types. It can be social or asocial, organized or unorganized as an activity. The long-term effects on joints and organs of regular, sustained, vigorous walking currently are unknown; physicians do report a lower incidence of the type of musculoskeletal damage resulting from the "pounding" effects of jogging.

Making time for exercising regularly is hard. What can I do to make it easier?

There are two major obstacles to overcome in undertaking and maintaining an exercise program: making exercise part of a life-style and avoiding injury. Suggestions for making exercise a safe part of a life-style include:

1. Start in small increments, and keep it fun.
2. Avoid exercising for 2 hours after a large meal, and do not eat for 1 hour after exercising.
3. Include at least 10 minutes of warm-up and cool-down exercises.
4. Use proper equipment and clothing.
5. Post goals, pictures of the ideal self, and notes of encouragement in a readily seen place for self-encouragement.
6. Use visualization daily to picture successful attainment of exercise benefit (e.g., looking toned or graceful or achieving an ideal weight).
7. Keep records of weekly measures of weight, blood pressure, and pulse.
8. Focus on the rewards of exercise; keep a record of feelings, and compare differences in relaxation, energy, concentration, and sleep patterns.
9. Work with a peer or join a structured exercise class, running club, or fitness center. Spend more time with people dedicated to wellness.
10. Stop exercising or at least slow down and consult with a practitioner if any unusual, unexplainable symptoms occur.
11. Reward yourself for working toward exercise goals as well as attaining them. For example, after a month in an exercise program, buy a new pair of running shoes or treat yourself to a special wish.

What does a walking (or "rhythmic walking") program entail?

Rhythmic walking consists of walking briskly, arms swinging, so your whole body is involved in the rhythm of your movement and your heart rate is increased. It is a regular program to benefit every system of your body.

A good exercise plan starts slowly, allowing your body time to adjust. It is important that you do something to exercise the whole body on a regular basis. *Regular* means every day, or at least every other day; build up to about 20 minutes 3 or more days a week. The right kind of exercise never makes you feel sore, stiff, or exhausted.

We repeat: *first check with your physician.* Before starting a program, it is important to know if there are precautions you need to take. This is especially important if you have high blood pressure, diabetes, joint or bone problems, or heart disease. People with these conditions can exercise, but they must follow certain guidelines to do it safely.

Rhythmic walking is inexpensive. It requires no special equipment or uniforms. Wear comfortable clothes in which you can move freely. You must have the right kind of shoes. Running or jogging shoes or the shoes specially designed for walking are good. The wrong shoes can cause painful damage, such as tendonitis. Select shoes designed for walking, jogging, or running; look for a shock-absorbent cushioning midsole. A watch with a second hand to measure your heart rate is also important.

Everyone who exercises outside the home should carry identification and change for a telephone call and money for a taxi. Some people like to carry a small water bottle such as a plastic soda bottle. To carry these items, a small backpack or hip pack leaves your hands free to swing.

If it is wet, slippery, or hot, or if you feel unsafe walking in your neighborhood, enclosed shopping malls can be great places for walking. Some malls open early, before the shopping crowds arrive, especially for people who want to walk.

How hard should I exercise?

Your heart rate is the best indicator of how hard your body is working. As you work harder, your heart rate increases; as you slow down, your heart rate decreases. You can take your pulse to measure your heart rate. To experience the benefits of exercise, you need to work hard enough to get your heart rate up to a certain point, called the *training heart rate,* and keep it there. Your nurse or doctor can tell you what your training heart rate should be and how to take your own pulse. Find these two things out before beginning your exercise regimen.

How long should I exercise?

It is important to start exercising slowly and build up gradually. If you have been very ill or have not been exercising on a regular basis, start with a 5- or 10-minute walk and add 2 minutes each week. If you are able to build up endurance without problems, work up to 45 minutes daily or every other day. More than 60 minutes of rhythmic walking daily is not necessary.

A good work-out consists of three phases: warm-up, training period, and cool-down. The warm-up is necessary to prepare the body for exercise. Warm up by walking slowly. Next, begin rhythmic walking. This is your training period. Work up to your target heart rate, and walk steadily for your set period of time. Finally, walk slowly to cool off. The cool-down is necessary to help your body recover and to prevent soreness or stiffness.

If you are exercising correctly, you should never feel exhausted after the cool-down. If you do, slow down and take it easier next time. If you feel fatigued for hours after exercise or if you feel sore and stiff, you have done too much or exercised incorrectly.

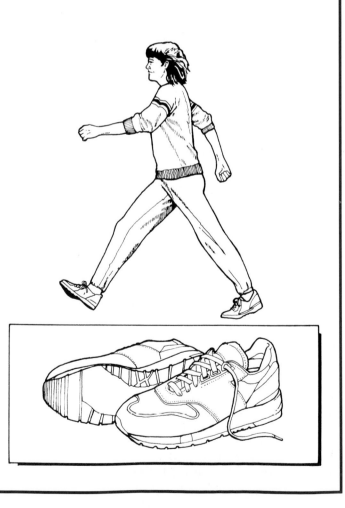

Dealing With Stress

Stress and stressors

Quick! Can you identify which of the following are causes of stress: the fender-bender during rush hour or getting a new car? Too much chocolate or a ringing telephone? Facing retirement or having a baby? Getting laid off or getting that incredible job you dreamed of? The correct answer: all of the above. In fact, the word "Quick!" at the beginning of this paragraph can cause stress in the tense, worried, or even enthusiastic reader. Stress is neither good nor bad. Stress is a general term used to describe change, and a stressor is anything that can cause a response in you, whether physically, mentally, or emotionally. Stressors, like stress, are neither good nor bad. They take on meaning only as you react to them. Stressors fall into three categories: environmental (that ringing telephone), physical (too much chocolate!), or psychological (having a baby or a fender-bender; both of these stressors tend to provoke an emotional response).

The stress response

So what happens when you're hit by a stressor? Physiologically, your body enters a state of arousal. For example, blood is diverted from the digestive functions to muscles to prepare the body for action. Nerve impulses signal the heart to beat harder and faster; blood pressure and pulse rate both rise. Changes occur in the movements of the stomach and intestines, and hormones secreted into the body mobilize sugar and blood, making more energy available to the brain and muscles. All of this is your body's effort to defend itself. Psychologically, you respond by trying to evaluate the emotional impact of the situation. This can calm you down or make you even more upset. This often depends, too, on the kind of stress you're experiencing: short-term or long-term. Short-term stress is a healthy kind of stress, because it represents a challenge or a threat, which causes an alarm reaction and elicits a response, which resolves the situation and eliminates the stress. Short-term stress is the kind of stress we were designed to deal with. Long-term stress is what causes the most trouble. All of us have a certain amount of long-term stress—experiences or situations that may never be resolved in our lifetime, such as coping with a chronic illness of a family member, financial problems, or conflict in the work site. But if this level of emotional arousal continues over a prolonged period, the body pays a price for the strain.

In a crisis, your doctor may prescribe therapy or medication. But for ongoing, daily stress situations, a variety of relaxation techniques or exercises can provide the individual in stress with nonmedical relief. These can range from passive or concentration responses (e.g., meditation, progressive relaxation, imagery, yoga, positive health promotion, vacations, and biofeedback) to active coping techniques (e.g., humor, reading, socializing with friends, exercising, and engaging in sports, music, art, or a craft). A few specific stress management techniques are outlined below. You can get more details on any of these from your physician or a stress management clinic or workshop.

Stress charting. A good first step is to "chart" or track down the stressors in your life, so that you are aware of where they come from. Sometimes the individual under stress discovers stressors that simply don't need to *be* stressors—causes that had simply not been noticed. The first step is to list all the stressors present and the area of life in which each stressor occurs (e.g., family members, friends, work, health, finances, social concerns, recreation, or church). Then each stressor is rated as to effect, using a scale of 1 to 5. Awareness gained from this exercise may motivate you to making decisions about life-style changes or in choosing relaxation techniques.

Progressive relaxation. A simple relaxation technique that can be done anywhere and at any time is progressive relaxation. Find a quiet, soothing, private place and, with eyes closed, concentrate on relaxing each part of the body, beginning with the toes and concentrating on each muscle and joint, moving up the body and ending with the head. Some people like to imagine all the stress or pain leaving each muscle as it relaxes, finally visualizing the stress leaving the body through the top of the head. Others like to incorporate deep-breathing exercises into this practice. However you choose to do it, try to allow yourself time after this exercise to sit quietly for a few minutes before resuming your daily activities.

Acupuncture, acupressure, shiatsu, and reflexology. *Acupuncture* is based on the Chinese philosophy that all life is a microcosm of a vast, constantly changing, flowing circle of energy. The body can reach a balanced state only if both the "rising" energy (yang) and "descending" energy (yin) are flowing smoothly. *Acupressure,* the predecessor of acupuncture, is the term applied to a number of techniques of applying pressure to stimulate acupuncture points on the body. Both techniques release tension and relieve pain and are used to balance energy by applying needles or pressure to specific points. *Shiatsu* is an ancient form of manipulation administered by the thumbs, fingers, and palms, without any instruments, to correct internal malfunctioning, maintain health, and treat disease. *Reflexology* is a technique based on the premise that body organs have corresponding reflex points on other parts of the body.

Biofeedback. Biofeedback is a means of receiving feedback or a message from the body about internal physiologic processes, using specific techniques or equipment to read tension and to learn ways of releasing that tension when cues of stress response are identified.

Massage is a systematic manipulation of the body tissue that benefits the nervous and muscular systems, local and general circulation, the skin, viscera, and metabolism. During massage the hands stimulate the sensory receptors of the skin and subcutaneous tissues, causing a series of reflex effects, including capillary vasodilation or constriction, relaxation or stimulation of voluntary muscle contraction, and possible sedation or stimulation of pain in an area far from the area touched.

Yoga is an Indian philosophic system that emphasizes the practice of special techniques to attain the highest degree of physical, emotional, and spiritual integration. Its practice can reduce blood pressure, lower pulse rate, reduce serum cholesterol, regulate menstrual flow and thyroid function, increase range of motion, reduce joint pain, and increase the feeling of well-being.

Self-hypnosis allows the individual to induce the feeling of warmth and heaviness associated with a trance state. The exercises can be used to increase resistance to stressors, reduce or eliminate sleep disorders, and modify pain reactions. The system has been found effective in treating disorders of the respiratory and gastrointestinal-tracts and the circulatory and endocrine systems, and also in alleviating anxiety and fatigue.

Thought stopping is a behavioral modification technique useful when nagging, repetitive thoughts interfere with behavior and wellness. Such unwanted thoughts are interrupted with the command "Stop," and a positive thought is substituted.

Refuting irrational ideas. Everyone engages in almost continuous self-talk during waking hours. When this internal dialogue is accurate and realistic, wellness is enhanced; when it is irrational and untrue, stress occurs. Refuting these irrational ideas requires a series of steps: identifying what brought on the stress-inducing thought; writing down and identifying the negative thought and the emotion it brought on; writing down all evidence that the idea is false; predicting both the worst and best possible outcomes if the negative, irrational idea *were* true; and, finally, substituting alternative self-talk with positive, rational statements.

Centering refers to separating from outside influences to gain an inner reference or thought of stability, calm, and self-awareness; a sense of self-relatedness, a quiet place within self where the individual can feel integrated, unified, and focused. Centering reduces fatigue, stress, depression, or anger when working with others and increases self-control. It involves sitting quietly, relaxing tense spots in the body as you inhale and exhale, and concentrating on that breathing until you feel calm.

Assertive communication/behavior. Assertiveness means expressing personal thoughts, feelings, and desires, defining and making known personal rights that are reasonable while respecting the other person. Workshops frequently help people learn this way of behaving. Assertive techniques are particularly helpful in the face of criticism and other negative reactions. These include admitting mistakes, without defensiveness but without agreeing to a specific change that you may not want; asking what specifically is bothersome about a behavior for which you are criticized; shifting the conversation back to the subject and away from an intense expression of negative emotions; postponing a conversation when it reaches an impasse; not responding to an inappropriate or irrational attack; and using humor or deflection.

Guided imagery can be defined as focused attention on an inner, mental picture or a statement of belief of what the individual wants to accomplish by being open to and responding to the language of the unconscious or the deeper body levels. It is similar to self-hypnosis in that it involves sitting in a quiet place, relaxing, and envisioning a peaceful, soothing scene that can maintain relaxation and a positive attitude. Guided imagery promotes emotional health by building self-awareness and increasing coping resources.

Quitting Smoking

Your doctor has told you to quit smoking. You want to, but you aren't sure of the best way. Perhaps you've tried before. Or you're afraid you'll gain weight.

What's the best way to quit?

There are many ways to quit smoking, but you need only one thing—*the desire to quit.* Once you have that all-important ingredient, you will succeed.

You can quit "cold turkey," or you can set a quit date and taper off gradually over a 2-week period. Some people find it helpful to have support from others who are quitting at the same time. Your local chapter of the American Lung Association, the American Cancer Society, or the American Heart Association, or a hospital in your community can help you locate a smoking cessation class. Or, you can use the "buddy system"—make a pact with a friend who wants to quit and provide support for each other.

Many people find chewing nicotine gum or using a nicotine patch helpful for the first few weeks. Talk to your doctor about prescribing one of these for you.

Adopt as many techniques as you think will work for you, and use them all.

What about withdrawal symptoms?

Keep in mind that most smokers actually have a double addiction: physical and psychological. You will need to deal with both aspects.

Physical withdrawal can be a problem for heavy smokers (more than one pack a day). The symptoms vary from one person to another, but common complaints are headaches, constipation, irritability, nervousness, trouble concentrating, and insomnia. You may even cough more for the first week after quitting as your cilia become active again. This is actually a sign that your body is healing itself.

You can do several things to ease the withdrawal symptoms. Although you may fear that you'll be craving a cigarette all the time, each urge actually lasts only 2 or 3 minutes. When it hits, do a minute or two of deep-breathing exercises to calm the urge; close your eyes, take a deep breath, and slowly let it out. If you still feel a craving, change your activity—walk around or do something that requires both hands, or do something that you especially enjoy.

Drink lots of water to help flush the toxins from your body. Eat a healthy, well-balanced diet. Many authorities say that eating less meat and more fresh vegetables and fruits helps reduce withdrawal symptoms. To combat aftermeal cravings, leave the table immediately and brush your teeth. Sugarless gum or hard candy, a toothpick, or unsalted, shelled sunflower seeds satisfy the oral craving without adding calories.

Daily exercise (unless your doctor advises you not to) will help relax you and hasten recovery from the effects of nicotine.

Try to avoid situations that you associate with smoking, such as a morning cup of coffee or a before-dinner drink. You may need to modify your habits for a while until the withdrawal period is over. This also means avoiding spending much time around other smokers.

Write down all your reasons for quitting smoking to remind yourself whenever you're discouraged or tempted to smoke. Keep the list handy, and look at it often. And feel proud of yourself for quitting.

Won't I gain weight?

According to recent studies, only about one third of ex-smokers gain some weight; one third lose weight, and one third stay the same. The key to not gaining weight is not to eat every time you crave a smoke. As long as you maintain a well-balanced diet, don't snack between meals, and exercise, you shouldn't experience any weight problems.

What if I fail?

Many people who have successfully quit smoking failed the first time they tried. Often they describe these "failures" as valuable learning experiences that helped them succeed the next time. Whatever you do, don't give up. More than 36 million Americans have already quit. You can, too.

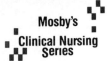

Anticoagulant Therapy

How to take the medication

If your doctor has given you a prescription for an anticoagulant, this is to prevent clots from forming in your blood. It is important to take the medication exactly as ordered, since too much of the drug can cause bleeding and too little can cause clotting. For this reason, you must have blood tests done periodically to ensure that your blood is clotting properly. If it is not, your doctor will change the dosage. Here are important guidelines for taking your medication:

1. Take your anticoagulant at the same time of day. If you are supposed to take it on alternate days, marking a calendar can help.
2. If you forget to take a dose, do not double up next time. Just take the next dose as scheduled. If you miss two doses, call your doctor.
3. Keep your appointments for blood tests.
4. Refill your prescription 1 week ahead so you don't run out.
5. Keep anticoagulants away from heat and cold.

Helping the medication work

Your diet and health, as well as other drugs, can affect the way anticoagulants work in your body. For this reason, follow these guidelines:

1. Eat only normal amounts of green leafy vegetables (spinach, broccoli, etc.). These foods are high in vitamin K, which helps your blood clot. However, too much vitamin K can interfere with the anticoagulant.
2. If you drink alcohol, limit the amount to one drink per day. Excessive alcohol can affect blood clotting.
3. **Do not take aspirin** or any drugs containing aspirin. Check with your doctor or pharmacist before taking over-the-counter drugs to be sure they do not contain aspirin or other substances that might affect blood clotting.
4. Do not take any supplements that contain vitamin K. If you take multivitamins or other supplements, check with your doctor or pharmacist to be sure that they are safe.
5. Many prescription drugs can interfere with anticoagulants. Take other prescription medications only as prescribed by your doctor.
6. If you develop diarrhea, vomiting, or a fever that lasts longer than 24 hours, call your doctor.

Safety first

While you are taking anticoagulant medication, your blood will clot more slowly if you are injured. Therefore you should take precautions against even minor cuts and bruises. In addition, you must be alert for signs that you may be bleeding internally. The following safety measures will help prevent problems:

1. Use a toothbrush with soft bristles.
2. Avoid putting toothpicks or other sharp objects in your mouth.
3. Protect your feet from injury. Don't walk barefoot, and don't trim corns or calluses yourself. See a podiatrist if necessary.
4. Inform all doctors (e.g., dentist, gynecologist) that you are taking anticoagulants *before* receiving any treatment.
5. Avoid using cutting tools or other sharp objects that could result in injury.
6. Avoid rough sports.
7. Protect yourself from falling. Put a nonskid mat in your bathtub or shower, remove hazardous throw rugs, and wear low-heeled shoes with nonslip soles.
8. If you cut yourself, keep pressure on the injury for 10 minutes. If the bleeding doesn't stop, call your doctor immediately.
9. If you are bruised, draw a line around the margin. If the bruise enlarges, call your doctor.
10. Check urine and stools daily. Call the doctor if you see pink or red urine or black stools.
11. Call your doctor if you suddenly develop excessive nosebleeds, bleeding gums, purplish or reddish spots on your skin, unusual vaginal bleeding or excessive menstrual flow, or bleeding hemorrhoids.
12. Carry either an identification card or a Medic-Alert bracelet at all times. It should include the name of the anticoagulant you're taking and your doctor's name and phone number.
13. If you are planning a long trip, inform your doctor so he or she can arrange for the blood tests to be done while you are away.

FOR WOMEN: Coumadin is a drug that crosses the placenta and can cause serious birth defects. Therefore you should take precautions to avoid pregnancy while taking this drug. If you suspect that you are pregnant, notify your doctor **immediately.**

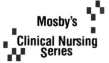
Subcutaneous Heparin Self-Injection

What are some of the general guidelines I should follow in learning to give myself injections?

Be sure you know and understand:

1. The name of your medication and its dosage, time of administration, purpose, and side effects.
2. The importance of giving heparin injections at the exact time designated.
3. The importance of not skipping any doses; keep a record of all missed doses.

Check with your doctor before taking over-the-counter medication, and read labels on all medications. Do not take aspirin, laxatives, or vitamins before consulting your doctor, and do not drink alcoholic beverages while receiving heparin therapy.

Always have your laboratory work done as ordered.

Report to your doctor any signs of bleeding (e.g., bleeding gums, joint pain, nose bleed, blood in urine, tarry stools, increased menstrual flow, easy bruisability).

Certain safety precautions can help you prevent injury: Don't blow your nose too hard; don't brush your teeth too vigorously, and use a soft-bristled toothbrush; don't use sharp-edged instruments, such as razors, or water-jet tooth cleaners; don't engage in dangerous hobbies or contact sports.

It is crucial that you prevent pregnancy while taking this medication; report a suspected pregnancy to your physician immediately. Do not use an intrauterine device (IUD) for birth control.

How do I prepare a heparin subcutaneous injection?

Be sure to have a health care professional teach you the correct techniques for handwashing, sterile preparation of a syringe and needle, withdrawal of the exact heparin dosage from a vial, and the best way to maintain sterile technique throughout the procedure.

What should I watch out for at the site of my injections?

Always use subcutaneous fatty tissue and avoid bruised areas, hematomas, incisions, or scarred tissue, and the area within 5 cm (2 inches) of the umbilicus. Rotate the site of injection with every dose of heparin to prevent bleeding or tissue damage, and record the site of each injection.

The most convenient sites are along the lower abdominal fat pad (to avoid inadvertent intramuscular injection and hematoma formation). For instance, a common site is the fatty area to the front of the iliac ridge. Areas where the subcutaneous layer is thin should be avoided.

Once I have selected a good site for the injection, what next?

First, prepare the skin by cleaning it with alcohol. Do not rub! Rubbing might damage the tissue, and heparin would aggravate any bleeding. Next, hold the syringe filled with the correct heparin dosage like a pencil or a dart, and pinch up the skin, forming a fat roll between your fingers. Insert the needle at a 45-degree angle, and quickly push it into the subcutaneous tissue just into the subcutaneous fatty layer (up to the hub of the syringe). Once inserted, do not move the needle tip or pull back on the plunger; forcible aspiration can damage small blood vessels and lead to bleeding and hematoma formation, especially with high local concentrations of heparin. Inject the medication slowly, and then withdraw the needle, gently releasing the skin as the needle is removed to minimize tissue damage.

Press the area gently to minimize oozing or bleeding; do not rub or massage the area, since this would increase the likelihood of bleeding. Record the date, time, site, and dosage of each injection. This will be particularly helpful in ensuring rotation of sites. The box shows an example of how to keep a record of injections.

HEPARIN HOME RECORD*

Date	Time	Site	Dosage
1/22/88	6:30 AM	Right upper side	5,000 U
	2:30 PM	Left upper side	5,000 U
	10:30 PM	Right lower side	5,000 U
1/23/88			
1/24/88			

*Physician's order—5,000 U heparin injected every 8 hours.

Continued.

Subcutaneous Heparin Self-Injection—cont'd

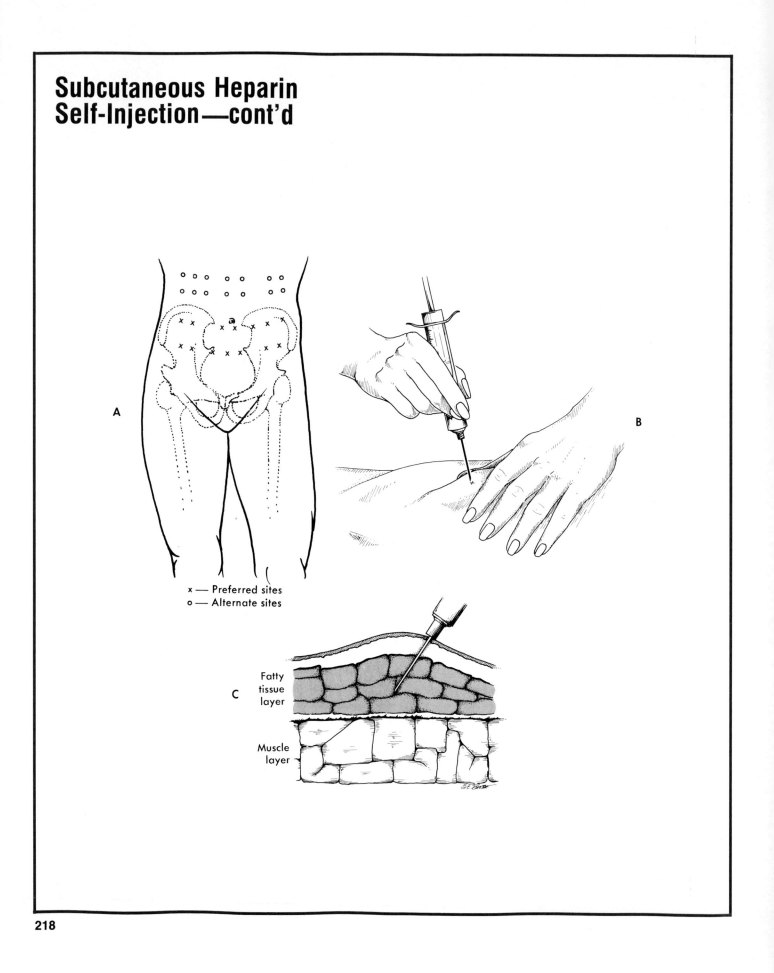

A

x — Preferred sites
o — Alternate sites

B

C

Fatty tissue layer

Muscle layer

Care of the Hickman-Broviac External Venous Catheter

An external venous catheter is a convenient way to deliver medications, including drugs for chemotherapy, and to take the many blood samples needed without having to insert a needle into your vein. The catheter is a soft, plastic tube that is implanted in your chest. One end of the tube is placed in a large vein close to your heart; the other end stays outside your body. The catheter has a cap that can be removed when blood samples are needed or drugs for chemotherapy must be given.

You will need to follow three procedures to care for your external venous catheter: changing the dressing, changing the cap, and flushing the catheter. Follow the procedures carefully to prevent infection and clotting of the tube.

Changing the dressing

You must change the dressing on your catheter frequently (at least every other day) until the wound site has healed. (After the site has healed, your doctor may allow you to clean around the wound site with soap and water while you shower; then dry the area and apply a small gauze pad or adhesive bandage to the exit site.)
Assemble the following equipment:
Hydrogen peroxide
Small container to pour hydrogen peroxide in
Alcohol wipes
Antibiotic ointment
Dressing
Tape
Cotton-tipped ear swabs
1. Wash your hands.
2. Remove the old dressing, and wash your hands again.
3. Pour the hydrogen peroxide into the container, and dip a cotton swab into the hydrogen peroxide. Starting at the wound site and using a circular motion, clean the skin around the wound site, working your way out. Use a new cotton swab whenever you need more hydrogen peroxide.
4. Clean the length of the catheter with an alcohol wipe.
5. Apply antibiotic ointment to the wound site with a cotton swab.
6. Tape a new dressing over the wound site.

Changing the catheter cap

Catheter caps should be changed every 7 days.
Assemble the following equipment:
Catheter cap
Catheter clamp
Alcohol wipes
1. Wash your hands.
2. Clamp the catheter.
3. Unscrew the old cap. Wipe around the end of the catheter with alcohol wipes. Screw on a new cap. Unclamp the catheter.

Flushing the catheter

You need to flush your catheter as directed by the nurse (as often as once a day) to prevent blood clots from forming inside it.
Assemble the following equipment:
Vial of heparin-saline solution
Disposable syringe and needle
Alcohol wipes
1. Wash your hands.
2. Open the bottle of heparin-saline solution; wipe the vial opening with an alcohol wipe.
3. Remove the needle guard from the syringe, and pull back the plunger. Insert the needle into the vial, turn the vial upside down, and pull back on the syringe to fill it (tap on the side of the syringe to remove air bubbles).
4. Clean the catheter cap with an alcohol wipe. Insert the needle into the cap, and push down on the plunger to inject solution into the catheter.
5. Remove the needle, and carefully discard it and the syringe.

Catheter maintenance

Be sure to buy a catheter repair kit to use when a leak occurs. If the catheter continues to leak despite your repairs, call your doctor or nurse.

Call your doctor or nurse if:

Pain, redness, or puffiness develops around the catheter site.
You notice drainage from the catheter site.
Your temperature is above 100° F.
The catheter slips.
There is blood in the catheter.
You are unable to flush the catheter.

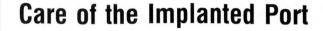
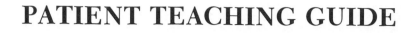
Care of the Implanted Port

An implanted port is a convenient way to deliver medications, including drugs for chemotherapy, and to take the many blood samples needed without damaging your veins. The implanted port consists of a soft, plastic catheter that is placed in a large vein close to your heart and a port with a metal base and rubber top through which medications will be administered and blood will be drawn. The implanted port is surgically placed in your chest or abdomen, and there are no external parts.

Because an implanted port is completely under the skin, it doesn't require a lot of care. You must watch for signs of infection, protect the needle during ambulatory infusion pump treatments, and prevent the skin over the port from becoming irritated.

Watching for signs of infection

Call your doctor if:
Redness, pain, or puffiness develops around the port.
You notice drainage from the incision site.
Your temperature is above 100° F.
You become short of breath.
You have chest pain.

Protecting the needle during infusion

Sometimes you may need to receive treatments over an extended period. For these occasions, a bent needle (Huber needle) is inserted into the port and connected to an ambulatory infusion pump. The needle is left in the port until the treatment is finished, sometimes for several days. The pump is attached to your body by a belt or pouch and is worn for the duration of the treatment.

During this time you will need to prevent the needle from becoming dislodged. A dressing will be taped over the needle, and you must check it to make sure the tape is holding the dressing and the needle hasn't slipped. You may need to change this dressing periodically.

Protecting the skin over the port

It is important that you prevent irritation of the skin over and around the port. Do not wear any bra straps or clothing that may rub the port site. Adjust your seat belt if it rubs the port site.

Unless you are receiving an infusion, you may shower, bathe, and swim without worry. When re-

ceiving an infusion, you need to keep the site dry and protected.

Changing the drug reservoir bag

If you are receiving treatment over several days, you may be taught to change the drug reservoir bag. Directions for changing the bag vary with the type of pump. Your nurse will provide you with a diagram and complete instructions.

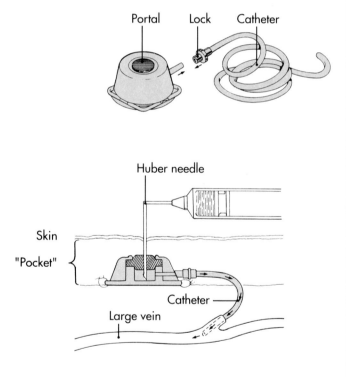

Portal   Lock   Catheter

Huber needle

Skin

"Pocket"

Catheter

Large vein

Dealing with Loss of Appetite, Nausea and Vomiting, and Stomatitis

Loss of appetite, nausea and vomiting, and stomatitis are common symptoms of cancer and cancer treatment, although not everyone has them. There are a variety of ways to relieve nausea and vomiting and help increase appetite.

Loss of appetite

Loss of appetite can be a serious problem; it can lead to malnutrition and severe weight loss. When your body is trying to fight cancer, it needs nutrition. It needs enough protein and calories to function at its best, to give you energy, and to help reduce the effects of the cancer and its treatment.

Eating enough of the right kinds of foods can be difficult when you don't feel like eating at all. Here are some tips to help you increase your appetite:

Take a walk before mealtime. Mild exercise can stimulate your appetite.

Avoid drinking liquids before a meal, because they can fill you up. If you want to drink, then drink juices or milk—something nutritious.

Eat with family or friends if possible. If eating is a social event, it will seem less of a chore.

Eat a variety of foods. Spice up your food with herbs, spices, and sauces. Use butter, bacon bits, croutons, wine sauces, and marinades to provide taste-pleasing meals.

Don't fill up on salads or "diet" foods. Eat vegetables and fruits along with meats, poultry, and fish to make sure you get enough calories and nutrition.

Eat smaller meals more often, especially if you fill up before you've eaten all your dinner.

If you still are not getting enough calories or protein, your doctor may recommend dietary supple ments that can be added to milk, soup, or pud ding.

Nausea and vomiting

Nausea and vomiting are common side effects of chemotherapy and radiation therapy. Doctors frequently prescribe an *antiemetic* to combat this. The antiemetic usually is given a few hours before the treatment and then every 3 or 4 hours after the treatment for a day or two. It may take some experimenting with dosage and timing to come up with the best schedule for you.

The following are other remedies and preventive measures you can try to help prevent or alleviate nausea and vomiting:

Eat soda crackers and suck on sour candy balls throughout the day to relieve queasiness.

Choose cold or room-temperature foods instead of hot ones; hot and warm foods seem to cause nausea.

Avoid salty, fatty, and sweet foods or any food with strong odors—opt instead for bland, creamy foods such as cottage cheese, toast, and mashed potatoes.

Stay away from nauseating odors, sights, and sounds. Get as much fresh air as possible. A leisurely walk can help alleviate nausea.

Don't eat right before your cancer treatment. Eat lightly for a few hours after your treatment.

Try relaxation therapy, self-hypnosis, or imagery to alleviate nausea-inducing tension.

Distract yourself with a book, TV, or activity.

Sleep during episodes of nausea if possible.

If vomiting does occur, eat or drink nothing until your stomach has settled, usually a few hours after the last vomiting episode. Then begin sipping clear liquids or sucking on ice cubes. If you tolerate the liquids, you may begin eating bland foods a few hours after you started the liquids.

Stomatitis

Stomatitis is an inflammation of the lining of the mouth. It may occur 7 to 14 days after beginning chemotherapy or radiation therapy to the mouth, or earlier if other problems were already present. A dentist should assess the status of your mouth and teeth before you begin therapy.

Stomatitis often can be prevented or alleviated by using a soft toothbrush and rinsing with a solution of 1 pint of water with ½ teaspoon of salt and ½ teaspoon of baking soda after meals and at bedtime. Flossing with unwaxed floss, drinking water or nonacidic juices (e.g., apple or grape), eating artificially sweetened candy or gum, and using artificial saliva sprays for dry mouth can also help.

Watch for signs and symptoms of possible stomatitis: a burning feeling in the mouth; a red, irritated oral lining; a swollen, inflamed tongue; and sores in the mouth. Treatment is based on the extent and seriousness of the stomatitis; measures include rinsing with the solution described above; loosening thick mucus and crusted drainage with Milk of Magnesia, Maalox, or another antacid; and using an analgesic rinse before meals to lessen painful swallowing. If you have dentures, they should be worn only during meals. Avoid spicy, acidic, and crusty or rough foods and hot or cold foods and beverages.

Report signs of infection to your doctor: soft, white patches; dry, brownish yellow areas; moist, creamy white areas; painless, dry, yellow ulcers with well-defined edges; or open areas on the lips or mouth.

Dealing with the Effects of Bone Marrow Suppression

Preventing infection

Cancer and cancer treatments impair your immune system and leave you susceptible to infection. The most common sites of infection are the bladder and urinary tract, the skin, the lungs, and the blood. Infection is a serious problem, and you should do everything possible to prevent it by following these guidelines:

Eat nutritious meals, drink plenty of fluids, get enough rest, and avoid stress as much as possible.

Keep your mouth, teeth, and gums clean. Use a soft toothbrush and salt-water rinse.

Wash your hands frequently with soap and water, especially before eating and after using the toilet.

Shower rather than take a bath.

Cleanse your perianal area after each bowel movement.

Women should avoid bubble baths, douches, and feminine hygiene products such as tampons. Sanitary napkins should be changed frequently. Use a commercial lubricant during sexual intercourse. Urinate before and after intercourse.

Avoid the following:

People who are ill.

People vaccinated recently with a live virus.

Crowded places (waiting rooms, malls).

Raw fruits and vegetables, raw eggs, and raw milk; eat only cooked food and pasteurized milk and milk products.

All sources of stagnant water (water in flower vases, pitchers, denture cups, humidifiers, and respiratory equipment). Water in these containers should be changed daily.

Dog, cat, and bird feces. Let someone else change bird cages or litter boxes.

Even if you follow these guidelines carefully, an infection may occur. Call your doctor immediately if you develop any sign of infection:

Fever over 100° F

Redness, swelling, or pain around any wound

Coughing, sore throat, and stuffy or runny nose

Nausea, vomiting, or diarrhea

Chest pain or shortness of breath

Burning or frequency of urination, or a change in the color or odor of urine

Sores or white patches in the mouth

Even if your symptoms seem mild, they may indicate a life-threatening infection.

Preventing bleeding

A person with cancer runs a greater risk of bleeding from the skin and mucous membranes or internally. The bleeding results because the bone marrow is producing few or no platelets (special blood cells that cause the blood to clot), or because platelets already in the blood are being destroyed. Cancer itself, allergic reactions to medication, radiation therapy, or chemotherapy can reduce the number of platelets; this condition is called **thrombocytopenia.**

Because the lack of platelets makes bleeding hard to stop once it has begun, it is *very* important that a person with thrombocytopenia take great care to prevent bleeding. Check your skin each day for bruises, and call the doctor if any get larger after you first notice them.

To prevent bleeding from the skin:

Avoid physical activities that could cause injury.

Shave with an electric razor.

Keep your nails short; file rough edges.

If bleeding does occur, apply pressure to the site for 5 minutes and elevate. If the bleeding lasts longer than 5 minutes, call your doctor.

To prevent bleeding from the mucous membranes of the mouth, nose, gastrointestinal system, and genitourinary tract:

Brush with a soft toothbrush. If you still have trouble with bleeding gums, use sponge-tipped applicators. Do not floss. Keep your lips moist with petroleum jelly. Check with your doctor before having dental work.

Avoid hot foods that might burn your mouth.

Blow your nose gently. Humidify your house if the air is too dry, because dry air can cause nose bleeds. If your nose does bleed, pinch your nostrils shut for a few minutes. If the bleeding persists, put an ice bag on the back of your neck. Call your doctor if the bleeding does not stop.

Use stool softeners and drink plenty of water if you are constipated. Do not use enemas or suppositories.

Take acetaminophen (e.g., Tylenol) or ibuprofen (e.g., Advil) instead of aspirin, which can cause stomach bleeding.

Avoid douches and vaginal suppositories. Use a lubricating jelly before sexual intercourse.

To prevent internal bleeding:

Try to arrange furniture so you won't bruise yourself on it. Keep clutter off floors.

Avoid tight-fitting clothing and any buttons or ornaments that could bruise or chafe your skin.

Do not lift heavy objects.

Any bleeding that does not stop after 5 minutes should be reported to your doctor.

Preventing anemia

In anemia there are not enough red blood cells to carry oxygen to the cells and take away carbon dioxide. (With bone marrow suppression the marrow is producing fewer red blood cells.) You may tire easily and need to rest more often.

To lessen the effects of anemia:

Schedule activities with frequent rest periods.

Eat a diet high in protein. Take a multivitamin supplement with minerals.

Be alert for any of these signs: pallor, dizziness, ringing in the ears, chest pain, or shortness of breath. Report these problems to your doctor.

Skin Care During External Beam Radiation Therapy

Radiation therapy can cause mild to severe skin reactions. The severity of the reaction depends on how much radiation is given and how frequently, how much skin area is irradiated, and the type of radiation used. In the first 2 weeks of treatment, the skin being irradiated may turn pink or red, become sensitive to sun, lose hair, or develop a rash. As treatment progresses, a condition called dry desquamation may develop (i.e., the skin becomes dry, itchy, and flaky). Moist desquamation may then set in, and the skin may peel and become painful and weepy. Skin reactions are most noticeable 10 days to 2 weeks after therapy is completed. Hair loss from irradiated scalp begins 10 days after the first treatment.

Preventing skin reactions

The following skin care guidelines may prevent reactions or lessen their severity:

Cleanse the skin with warm water, not hot. After washing, rinse with tepid water and pat dry with a soft towel. Do not soak in a tub. Do not remove the treatment field markings during bathing. Avoid soap as much as possible. If soap becomes necessary, use Aveeno, Dove, or some other mild, unscented soap that will not dry the skin.

Do not use heating pads, hot packs, or ice on the area.

Do not use perfumed or powdered products on the treated skin.

If necessary, use a light dusting of cornstarch to prevent itching and to eliminate moisture in neck creases, armpits, and beneath the breasts.

Do not use ointments or menthol rubs.

Shave with an electric razor.

Protect your skin from heat, cold, and sunlight. Use a sunscreen with a sun protection factor (SPF) of 15 or higher (the SPF is shown on the bottle). Shield your face and neck with a scarf or wide-brimmed hat.

Wear loose-fitting clothing. Tight clothing and belts rub and chafe already sensitive skin.

Do not put adhesive bandages (e.g., Band-Aids) on irradiated skin.

Treating skin reactions

If your skin is dry, ask your doctor or nurse to recommend a lotion to apply. For dry desquamation you may be encouraged to use pure aloe vera gel, vitamin A and D ointments (e.g., Desitin), Lubriderm, or other water-soluble, nonirritating substances.

For moist desquamation you may be allowed to apply cool compresses moistened with water or normal saline. Sometimes a special ointment is prescribed. You may be taught to apply moisture-vapor—permeable film or other sterile dressings (e.g., OpSite, Tegaderm) to the area to protect it while it heals. Moist desquamation usually resolves 1 to 2 weeks after treatment ends. If you have pain, your doctor may suggest that you take an over-the-counter analgesic such as aspirin, acetaminophen (e.g., Tylenol), or ibuprofen (e.g., Motrin).

Even after your skin heals, it may still be sensitive to heat, cold, and sunlight. Some chemotherapeutic agents cause "radiation recall," which is a reappearance of the previous skin reaction, usually seen as redness.

If hair loss is likely to occur, select scarves, hats, wigs, or hairpieces before the loss begins. This loss usually is temporary, but this depends on the dose of radiation received, the patient's sex and age, and whether adjuvant chemotherapy was used.

Mosby's
Clinical Nursing
Series

Managing Pain Without Drugs

There are several techniques you can use to relieve pain without taking drugs or to enhance the effect of your pain medication—**relaxation, imagery, distraction,** and **skin stimulation.**

Relaxation

Relaxation relieves pain by easing muscle tension. Easing muscle tension can also help you feel less tired and anxious and help other pain-relieving methods work better.

How to relax. Sit or lie down, preferably in a quiet place. Be sure you are comfortable. Do not cross your legs or arms.

Take a deep breath, and tense your muscles (you may tense up your whole body or concentrate on one set of muscles at a time, such as your facial muscles or those in your arms and hands).

Hold your breath, and keep your muscles tense.

Release your breath and your muscles at the same time. Let your body go limp (repeat for other muscle areas if you are concentrating on one set at a time).

You can add imagery (see below) or music to help you relax. Relaxation tapes are also available.

Don't be discouraged if relaxation doesn't help immediately. Practice the relaxation technique for 2 weeks before you give it up. If you find that it aggravates your pain, try another method.

Imagery

Imagery involves using your imagination to create mental scenes that use all your senses: sight, sound, touch, smell, and taste. You can imagine exotic locations or revisit one of your favorite places. You can create stories and characters to add to your scenes. Imagery can take your mind off your anxiety, boredom, and pain.

How to use imagery. Close your eyes. A few moments of the relaxation technique (see above) will help your body and mind prepare for imagery.

Let your mind begin forming its image. The following is an example of imagery:

Imagine that you are at the seashore. You are sitting in the wet sand; the afternoon sun is warm on your shoulders. The ocean rolls into the shore in gentle waves, and the water laps teasingly at your toes. A hungry pair of seagulls cry overhead and take swift, darting dives at a dog that is scavenging along the shore. Your tension lessens with each wave that touches your toes and retreats. You close your eyes and take a deep, slow breath of salt-filled air. You are completely relaxed. Stay on the beach as long as you like.

To end the image, count to three and open your eyes. Resume your regular activities slowly.

Distraction

A distraction is any activity that takes your mind off your pain and focuses your attention elsewhere. Doing crafts, reading a book, watching television, or listening to music through headphones can all help distract your mind. Distraction works well when you are waiting for drugs to take effect or if you have brief bouts of pain. Sometimes people can take their minds off their pain for long periods, especially if the pain is mild.

Skin stimulation

Skin stimulation is used to block pain sensation in the nerves. Pressure, massage, hot and cold applications, rubbing, and mild electrical current are all ways to stimulate the skin. However, if you are undergoing radiation treatment, consult your doctor before applying any skin stimulation.

You can do skin stimulation at the site of the pain, near it, or on the opposite side of pain. For example, stimulating the left wrist when the right wrist is in pain can actually ease the pain in the right wrist.

Pressure. Using your entire hand, the heel of your hand, your thumb, your knuckles, or both hands, apply at least 15 seconds of pressure at the point where you feel pain. Keep trying spots around the painful area if you find no relief the first time. You may extend the time you apply pressure to 1 minute.

Massage. You or someone else can perform the slow, circular motions of massage. The feet, back, neck, and scalp can be massaged to relieve tension and pain anywhere in the body. Some people prefer to use oils or lotions during the massage. If deep massage is too uncomfortable, try light stroking. Do not massage red, raw, or broken skin.

Heat and cold. Some people prefer cold; others prefer heat. Use whichever works best for you. A convenient way to use cold is to freeze gel-filled packs and wrap them in towels. Ice cubes can also be used. Heat can be applied with a heating pad; hot, moist towels; or a hot water bottle or by taking a hot bath. Be careful not to burn your skin with water that is too hot or to go to sleep with a heating pad on. Don't expose your skin to intense cold for very long.

Transcutaneous electrical nerve stimulation (TENS). TENS can be used to eliminate or ease pain. A TENS unit is a pocket-sized, battery-operated device that provides a mild, continuous electrical current through the skin by the use of two to four electrodes, which are taped onto the skin. Lead wires connect the electrodes to the device. It is this mild electrical current that blocks or modifies the pain messages and replaces them with a buzzing, tingling sensation. It is also thought that TENS may stimulate the body's production of endorphin, a natural pain reliever.

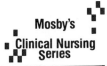
Bone Marrow Harvest

One of the newer treatments for some cancers and metabolic and immunologic diseases is **bone marrow transplantation.** Bone marrow transplantation has the potential to cure patients with these otherwise fatal diseases.

The patient's bone marrow is first destroyed by high doses of chemotherapy or radiation and then replaced with healthy bone marrow donated by a family member or the patient herself. The transplanted bone marrow begins making new blood cells within 10 to 14 days after transplantation.

How bone marrow is harvested

Whether a family member or the patient, the bone marrow donor must understand the process of harvesting bone marrow. The following is a step-by-step description of this procedure.

Preparation. Before the bone marrow harvest even begins, you will have gone through a series of blood tests to make sure your bone marrow matches the recipient's. (If you are donating your own marrow, there is no problem with matching.) You will also undergo a physical examination, a chest x-ray, an electrocardiogram, and urinalysis to ensure that you are in good health. The evening before the harvest, you will take a shower with an antiseptic solution. You will not be allowed to eat or drink after midnight.

The day of the procedure. The morning of the harvest, a nurse will come to your room and insert an intravenous line (IV) into your arm. Just before you are taken to the operating room, the nurse will give you a shot to help you relax and make you drowsy.

A team consisting of doctors, nurses, and an anesthesiologist will be waiting in the operating room. The anesthesiologist will give you a drug through your IV to make you sleep.

The bone marrow will be harvested from your hip. The doctor will insert a needle several times into the rear portion of your hip bones and withdraw a total of 1 to 2 quarts of bone marrow and blood. (You will receive a blood transfusion to make up for the loss of blood.) A pressure dressing will be applied over the harvest sites to help prevent bleeding. The entire harvest procedure takes about 2 to 3 hours.

After the procedure. You will wake up in the recovery room after the anesthetic has worn off. A nurse will check on you every 15 minutes to record your vital signs (pulse, blood pressure, temperature, and respirations) and make sure that you are not bleeding from the harvest sites.

While you recover, the bone marrow that you donated will be filtered to remove fat and bone particles. If the marrow is for your future use, it will be frozen until you are ready for it. If it is for someone else, it will be immediately given to that person through an IV transfusion.

Within a day you will be able to eat solid food and begin walking around. The pressure dressing will be removed, but you will have to keep the harvest sites clean and covered with a bandage for 3 days. If you have pain, your doctor can prescribe medication to relieve it.

You will be able to leave the hospital after 1 or 2 days. You should be able to resume your normal activities soon after.

If you have any questions before or after the bone marrow harvest, don't hesitate to ask your doctor or nurse.

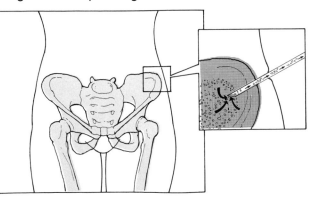

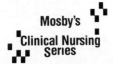

Clinical Trials—What Are They?

Research studies that use patients are called clinical trials. As a person with cancer, you may be asked to help evaluate a new treatment.

What are clinical trials?

When a new cancer treatment becomes available, it must first go through rigorous testing in a laboratory and then in a clinical setting. The testing is carefully monitored, and the results are evaluated and published in medical journals, where other researchers and clinicians further evaluate the data.

There are three types of clinical trials: phase I trials, phase II trials, and phase III trials. Each of these trials is a carefully controlled, highly ethical human experiment designed to test a new drug or procedure that could cure or halt the spread of a cancer. The drug or procedure usually is tested in all three phases before it can be accepted as a treatment.

Phase I trials determine the best way to provide a new treatment and how much can be given safely. These trials involve cancer patients with advanced disease who have tried every possible treatment with no long-term success. These patients are willing to undergo treatments that probably will not cure their cancer but that give them some hope and that might help a cancer patient in the future. Any treatment given these patients has first undergone testing on animals and has been approved for human trials.

Phase II trials study the effect of a new treatment on patients whose cancer has not been cured by standard treatments. There is some possibility that the treatment may benefit these patients. A treatment reaching phase II trials has gone through phase I trials.

Phase III trials compare a new treatment to current treatments. These trials require large numbers of patients to control the effects that age, race, gender, and other factors may have on the experimental treatment.

One group of patients receives the experimental treatment, and another is given a standard treatment. Randomization (selection by chance to be in one group or the other) is used to keep bias out of the trial.

Informed consent

Informed consent means that you have been given the information you need to decide whether to participate in a clinical trial. This information includes what is involved, possible benefits and risks, the length of the study, the cost (if any), and how your anonymity and the confidentiality of your participation will be protected. Ask any questions you have. Then, if you wish to be a part of the study, you can sign the form. You can refuse to participate or withdraw from the study at any time without penalty.

Should you participate in a trial?

Those who participate in clinical trials have the opportunity to receive the latest in cancer treatments or a new, experimental treatment that could be even more effective. In fact, according to published studies, patients who participate in trials often have a better survival rate.

You and your doctor should discuss the possibility of your participating in a clinical trial. If you are interested, your doctor should be aware of the different trials being conducted so he or she can recommend the best one for you. Many patients benefit both physically and mentally from participating in clinical trials.

For more information, write to the Office of Cancer Communications, National Cancer Institute, Bethesda, Maryland 20205, or call the Cancer Information Service at 1-800-4-CANCER. Ask for *What Are Clinical Trials? A Booklet for Patients with Cancer.*

Genetic Counseling

My doctor suggested that I get genetic counseling now that my husband and I are considering having a family. Obviously, there is bad news, right?

No, not necessarily. A common myth is that genetic counseling is a gloomy experience. But in many instances, genetic counseling gives couples better chances than they'd expected that a child will be free of the family's inherited disorder. Also, genetic counselors frequently find that they give couples who have had a child with a birth defect a much better chance than they expected of having a subsequent normal child. Genetic counseling is not just for potential parents. Genetic counseling can tell you how likely you are to develop a disorder that runs in your family. Often that's good news, too.

What is genetic counseling?

The American Society of Human Genetics defines genetic counseling as a communication process, an exchange of information in which a well-informed medical professional thoroughly explains the disease or birth defect for which the patient or the offspring is at risk. It is important that all of the medical, social, and economic aspects of these conditions be discussed, along with all reproductive options. Remember: Any reproductive decision is up to you; it is always your choice. With genetic counseling, you can make your own, well-informed decisions in accordance with your ethical or moral standards.

Isn't genetic counseling a relatively new field? How do I know I can trust it?

This, like the "bad news" theory above, is another myth about genetic counseling. Like most aspects of health care, the science of genetic counseling is quite new. Many techniques used have been available for only a few decades. However, the art of genetics itself is ancient. For instance, more than 1,000 years ago, the Talmud recommended that parents avoid circumcising an infant whose maternal uncle had "the bleeding disease." The Egyptians wrote the first known account of prenatal diagnosis (sex identity) of an infant more than 3,500 years ago!

When is the best time to get genetic counseling?

You should get counseling at any time during health care when an at-risk situation becomes evident. Pediatric care, obstetrical care, and premarital examinations are common opportunities for genetic counseling. Unfortunately, genetic counseling is most often sought after the birth of a child with a birth defect or genetic disease. The disadvantage in such cases is twofold. When the risk is high and the burden serious, many couples elect not to have children if they receive counseling before conception takes place. On the other hand, many parents feel ready for the challenges and unique rewards of raising a child born with a birth defect or genetic disease, but without prenatal counseling they begin their new life with their child less prepared. Prenatal genetic counseling enables such parents to welcome the new child mentally prepared and with a network of support systems already in place.

If you do find yourself the parent of a new baby with an unexpected birth defect or disorder, allow yourself time to go through the natural "mourning process" associated with that experience. All parents in this situation feel anger, guilt, depression and, in some instances, rejection of the baby. Allow yourself time to work through these feelings with support from family and health care professionals or community resources before diving into the more technical aspects of genetic counseling.

CHAPTER 12

Pharmacologic Agents for Blood Disorders

Hemostatic Agents

AMINOCAPROIC ACID

Amicar

Aminocaproic acid is a synthetic monoaminocarboxylic acid with antifibrinolytic action. It inhibits plasminogen activator substance and, to a lesser degree, plasmin (fibrinolysin) activity. Aminocaproic acid does not control bleeding caused by thrombocytopenia or most other coagulation defects, although it has proved very beneficial in individuals with hemophilia when used before and after tooth extraction and for other traumatic bleeding in the mouth and nasopharynx.

Indications: Used to control excessive bleeding caused by systemic hyperfibrosis, a pathologic condition that may accompany heart surgery, portacaval shunt, abruptio placentae, aplastic anemia, or various carcinomas. Also used to treat urinary fibrinolysis associated with severe trauma, anoxia, shock, urologic surgery, or neoplastic diseases of the stomach.

Usual dosage: (PO; IV, slow infusion): initial priming dose of 4-5 g PO or by slow IV infusion (in 250 ml of physiologic sodium chloride, sterile water, 5% D_5W, or Ringer's solution) over 1 hour, followed by 1-1.25 g at hourly intervals for about 8 hours until bleeding has been controlled. Do not exceed 30 g in 24 hours.

Precautions/contraindications: *Cautious use:* cardiac, renal, or hepatic disease; history of pulmonary embolus or other thrombotic disease. *Contraindicated:* severe renal impairment, active disseminated intravascular coagulation (DIC), upper urinary tract bleeding. Safe use during pregnancy has not been established.

Side effects/adverse reactions: *CNS:* dizziness, malaise, headaches, weakness, hallucinations, psychotic reactions. *CV:* orthostatic hypotension, bradycardia and other dysrhythmias, thrombophlebitis. *ENT:* tinnitus, nasal stuffiness. *Ophthalmic:* conjunctival erythema. *GI:* nausea, vomiting, cramps, diarrhea. *GU:* diuresis, dysuria, inhibition of ejaculation, prolonged menstruation with cramping. *Dermatologic:* rash, pruritus, erythema. *Other:* myopathy.

Pharmacokinetics: Rapidly absorbed from the GI tract after oral administration; peak plasma levels are achieved in about 2 hours. Concentrated in the urine and excreted largely unchanged by the kidneys. Widely distributed throughout the body.

Interactions: May increase the potential for thromboses in women taking oral contraceptives or estrogens.

Nursing considerations:

- Check IV for extravasation. Observe for signs of thrombophlebitis (redness, warmth, tenderness, swelling).
- Caution patient to avoid rapid positional changes that might cause orthostatic hypotension.
- Monitor vital signs.
- Monitor input/output ratio.
- Tell patient that urine will have a reddish brown color.

- Monitor for and report signs of myopathy.
- Monitor for and report signs of thrombotic complications (arm or leg pain, tenderness or swelling, Homans' sign, prominence of superficial veins, chest pain, breathlessness, dyspnea).

THROMBIN
Thrombinar, Thrombostat

Thrombin is a sterile plasma protein prepared from bovine prothrombin. It induces clotting of whole blood or a fibrinogen solution without the addition of other substances. The mechanism of action is the conversion of fibrinogen to thrombin.

Indications: Used to stop the oozing of blood from capillaries and small venules such as those involved in dental extraction, plastic surgery grafts, and epistaxis. Also used to shorten bleeding time at puncture sites in patients undergoing heparin therapy (i.e., after hemodialysis).

Usual dosage: (Topical administration): 100-2,000 NIH U/ml. May be used in dry form or mixed with blood plasma to form a fibrin glue. Can also be used with absorbable gelatin sponge.

Precautions/contraindications: Known hypersensitivity to any component or material of bovine origin. Do not administer parenterally, and avoid infiltration into large blood vessels. Safe use during pregnancy has not been established.

Side effects/adverse reactions: *Sensitivity:* allergic and febrile reactions. Intravascular clotting and death result if thrombin enters the larger blood vessels.

Pharmacokinetics: None.
Interactions: None.
Nursing considerations:

- Be prepared for a possible hemorrhage by having cross-matched blood available.
- Sponge area clean of blood before and after applying thrombin.
- Use extreme care to ensure that thrombin does not enter large blood vessels.

ANTIHEMOPHILIC AGENTS

HUMAN ANTIHEMOPHILIC FACTOR (SYNTHETIC FACTOR VIII)

Synthetic factor VIII is a stable, lyophilized concentrate of antihemophilic factor (AHF) obtained from large pools of fresh, normal human plasma. Commercial factor VIII preparations are now subjected to heat treatment to reduce the potential for transmitting the human immunodeficiency virus (HIV) and viral hepatitis.

Indications: Used in the treatment of hemophilia A, a genetic deficiency of factor VIII, and in patients with acquired circulating factor VIII inhibitors.

Usual dosage: (IV): 10-20 U/kg by slow IV injection or infusion q 8-12 h. Dosage is individualized according to weight, severity of bleeding, and coagulation studies (patient <50 kg, 250 U daily in AM; patient >50 kg, 500 U daily in AM).

Precautions/contraindications: *Cautious use:* hepatic disease, large or frequently repeated doses in patient with blood type A, B, or AB. *Contraindicated:* von Willebrand's disease (not effective in controlling bleeding with this disorder). Safe use during pregnancy has not been established.

Side effects/adverse reactions: Generally related to rate of administration. *CNS:* headaches, paresthesia, somnolence, lethargy, clouding or loss of consciousness. *CV:* hypotension, tachycardia. *Hypersensitivity:* anaphylactic or febrile reaction. *Other:* dizziness, nausea, vomiting, transient chest discomfort, cough, altered vision, viral hepatitis, jaundice.

Pharmacokinetics: Rapidly cleared from the plasma after IV administration. Half-life ranges from 4 to 24 hours (average is 12 hours). Does not readily cross the placenta.

Interactions: None.
Nursing considerations:

- Infuse at prescribed rate (rate for preparations containing more than 34 U/ml should not exceed 2 ml/min).
- Monitor vital signs; closely observe for vasomotor or hypersensitivity reactions.
- Some patients have an acute, transient allergic reaction (erythema, urticaria, backache, fever).
- Monitor for hepatitis.

FACTOR IX COMPLEX
Konyne

Factor IX complex is a dried, purified concentrate of vitamin K–dependent blood coagulation factors II, VII, IX, and X derived from fresh pooled plasma from healthy donors. Although the drug is tested for the hepatitis and HIV viruses, some risk of transmission exists.

Indications: Used primarily to control bleeding in patients with factor IX deficiency (hemophilia B, or Christmas disease). Also used to reverse the effects of coumarin anticoagulants and to control bleeding in patients with hemophilia A who have factor VIII inhibitors.

Usual dosage: (IV): dosing is individualized. *Bleeding in patient with hemophilia A with factor VIII inhibitors:* 75 U/kg ideal body weight, second dose if necessary after 8 to 12 hours. *Prompt reversal of coumarin anticoagulant effect:* 15 U/kg. *Prophylaxis to reduce in-*

cidence and severity of spontaneous bleeding: 500 U weekly, or 500-1,000 U q 2 wk.

Precautions/contraindications: *Cautious use:* liver disease, possible signs of disseminated intravascular coagulation (DIC), fibrinolysis. Also in patients with mild factor IX deficiency who could be treated effectively with fresh frozen plasma; patients with little exposure to blood products; and patients undergoing elective surgery. Safe use during pregnancy has not been established.

Side effects/adverse reactions: Generally well tolerated. *With large doses:* chills, fever (pyrogenic reaction), DIC, thromboses, myocardial infarction. *With rapid infusion:* vasomotor reactions, transient fever, chills, vomiting, somnolence. *Other:* severe hypersensitivity reactions, viral hepatitis.

Pharmacokinetics: Rapidly cleared from the plasma; half-life is biphasic (first phase, 4 to 6 hours; terminal phase, 22½ hours).

Interactions: None.

Nursing considerations:

- Type and cross-match blood to reduce the risk of intravascular hemolysis in patient with type A, B, or AB blood.
- Some health care providers recommend immunization for hepatitis B if several administrations of factor IX are planned.
- Do not allow infusion rate to exceed 10 ml/min, to prevent vasomotor reactions.
- Ensure that coagulation tests are done during therapy to guide adjustment of dosage.
- Monitor vital signs and input/output ratio.
- Monitor for signs of disseminated intravascular coagulation (risk increases with repeated administration).
- Monitor for hypersensitivity reaction and signs of hepatitis.

THROMBOLYTIC AGENTS

STREPTOKINASE

Streptase

Streptokinase is extracted from purified beta-hemolytic streptococci filtrates. It promotes thrombolysis by activating the conversion of plasminogen to plasmin, an enzyme that degrades fibrin, fibrinogen, and other procoagulant proteins into soluble fragments.

Indications: Used in the treatment of extensive deep vein thrombosis, acute arterial thrombosis or embolism, acute pulmonary embolus, and coronary artery thrombosis. Also used to clear an occluded arteriovenous cannula.

Usual dosage: (IV): *Pulmonary embolism and deep vein thrombosis:* loading dose of 250,000 U over 30 minutes, followed by continuous infusion of 100,000 U/h; continue for 24 to 72 hours. *Intracoronary thrombosis:* initial loading dose of 10,000-20,000 U, followed by 2,000-4,000 U/min until lysis occurs, then 2,000 U/min for 1 hour. *Occluded arteriovenous cannula:* 25,000 U.

Precautions/contraindications: *Cautious use:* preexisting hemostatic deficits, hepatic failure. *Contraindicated:* active internal bleeding, recent (2 months) cerebrovascular accident, intracranial or intraspinal surgery, intracranial neoplasm, uncontrollable hypertension, severe allergic reaction to the drug. Safe use during pregnancy has not been established.

Side effects/adverse reactions: *Allergic:* ranges from mild (e.g., urticaria, nausea) to major (e.g., anaphylaxis). *Hematopoietic:* phlebitis, spontaneous bleeding, unstable BP.

Pharmacokinetics: Plasminogen activation begins immediately; drug is rapidly removed from circulation by antibodies and the mononuclear phagocytic system. Half-life is biphasic (initial phase, 18 minutes; terminal phase, 83 minutes). Drug does not cross placenta, but antibodies do. Anticoagulation effect may persist 12 to 24 hours after the infusion is discontinued. Mechanism of elimination is unknown, and no metabolites have been identified.

Interactions: Inhibits streptokinase-induced activation of plasminogen; concomitant infusion with anticoagulants and antiplatelet agents increases risk of hemorrhage.

Nursing considerations:

- Because spontaneous bleeding often occurs, protect patient from invasive procedures and IM injections.
- Ensure that the thrombin time (TT) is kept at about two times the baseline value during treatment.
- Monitor for and report signs of spontaneous bleeding.
- Check infusion site for thrombosis.
- Keep patient on complete bed rest for entire treatment.
- Monitor for allergic reaction; minor reaction requires treatment with steroids or antihistamines.
- Monitor temperature; treat with acetaminophen, not aspirin.
- Check pulse and cardiac rhythm; dysrhythmias are a sign to discontinue therapy.

UROKINASE

Abbokinase

Urokinase is an enzyme produced by the kidneys and isolated from human kidney tissue cultures. It promotes thrombolysis by stimulating the endogenous fibrinolytic system to convert plasminogen to the enzyme plasmin.

Indications: Used to lyse acute massive pulmonary emboli and peripheral emboli and to restore patency in occluded IV catheters, including central venous catheters.

Usual dosage: *Thrombotic occlusions:* (IV infusion via constant infusion pump): initial dose of 4,400 IU/kg as an admixture at 90 ml/h over 10 minutes, followed by continuous infusion of 4,400 IU/kg/h for 12 hours. *Occluded coronary artery:* precede urokinase with a bolus of heparin (2,500-10,000 U IV), then infuse urokinase at 6,000 IU/min for periods of up to 2 hours; continue until artery is maximally opened. *Occluded central venous catheter:* 5,000 IU.

Precautions/contraindications: Safe use during pregnancy or in nursing mothers has not been established. (See also Precautions/contraindications for streptokinase.)

Side effects/adverse reactions: Side effects/adverse reactions for streptokinase.

Pharmacokinetics: Rapidly cleared by the liver; serum half-life is 20 minutes or less (impaired liver function prolongs half-life). Small amounts are excreted in the bile and urine. Fibrinolytic effects usually disappear within a few hours after treatment is discontinued, but increased thrombin time, decreased fibrinogen and plasminogen levels, and an increase in degradation products may persist for 12 to 24 hours.

Interactions: May exacerbate risk of bleeding complications; monitor patient closely during treatment.

Nursing considerations:

- Clinical response is observed 6 to 8 hours after starting therapy.
- Because severe spontaneous bleeding can occur, observe same precautions as with streptokinase (see page 230).
- Urokinase is more expensive than streptokinase.
- When clearing a central venous catheter with urokinase, instruct patient to exhale and hold his breath any time the catheter is not connected to IV tubing or a syringe to prevent air from entering the open catheter.

TISSUE PLASMINOGEN ACTIVATOR

RECOMBINANT ALTEPLASE
Activase

Tissue plasminogen activator (TPA), also known as recombinant alteplase, is a serine protease enzyme derived from a human melanoma cell line and produced in large quantities by recombinant DNA technology. Its fibrinolytic activity is almost identical to that of the natural activator.

Indications: Used in the treatment of coronary artery thrombosis associated with acute myocardial infarction.

Usual dosage: (IV): Doses are individualized. Initial bolus of 6-10 mg over 1 to 2 minutes; then 100 mg over 3 hours, given as 60 mg over the first hour, 20 mg over the second hour, and 20 mg over the third hour.

Precautions/contraindications: *Cautious use:* severe liver disease, elderly patient. *Contraindicated:* severe, uncontrolled hypertension; predisposition to bleeding; active bleeding; cardiogenic shock; history of cardiovascular accident.

Side effects/adverse reactions: *CV:* hemorrhage, especially at arterial or venous access site; GI bleeding; reocclusion of coronary artery; cardiac dysrhythmias with reperfusion.

Pharmacokinetics: Disappears rapidly from plasma; activity phase half-life lasts 5 to 8 minutes, terminal phase half-life may last up to 1.3 hours. Changes in plasminogen and fibrin activity, and prothrombin time, peak within 5 to 10 minutes; baseline values are restored within 3 hours. Drug is metabolized in the liver and excreted in the urine.

Interactions: Increased risk of bleeding with any drug that alters platelet function (e.g., aspirin, dipyridamole). Heparin, given either before or after TPA to reduce risk of clotting, may exacerbate bleeding complications. Monitor patient closely for bleeding, especially at infusion site.

Nursing considerations:

- Administer TPA as soon as possible after an acute myocardial infarction (within 3 to 4 hours).
- Keep patient on complete bed rest during drug infusion.
- Observe infusion site for bleeding.
- Hematologic effect of drug may be prolonged in patients with severe hepatic impairment.

VITAMINS

CYANOCOBALAMIN (VITAMIN B$_{12}$)
Betalin 12, Rubramin PC

Cyanocobalamin (vitamin B$_{12}$) is a cobalt-containing, B-complex vitamin that is essential for normal growth, cell reproduction, maturation of RBCs, and nucleoprotein and myelin synthesis. It is a coenzyme in the synthesis of nucleic acids and proteins and acts with folic acid in the formation of RBCs.

Indications: Used in the treatment of vitamin B$_{12}$ deficiency caused by a variety of conditions (e.g., malabsorption syndrome, as seen in pernicious anemia

Table 12-1

DRUG INTERACTIONS WITH CYANOCOBALAMIN

Drugs	Effect
Neomycin, colchicine, paraaminosalicylic acid, time-release potassium, excessive alcohol intake	Malabsorption of vitamin B_{12}
Cimetidine and other H_2-antagonists	Reduced absorption of vitamin B_{12}
Chloramphenicol and other drugs that suppress bone marrow	Suppressed therapeutic response to vitamin B_{12}

[Addison's anemia]; GI disorders caused by dysfunction or surgery; fish tapeworm infestation; pancreatic or bowel malignancies; gluten enteropathy or sprue; small bowel bacterial overgrowth). Also given for vitamin B_{12} deficiency caused by increased physiologic requirement or inadequate dietary intake.

Usual dosage: (IM, deep SC, PO): Dosing schedules are individualized. *Vitamin B_{12} deficiency:* (IM, deep SC) 30 µg daily for 5 to 10 days. Maintenance dosage of 100-200 µg monthly. *Pernicious (Addison's) anemia:* Parenteral therapy is required for life, because absorption from oral therapy is not dependable; dosage is 100 µg daily for 6 to 7 days by IM or deep SC injection. If clinical improvement and a reticulocyte response ensue, give the same amount on alternate days for seven doses, then q 3-4 days for another 2 to 3 weeks (by this time hematologic values should be normal). Maintenance dosage is 100 µg monthly for life. Folic acid may be administered concomitantly if needed. *Nutritional supplement:* Patients with normal intestinal absorption can take a daily oral multivitamin preparation containing 15 µg of vitamin B_{12}. Oral therapy is not usually recommended for vitamin B_{12} deficiency because the maximum amount absorbed from a single oral dose is 2-3 µg. The percentage absorbed decreases with increasing doses. *Schilling test (vitamin B_{12} absorption test):* flushing dose is 1,000 µg IM.

Precautions/contraindications: *Cautious use:* heart disease, folic acid deficiency. *Contraindicated:* history of hypersensitivity to vitamin B_{12} or cobalt. Safe use of parenteral form during pregnancy or in nursing mothers has not been established.

Side effects/adverse reactions: *Hypersensitivity:* anaphylactic shock, death. *CV:* pulmonary edema, congestive heart failure early in treatment, peripheral vascular thrombosis. *Dermatologic:* itching, transitory exanthema, urticaria, pain at injection site. *Ophthalmic:* severe, swift optic nerve atrophy. *Other:* feeling of swelling of entire body; hypokalemia; mild, transient diarrhea; polycythemia vera.

Pharmacokinetics: When administered PO, absorption depends on the presence of sufficient intrinsic fac-

tor and calcium. In general, absorption is inadequate in malabsorption states and pernicious anemia unless intrinsic factor is administered simultaneously.

When administered IM or SC, vitamin B_{12} is excreted in bile and then undergoes enterohepatic recycling, with wide distribution in most tissues. Principal storage site is the liver, with some storage in the kidneys and adrenals. With a dose of 100 µg or more, 50% to 95% is excreted in the urine within 48 hours; most of the dose is eliminated during the first 8 hours. Vitamin B_{12} crosses the placenta and enters breast milk.

Interactions: See Table 12-1.

Nursing considerations:

- Give oral vitamin B_{12} with food to enhance absorption.
- Before therapy is started, obtain Hb, Hct, vitamin B_{12}, and serum folate values.
- Monitor potassium level during first 48 hours of therapy.
- Use parenteral route when treating pernicious anemia (preferred technique for this disorder).
- Inform patient that pernicious anemia requires lifelong treatment.

FOLIC ACID (VITAMIN B₉)
Folvite

Folic acid (vitamin B_9) is also a member of the B-complex group of vitamins. Its role in nucleoprotein synthesis and the maturation of RBCs is similar to that of vitamin B_{12}.

Indications: Used in the treatment of megaloblastic anemia associated with malabsorption syndromes, alcoholism, inadequate dietary intake, pregnancy, infancy, or childhood.

Usual dosage: (Usually administered PO except with severe intestinal malabsorption; given IM, IV, or SC if GI absorption is very severely impaired). Usual therapeutic dosage is up to 1 mg daily PO, deep IM, or IV (resistant cases may require more). Maintenance dosage of 0.4 mg daily is started when clinical symptoms have improved. For pregnant women or nursing mothers, the daily dosage is 0.8 mg.

Table 12-2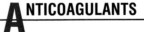

DRUG INTERACTIONS WITH FOLIC ACID

Drugs	Effect
Oral contraceptives	May impair folate metabolism and cause folate depletion (effect is mild)
Phenytoin	May produce subtherapeutic level of phenytoin, precipitating seizures
Pyrimethamine, trimethoprim, or triamterene	May interfere with folic acid utilization
Antimicrobial drugs	May interfere with the antimicrobial treatment of toxoplasmosis
Chloramphenicol and other drugs that suppress bone marrow	May suppress therapeutic response to folic acid

Precautions/contraindications: *Contraindicated:* pernicious anemia, aplastic or normocytic anemia. Dosages above 0.1 mg daily may obscure diagnosis of pernicious anemia.

Side effects/adverse reactions: Relatively nontoxic; some allergic sensitization has been reported.

Pharmacokinetics: Oral doses are readily absorbed from the small intestine, with wide distribution to all body tissues. Peak activity is seen in 30 to 60 minutes. Drug is metabolized in the liver to active forms of folate. Traces of unchanged drug are found in the urine with therapeutic dosages; this amount increases with larger doses. Drug is also found in breast milk.

Interactions: See Table 12-2.

Nursing considerations:

- Obtain history of dietary patterns and drug and alcohol use before therapy is begun.
- Drugs such as oral contraceptives, alcohol, barbiturates, methotrexate, phenytoin, primidone, and trimethoprim can cause folic acid deficiency; relate this to drug history. Deficiency may also be the result of dialysis.
- Monitor for symptoms of folic acid deficiency (glossitis, diarrhea or constipation, weight loss, depression, fatigue, diffuse muscular pain).

AGENTS FOR TREATING METAL DEFICIENCIES THAT MANIFEST AS ANEMIA

COPPER AND COBALT

Copper and cobalt deficiencies are rare. Because copper metabolism and cobalt metabolism are interrelated, suspected copper-deficiency anemia responds to iron therapy with or without copper. Although primary cobalt deficiency has not been reported in people, supplemental doses of the metal may improve Hct, Hb, and erythrocyte values in refractory anemia that does not respond to conventional therapy.

VITAMINS FOR DEFICIENCIES THAT MANIFEST AS ANEMIA

ASCORBIC ACID (VITAMIN C)

Although rare, severe vitamin C deficiency may be associated with hypochromic anemia, which can be microcytic with chronic blood loss or macrocytic when associated with folic acid deficiency.

PYRIDOXINE (VITAMIN B₆)

Pyridoxine produces a beneficial hemoglobin response in individuals with a form of sideroblastic anemia characterized by abnormally large amounts of nonhemoglobin iron in erythrocyte precursors, hypochromic-microcytic anemia, and other signs of severely disturbed blood regeneration. This pyridoxine-responsive anemia occurs sporadically in men, possibly as a genetic condition.

ANTICOAGULANTS

The coagulation of blood requires a cascade of proteolytic reactions involving the interaction of clotting factors, platelets, and tissue materials. Many substances can prevent the formation of clots, but only those drugs that can be administered without undue toxicity are clinically useful. Depending on their mechanism of action, these drugs can be divided into two classes: direct-acting and indirect-acting anticoagulants. Direct-acting anticoagulants affect the blood components that play a role in coagulation, preventing them from interacting normally. Indirect-acting anticoagulants interfere with the synthesis of clotting factors.

ASPIRIN (VARIOUS TRADE NAMES)

Aspirin has a powerful antiplatelet action in addition to its antiinflammatory, analgesic, and antipyretic actions. Measurable antiplatelet effect can persist for 3 to 8 days after a single dose. At higher doses aspirin impairs hepatic synthesis of coagulation factors VII, IX, and X, possibly by inhibiting the action of vitamin K.

Indications: Used to reduce the recurrence of transient ischemic attacks (TIA) caused by fibrin platelet emboli and the risk of stroke. Also used to prevent recurrence of myocardial infarction (MI) and as prophylactic therapy in men with unstable angina. Low doses are used to prevent first or subsequent heart attacks and thromboembolic disorders.

Usual dosage: (PO): *Thromboembolic disorders:* 325-650 mg once or twice a day. *TIA prophylaxis:* 650 mg bid, or 325 mg qid. *Prophylaxis (as in recurrent MI):* 325 mg once a day.

Precautions/contraindications: *Cautious use:* otic disease, gout, hyperthyroidism, renal or hepatic impairment. *Contraindicated:* history of hypersensitivity to salicylates, patient with "aspirin triad" (aspirin sensitivity, nasal polyps, asthma), GI ulceration, bleeding disorders. Do not give to pregnant women or nursing mothers. Do not give to children or teenagers with chickenpox or influenza-like disease.

Side effects/adverse reactions: Mild, chronic intoxication (salicylism). *CNS:* dizziness. *CV:* flushing, increased heart rate. *ENT:* ringing in the ears. *Eye:* dimness of vision. *GI:* nausea, vomiting, bleeding. *Hypersensitivity:* urticaria, bronchospasm. *Skin:* petechiae. *Other:* sweating, hypoglycemia.

Pharmacokinetics: Partly absorbed from the stomach, but mainly from the small intestine. Administration with food retards rate of absorption but not amount. Peak plasma level is achieved in 1 to 2 hours. Half-life is 15 to 20 minutes; converted to salicylic acid about 2 to 3 hours after a 600 mg dose and 6 to 12 hours after larger doses. Aspirin is rapidly hydrolyzed to salicylic acid by enzymes found in the GI mucosa, plasma, erythrocytes, and synovial fluid before it is further metabolized; the metabolites and a small amount of salicylic acid are excreted in the urine. Enteric-coated preparations are erratically absorbed and can produce variable blood serum levels. Aspirin crosses the placenta and is distributed in breast milk.

Interactions: Use with oral anticoagulants or heparin can lead to hemorrhage. About 80% of salicylic acid is bound to plasma proteins. Other drugs that also bind to plasma proteins (e.g., sulfonamides) can be displaced, increasing the concentration of free drug. Similarly, infants with incompletely developed bilirubin-conjugating enzyme systems may develop kernicterus if given aspirin. Aspirin increases the toxicity of methotrexate. It may antagonize the uricosuric actions of sulfinpyrazone and probenecid. Blood loss may be increased by simultaneous consumption of aspirin and alcohol. Any agent that can acidify urine (e.g., ascorbic acid) increases reabsorption of salicylic acid. Antacids may reduce absorption of aspirin. When aspirin and oral hypoglycemic agents are given together, the plasma levels of both are elevated. Aspirin increases the half-life of penicillin.

Nursing considerations:

- Monitor for bleeding (petechiae, bruising).
- Minimize gastric irritation by administering with food or milk.
- Enteric-coated or extended-release formulations can reduce gastric irritation.
- Discontinue 1 week before surgery to reduce bleeding risk.
- Do not give to patients with asthma, nasal polyps, or hay fever (aspirin triad).
- Advise patients to report any hearing changes; tinnitus and muffled hearing are symptoms of chronic salicylate overdose.
- Do not give aspirin for flu or chickenpox, to prevent Reye's syndrome.
- **Overdose treatment:** Acute salicylate toxicity requires immediate induced emesis or gastric lavage. Further treatment is designed to maintain hydration and electrolyte and acid-base balance, to correct hypoglycemia and hyperthermia, to reduce excitation or convulsions, and to force excretion of salicylates by alkalinizing the urine.

HEPARIN CALCIUM, HEPARIN SODIUM

Commercial preparations of heparin are derived from bovine lung or porcine intestinal mucosa. There are chemical and biologic differences between the two but no clinical difference in their anticoagulant actions. Heparin directly affects blood coagulation by enhancing the inhibitory actions of antithrombin III. This blocks the conversion of prothrombin to thrombin and fibrinogen to fibrin. Heparin does not lyse clots already formed; however, it may prevent extension of such clots and the formation of new ones.

Indications: Used for prophylaxis and treatment of venous thrombosis and its extension, pulmonary embolism, peripheral arterial embolism, and atrial fibrillation with embolization. Also used in the diagnosis and treatment of acute and chronic consumption coagulopathies (e.g., disseminated intravascular coagulation, atrial fibrillation with embolization) and as an anticoagulant in blood transfusions, extracorporeal circulation, and dialysis procedures. In a low-dose regimen, drug is used to prevent postoperative deep vein thrombosis and pulmonary embolism in patients undergoing major abdominothoracic surgery or in patients at risk of developing thromboembolic disease after surgery.

Usual dosage: (SC): Adjusted according to results of coagulation tests done before each injection. Dosage is adequate when activated coagulation time (ACT) is approximately two and one half to three times the control value or when the activated partial thromboplastin time (APTT) is one and one half to two times normal. *Low-dose prophylaxis:* usually 5,000 U SC 2 hours before surgery and 5,000 U q 8-12 h for 7 days after surgery or until patient is fully ambulatory. *Overdose:* See Nursing considerations.

Precautions/contraindications: *Cautious use:* history of alcoholism, atopy, or allergy; menstruating women; liver and/or renal disease. *Contraindicated:* hypersensitivity to heparin, active bleeding or bleeding tendencies (i.e., hemophilia), advanced liver or kidney disease. Safe use during pregnancy has not been established.

Side effects/adverse reactions: Chief complication is hemorrhage. *Hypersensitivity:* fever, chills, urticaria, pruritus. *Other (with prolonged administration of large doses):* osteoporosis, hypoaldosteronism, suppressed renal function, rebound hyperlipidemia (occurs after therapy has been terminated).

Pharmacokinetics: Is not absorbed from the GI tract and must be given IV or SC. An IV bolus produces an immediate anticoagulation effect. The duration of action is dose dependent. Peak plasma levels are reached 2 to 4 hours after SC administration. Once absorbed from this route of administration, drug is distributed in plasma and extensively protein bound.

Elimination curve is biphasic. The absence of a relationship between plasma half-life and pharmacologic half-life may reflect drug's extensive plasma protein binding. Heparin is rapidly cleared from plasma, with an average half-life of 30 minutes to 3 hours. Heparin is partly metabolized by liver enzymes and by the mononuclear phagocytic system. Half of it is excreted unchanged in the urine, and the rest is excreted as metabolites, some of which continue to have anticoagulant activity.

Interactions: Anticoagulant effect may be increased by aspirin, other nonsteroidal antiinflammatory drugs and salicylates, cephalosporins, and penicillins. Use with oral anticoagulants may prolong prothrombin time, which is used to monitor oral anticoagulant therapy. Action of heparin may be decreased by nitroglycerin.

Nursing considerations:

- Ensure that baseline blood coagulation tests are performed before administering heparin and at regular intervals during therapy.
- Do not use the IM route because of the risk of hematoma formation.
- Heparin calcium reportedly is less likely to cause local hematomas than heparin sodium; however, no differences in side effects or efficacy have been observed.
- The anticoagulant potency of heparin is expressed in "units" of activity.
- **Guidelines for deep SC intrafat injection:** The site of administration is either the fatty layer of the abdomen or just above the iliac crest. Use a 25- or 26-gauge, ½- to ⅝-inch needle to make the injection. Discard the needle used to withdraw the heparin dose from the vial. Wipe the injection site lightly with alcohol and allow to dry. Gently grasp a defined roll of tissue without pinching, quickly insert the needle perpendicularly, and slowly inject. **Do not withdraw plunger to check for entry into a blood vessel.** Pause before withdrawing the needle to prevent trailing the drug; then withdraw rapidly. Apply gentle pressure to puncture site; **do not massage.**
- **Overdose treatment:** Bleeding is the chief sign of overdose. Observe patient for nosebleeds, hematuria, tarry stools, easy bleeding, or formation of petechiae, all of which may precede frank bleeding. Treatment consists of administering the heparin antidote protamine sulfate as a 1% solution. About 100 U of heparin can be neutralized by 1 mg of protamine sulfate.

COUMARIN COMPOUNDS

Coumarin compounds, which include warfarin, are agents that interfere with the hepatic synthesis of vitamin K–dependent clotting factors II (prothrombin), VII, IX, and X. Oral anticoagulants have no direct effect on a clot already formed, nor do they reverse ischemic tissue damage. However, once the thrombosis is established, they may prevent extension of the formed clot and secondary thromboembolic complications.

WARFARIN
Coumadin

Indications: Used for prophylaxis and treatment of venous thrombosis and its extension; treatment of atrial fibrillation with embolization; and prophylaxis and treatment of pulmonary embolism. Also used as adjunct therapy in the prophylaxis of systemic embolism after myocardial infarction.

Usual dosage: (PO, IM, IV): initially 10-15 mg daily for 2 to 5 days; maintenance dosage depends on daily prothrombin time (PT) response. Dosages are individually adjusted according to results of one-stage PT.

Precautions/contraindications: *Cautious use:* alcoholism, allergic disorders, menstruating women. *Contraindicated:* hemorrhagic tendencies, bleeding disorders, vitamin K or vitamin C deficiency, active peptic ulcer, pregnancy.

Side effects/adverse reactions: May cause major or minor hemorrhaging from any tissue or organ. *GI:* anorexia, nausea, vomiting. *Hypersensitivity:* dermatitis, urticaria. *Other:* increased serum transaminase, hepatitis. *Overdose:* internal or external bleeding; paralytic ileus; skin necrosis of toes, tip of nose, and other fat-rich areas.

Pharmacokinetics: With PO administration, onset of action is 12 to 24 hours, but clinically significant anticoagulant effects cannot be expected before 30 to 60 hours. Peak effect lasts 1½ to 3 days, and the duration of action is 3 to 5 days after a single dose. Half-life is 1½ to 2½ days and is independent of dose. Approximately 99% of the drug is plasma protein bound. It accumulates primarily in the liver, where it is metabolized and excreted in the urine and feces. Significant individual differences in metabolism and excretion rates occur.

Interactions: Because all anticoagulant drugs have the potential to interact adversely with numerous drugs, consult a pharmaceutic reference before adding or withdrawing a drug in the therapeutic regimen. Also, warn the patient about the hazards of taking any drug, including over-the-counter medications, without the advice of a health care provider.

Nursing considerations:

- Be sure to obtain a detailed drug history because of the numerous drug interactions possible.
- Patient teaching is very important; be sure to include spoken and written instructions (see below).
- Dosing is highly individual and may have to be adjusted several times based on laboratory test results.
- Give patient a list of medications and foods to avoid.
- **Overdose treatment:** If excessive anticoagulation occurs with or without bleeding, discontinue warfarin and administer oral or parenteral vitamin K if necessary.

Patient teaching:

- Oral anticoagulants may give urine with an alkaline pH a red-orange color.
- Notify the physician if any of these signs occur:

unusual bleeding or bruising; red or dark brown urine, or red or tar black stools; diarrhea.

- Do not take products containing aspirin or *any* over-the-counter drugs without first checking with the physician.
- Do not make drastic changes in diet or alcohol consumption.
- Do not change from one brand of this medication to another without consulting the physician.
- Consult the physician before having any dental work or surgery.
- Use an electric razor and a soft toothbrush, and floss gently with waxed dental floss.
- Do not take the next dose of the anticoagulant medication and notify the physician promptly in the following circumstances: bleeding or signs of bleeding (blood in urine), hematuria, hypersensitivity reaction (itching or hives), liver damage, jaundice (yellow skin).

ANTINEOPLASTIC AGENTS

ANTINEOPLASTIC AGENTS FOR LEUKEMIAS

The leukemias are a group of neoplastic diseases characterized by abnormal proliferation of blood cells and their immature precursors. Leukemias may involve either lymphocytic or nonlymphocytic cell lines, and within each group the characteristic cell may be either relatively mature or immature in appearance. The leukemias characterized by immature cells are considered acute because of their short natural history (1 to 5 months if left untreated). Leukemias characterized by more mature cells are considered chronic because of their slower progressive course (2 to 5 years).

ACUTE LYMPHOCYTIC LEUKEMIA (ALL)
Two Remission Induction Regimens

Acronym: DVP	
Daunorubicin	45 mg/m² IV, days 1-3 and 14
Vincristine	2 mg/m² (maximum 2 mg) IV, weekly for 4 weeks
Prednisone	45 mg/m² PO, for 28 days

Cyclophosphamide	1,200 mg/m² IV, day 1
Daunorubicin	45 mg/m² IV, days 1-3
Prednisone	600 mg/m² PO, days 1-21
Vincristine	2 mg/m² (maximum 2 mg) IV, weekly for 4 weeks
ʟ-Asparaginase	6,000 U/m² IV, 3 times a week

CNS Prophylaxis Regimen

Even though induction therapy is effective in reducing leukemia blast cells, about half the patients will experience central nervous system relapse. CNS prophylaxis is begun 2 weeks after complete remission has been achieved.

Cranial irradiation

Methotrexate   12 mg/m^2 intrathecal twice a week for 5 doses

---

Maintenance Regimen

Acronym: MM

Mercaptopurine	50 mg/m^2 PO, daily
Methotrexate	20 mg/m^2 PO or IV, weekly

ACUTE NONLYMPHOCYTIC LEUKEMIA (ANLL)
Remission Induction Regimen

Acronym: DCT

Daunorubicin	60 mg/m^2 IV, days 1-3
Cytarabine	200 mg/m^2 IV daily as a continuous infusion, days 1-5
Thioguanine	100 mg/m^2 PO, q 12 h, days 1-5

Treatment During Remission

ANLL consolidation

Cytarabine   3,000 mg/m^2 IV, q 12 h, days 1-6

OR

Acronym: MC

Mitoxantrone	12 mg/m^2 IV daily, days 1-2
Cytarabine	100 mg/m^2 IV daily as a continuous infusion, days 1-5

Maintenance Regimen

Acronym: TC

Thioguanine	40 mg/m^2 PO, q 12 h, days 1-4 each week
Cytarabine	60 mg/m^2 SC, day 5 each week

CHRONIC LYMPHOCYTIC LEUKEMIA (CLL)

Chronic lymphocytic leukemia is seen primarily in older adults. In many cases the course of the disease is indolent, and survival rates of 5 to 10 years are not unusual. In other cases the disease progresses more rapidly, leading to death within a few years. The primary goal of therapy is to reduce the symptoms, although in some patients treatment may prolong life for a few months to years.

Treatment Regimen

Indolent phase:

- No therapy **or** chlorambucil (4 mg/m^2 PO daily) until the peripheral lymphocyte count falls to 10,000/mm^3; then 2 mg/daily or discontinue drug until WBC exceeds 50,000/mm^3.

Active phase:

- Chlorambucil (3-6 mg/m^2 PO daily) until WBC falls to 10,000/mm^3; maintain with 1-2 mg/m^2 PO daily.
- **OR**

Cyclophosphamide	300 mg/m^2 PO, days 1-5
Vincristine	1.4 mg/m^2 (maximum 2 mg) IV, day 1
Prednisone	100 mg/m^2 PO, days 1-5

Cycle is repeated q 21 days.

CHRONIC GRANULOCYTIC LEUKEMIA (CGL)

Chronic granulocytic leukemia is characterized by two phases, an early chronic phase and a late acute blastic crisis. The treatment goal in the chronic phase is to alleviate fatigue, weakness, abdominal pain, and other symptoms. The goal in the acute phase is complete remission.

Treatment Regimen

Chronic phase:

- Busulfan (3-4 mg/m^2 PO daily) until WBC is 50% of original level; then 1-2 mg/m^2 daily.

OR

- Hydroxyurea (1-2 g/m^2 PO daily) until WBC is 50% of original level; then 0.5-1 g/m^2 daily.

Acute phase:

- Therapy is guided by morphologic and biochemical markers.

POLYCYTHEMIA VERA

Polycythemia vera is a malignant-behaving disorder of blood cells characterized by overproduction of all cellular elements in the marrow. Treatment is directed toward controlling the overproduction or reducing the circulating red cell mass, or both.

Treatment Regimen

- Phlebotomy (performed as often as necessary to maintain Hct at 45% or less)
- Administration of radioactive phosphorus
- Chlorambucil (10 mg PO daily for 6 weeks, rest 1 month, then alternate 1 month on and 1 month off)

ANTINEOPLASTIC AGENTS FOR LYMPHOMAS

The Hodgkin's and non-Hodgkin's lymphomas constitute a spectrum of lymphoproliferative malignancies. Nevertheless, they share a number of important clinical features. Both may be present as solitary or generalized adenopathic conditions, and both require accurate clinical staging as the basis for therapeutic planning.

Hodgkin's Disease

Treatment: Drug therapy for Hodgkin's disease must be considered on a stage-by-stage basis. In general, early stages of Hodgkin's disease (stages IA and IIA) are treated with radiation therapy, and advanced stages (IVA and IVB) are treated with combination chemotherapy. Before drug therapy is begun, give the patient allopurinol (300 mg/daily PO) for 2 to 3 days with high fluid intake to prevent the hyperuricemia that may follow tumor lysis.

The following box lists several treatment regimens used in Hodgkin's disease.

Non-Hodgkin's Disease

The non-Hodgkin's lymphomas are a group of malignancies that involve lymphocytes. Although non-Hodgkin's disease often is considered a single disorder, it actually comprises several disorders that differ in many basic characteristics. When the disease is diagnosed, some types of lymphomas are almost always disseminated and have a high incidence of bone marrow and liver involvement (poorly differentiated lymphocytic lymphoma). Diffuse histiocytic lymphoma is lim-

---

CHEMOTHERAPY REGIMENS USED IN HODGKIN'S LYMPHOMA

Acronym: ABVD

Doxorubicin	25 mg/m² IV, days 1 and 15
Bleomycin	10 U/m² IV, days 1 and 15
Vinblastine	6 mg/m² IV, days 1 and 15
Dacarbazine	375 mg/m² IV, days 1 and 15
	Cycle is repeated q 28 days.

Acronym: MOPP

Mechlorethamine	6 mg/m² IV, days 1 and 8
Vincristine	1.4 mg/m² (maximum 2 mg) IV, days 1 and 8
Procarbazine	100 mg/m² PO, days 1-14
Prednisone	40 mg/m² PO, days 1-14
	Cycle is repeated q 28 days.

Acronym: MOPP/ABV hybrid

Mechlorethamine	6 mg/m² IV, day 1
Vincristine	1.2 mg/m² (maximum 2 mg) IV, day 1
Prednisone	40 mg/m² PO, days 1-14
Procarbazine	100 mg/m² PO, days 1-7
Doxorubicin	35 mg/m² IV, day 8
Vinblastine	6 mg/m² IV, day 8
Bleomycin	10 mg/m² IV, day 8
Hydrocortisone	100 mg/m² IV, day 8
	Cycle is repeated q 28 days.

Acronym: MVPP

Mechlorethamine	6 mg/m² IV, days 1 and 8
Vinblastine	6 mg/m² IV, days 1 and 8
Procarbazine	100 mg/m² PO, days 1-14
Prednisone	40 mg/m² PO, days 1-14
	Cycle is repeated q 42 days for 6 cycles.

ited to a single lymph node region or to two adjacent areas in up to 30% of cases.

Treatment Regimen

See the following boxes for information on combination chemotherapy regimens for clinically indolent lympho-mas and regimens for histologic lymphomas.

Before chemotherapy is begun, give the patient allopurinol (300 mg/daily PO) 2 to 3 days with high fluid intake to prevent the hyperuricemia that may follow tumor lysis.

COMBINATION CHEMOTHERAPY REGIMENS FOR CLINICALLY INDOLENT LYMPHOMAS

Acronym: CVP

Cyclophosphamide	400 mg/m^2 PO, days 1-5
Vincristine	1.4 mg/m^2 (maximum 2 mg) IV, day 1
Prednisone	100 mg/m^2 PO, days 1-5

Acronym: COPP

Cyclophosphamide	600 mg/m^2 IV, days 1 and 8
Vincristine	1.4 mg/m^2 (maximum 2 mg) IV, days 1 and 8
Procarbazine	100 mg/m^2 PO, days 1-14
Prednisone	40 mg/m^2 PO, days 1-14
	Cycle is repeated q 28 days.

Acronym: CHOP

Cyclophosphamide	750 mg/m^2 IV, day 1
Doxorubicin	50 mg/m^2 IV, day 1
Vincristine	1.4 mg/m^2 (maximum 2 mg) IV, day 1
Prednisone	100 mg/m^2 PO, days 1-5
	Cycle is repeated q 21 days.

CHEMOTHERAPY REGIMENS FOR NON-HODGKIN'S LYMPHOMAS

Acronym: BACOP

Bleomycin	5 U/m^2 IV, days 1 and 8
Doxorubicin	25 mg/m^2 IV, days 1 and 8
Cyclophosphamide	650 mg/m^2 IV, days 1 and 8
Vincristine	1.4 mg/m^2 (maximum 2 mg) IV, days 1 and 8
Prednisone	60 mg/m^2 PO, days 15-28
	Cycle is repeated q 42 days for 6 cycles.

Acronym: CHOP

Cyclophosphamide	750 mg/m^2 IV, day 1
Doxorubicin	50 mg/m^2 IV, day 1
Vincristine	1.4 mg/m^2 (maximum 2 mg) IV, day 1
Prednisone	100 mg/m^2 PO, days 1-5
	Cycle is repeated q 21 days.

Acronym: COMLA

Cyclophosphamide	1,500 mg/m^2 IV, day 1
Vincristine	1.4 mg/m^2 (maximum 2 mg) IV, days 15 and 18
Methotrexate	120 mg/m^2 IV, days 22, 29, 36, 43, 50, 57, 64, and 71
Leucovorin	25 mg/m^2 PO, q 6 h for 4 doses, given 24 hours after each methotrexate dose
Cytarabine	300 mg/m^2 IV, days 22, 29, 36, 43, 50, 57, 64, and 71
	Cycle is repeated q 21 days.

ANTINEOPLASTIC AGENTS FOR MULTIPLE MYELOMA

Multiple myeloma is a neoplasm of malignant plasma cells that invade bone and bone marrow and cause widespread skeletal destruction, bone marrow failure, and problems related to certain abnormal serum and/or urine proteins. Chemotherapy is used to improve the duration of survival and to prevent or diminish the serious manifestations of this disease (e.g., bone pain, pathologic fractures, severe anemia, renal failure, or hypercalcemia).

Standard Induction Regimen

Acronym: MP	
Melphalan	8 mg/m² PO, days 1-4
Prednisone	60 mg/m² PO, days 1-4
Cycle is repeated q 28 days for at least 1 year.	

Intensive Induction Regimen

Acronym: M-2	
Vincristine	0.03 mg/kg (maximum 2 mg) IV, day 1
Carmustine	0.5 mg/kg IV, day 1
Cyclophosphamide	10 mg/kg IV, day 1
Melphalan	0.25 mg/kg PO, days 1-4
Prednisone	1 mg/kg days 1-7, then taper over next 14 days Cycle is repeated q 35 days for 1 year.

There is no conclusive evidence that continuing chemotherapy beyond 1 year is beneficial.

Nursing considerations:

- Monitor patient's temperature at regular intervals; also note onset of chills or sore throat.
- Protect patient from infection and trauma during blood count nadir.
- Monitor patient for overgrowth of opportunistic organisms.
- Check patient's weight daily.
- Monitor ratio and pattern of intake and output.
- Administer antinausea medications before giving antineoplastic drugs to prevent nausea and vomiting.
- Remember: patient and family education is an integral part of treatment with antineoplastic drugs.

CHELATING AGENTS

DEFEROXAMINE MESYLATE
Desferal

Deferoxamine mesylate is a chelating agent with a binding affinity for ferric ions. The ferrioxamine complex is water soluble and readily excreted by the kidneys.

Indications: Used as an adjunct in the treatment of acute iron intoxication. Also used to promote iron excretion in patients with secondary iron overload from multiple blood transfusions.

Usual dosage: (IM, IV, SC): *Acute iron intoxication:* (adult dose) 1 g IM (preferred route) or IV (slow) followed by 500 mg at 4 hour intervals for two doses. Depending on clinical response, subsequent doses of 500 mg may be administered q 4-12 h (total 24-hour dosage should not exceed 6 g). *Chronic iron overload:* IM: 500 mg to 1 g IM daily. In addition, 2 g IV with each unit of blood transfused. IV: 1-2 g (20-40 mg/kg daily) given over 8 to 24 hours via continuous infusion pump.

Precautions/contraindications: *Cautious use:* history of pyelonephritis. *Contraindicated:* severe renal disease, anuria, pyelonephritis, primary hemochromatosis, pregnancy, woman of childbearing potential, child under 3 years of age.

Side effects/adverse reactions: *CV:* hypotensive shock, tachycardia. *ENT:* decreased hearing. *Eye:* blurred vision, decreased visual acuity. *GI:* abdominal discomfort. *GU:* dysuria, exacerbation of pyelonephritis. *Other:* leg cramps, pain and induration at injection site.

Pharmacokinetics: After parenteral administration drug is widely distributed throughout the body. It is metabolized primarily by plasma enzymes and excreted rapidly as iron chelate and unchanged drug in the urine.

Nursing considerations:

- IM route is preferred.
- Avoid rapid IV infusion; flushing of the skin, urticaria, hypotension, and shock have occurred with rapid infusion.
- Monitor vital signs during treatment.
- Have epinephrine 1:1,000 readily available in case of allergic reaction.
- Drug-iron complex imparts a reddish color to the urine.
- Ensure that baseline kidney function tests are done before treatment is begun.
- Monitor input/output ratio, and note any changes.
- Advise patient undergoing prolonged or high-dose therapy to have periodic vision and hearing tests.

DIMERCAPROL

BAL

Dimercaprol is a dithiol compound originally developed as an antidote for Lewisite, a chemical warfare agent that contained arsenic. Dimercaprol combines with ions of various heavy metals to form relatively stable, nontoxic, soluble chelates that can be excreted.

Indications: Used in the treatment of acute poisoning caused by arsenic, gold, or mercury. Also used as an adjunct to edetate calcium disodium in the treatment of lead encephalopathy.

Usual dosage: (Deep IM only): *Mild arsenic or gold poisoning:* 2.5 mg/kg qid for first 2 days; bid on third day; then once a day for 10 days. *Severe arsenic or gold poisoning:* 3 mg/kg q4h for first 2 days; qid on third day; then twice a day for 10 days. *Mercury poisoning:* initial dose of 5 mg/kg, followed by 2.5 mg/kg once or twice a day for 10 days. *Acute lead encephalopathy:* 4 mg/kg for initial dose; then q4h with edetate disodium for 2 to 7 days, depending on response.

Precautions/contraindications: *Cautious use:* hypertension or G6PD deficiency. *Contraindicated:* hepatic insufficiency (except with jaundice caused by arsenic poisoning), severe renal insufficiency, poisoning from cadmium, iron, selenium, or uranium. Safe use during pregnancy and in nursing women has not been established.

Side effects/adverse reactions: *CNS:* headaches, anxiety, muscle pain, weakness, paresthesia. *CV:* elevated BP with tachycardia (common). *ENT:* rhinorrhea, burning sensation, pain or constriction in throat. *Eye:* conjunctivitis, lacrimation, blepharospasm. *GI:* nausea, halitosis, salivation, abdominal pain, metabolic acidosis. *GU:* burning sensation in penis, renal damage. *Other:* transient fever, pain in chest or hands, sterile abscess at injection site.

Pharmacokinetics: Peak blood levels occur 30 to 60 minutes after injection. Drug is distributed mainly in intercellular spaces, including the brain; highest concentration is in the liver and kidneys. Uncomplexed dimercaprol is rapidly metabolized to inactive products and excreted in urine and feces via the bile. Metabolic degradation and urinary excretion are essentially complete within 4 hours.

Interactions: Forms toxic complexes with cadmium, iron, selenium, and uranium.

Nursing considerations:

- Administer by deep IM injection only (local pain, gluteal abscess, and skin sensitization have been reported).
- Monitor vital signs (elevated systolic and diastolic BP with tachycardia frequently occur within a few minutes of injection).

- Monitor for anxiety, weakness, and unrest, which often are relieved by antihistamines.
- Monitor input/output ratio (drug is potentially nephrotoxic).
- Urine should have an alkaline pH to reduce possible renal damage.
- Dimercaprol will give patient's breath a garlicky odor.

EDETATE CALCIUM DISODIUM (EDTA)

Edetate calcium disodium is a chelating agent that combines with divalent and trivalent metals to form stable, soluble complexes that can be readily excreted by the kidneys. Its action depends on the ability of heavy metal to displace the loosely bound calcium from the molecule.

Indications: Used mainly as an adjunct in the treatment of acute and chronic lead poisoning. Usually used in combination with dimercaprol for the treatment of lead encephalopathy.

Usual dosage: (IV, IM): *IV:* 1 g diluted in 250-500 ml 5% dextrose (D_5W) or normal saline. *Asymptomatic patient:* administer over at least 1 hour bid (q 12 h) for up to 5 days. Interrupt for 2 days, then resume for 5 days. *Symptomatic patient:* increase administration time to 2 hours. Give a second daily dose 6 hours or more after the first. *IM:* Do not exceed 35 mg/kg bid. In mild cases do not exceed 50 mg/kg/day; procaine may be added (0.5% final concentration) to minimize pain at injection site.

Precautions/contraindications: *Cautious use:* renal dysfunction, active tubercular lesions, history of gout. *Contraindicated:* severe renal disease, anuria, IV administration in patients with lead encephalopathy. Safe use during pregnancy and in women of childbearing age has not been established.

Side effects/adverse reactions: *CNS:* numbness, paresthesia, headaches, malaise, cramps. *CV:* hypotension, cardiac dysrhythmias, thrombophlebitis. *GI:* anorexia, nausea, vomiting, diarrhea, cheilosis. *Hematologic:* transient bone marrow depression, depletion of blood metals. *Renal:* nephrotoxicity (renal tubular necrosis is the principal toxicity). *Other:* febrile reaction accompanied by histamine reaction.

Pharmacokinetics: Plasma half-life is about 20 to 60 minutes after IV administration, 1½ hours after IM injection. After IV administration, drug is distributed to extracellular fluid only. Edetate calcium disodium is not metabolized. Approximately 50% of chelated lead is excreted within 1 hour, and more than 95% of chelates are excreted within 24 to 48 hours.

Nursing considerations:

- Avoid excessive fluids in patients with lead encephalopathy.
- Establish urine flow in dehydrated patients to facilitate excretion of chelated metal.
- Closely monitor infusion rate as prescribed (rapid infusion in patients with cerebral edema can be fatal).
- Closely monitor input/output ratio.
- Ensure that routine urinalysis and BUN test are done during treatment.
- Observe for febrile reaction, which occurs 4 to 8 hours after infusion.
- Watch for paresthesia and signs of impending convulsion (twitching, anxiety, disorientation).

DETATE DISODIUM

Although detate disodium is structurally different from edetate calcium disodium, it also forms chelates with many bivalent and trivalent metals (e.g., magnesium and zinc). However, it has a particular affinity for calcium, with which it forms a stable, soluble complex that can be easily excreted by the kidneys.

Indications: Used in selected patients for emergency treatment of hypercalcemia and to control ventricular dysrhythmias and heart block associated with digitalis toxicity when other drugs such as phenytoin and potassium are contraindicated.

Usual dosage: (IV): *Hypercalcemia:* 50 mg/kg daily up to 3 g a day. Dose should be added to 500 ml of 5% dextrose (D_5W) or normal saline and infused over 3 to 4 hours. *Digitalis-induced ventricular dysrhythmias:* 15 mg/kg, to a maximum of 60 mg/kg a day, by IV infusion in 5% dextrose.

Precautions/contraindications: *Cautious use:* limited cardiac reserve, incipient congestive heart failure, potassium deficiency. *Contraindicated:* significant renal disease, hypocalcemia, history of seizure disorder, intracranial lesions. Safe use during pregnancy and in women of childbearing age has not been established.

Side effects/adverse reactions: *Skin:* exfoliative dermatitis and other skin mucous membrane lesions similar to those in pyridoxine deficiency. *Other:* fever, chills, anemia, glycosuria, hyperuricemia, severe hypocalcemia, tetany, hypomagnesemia. *Local reactions:* pain, erythema, and dermatitis. CNS, cardiovascular, GI, and renal side effects are similar to those for edetate calcium disodium.

Pharmacokinetics: About 95% of administered dose is excreted rapidly from urine following IV administration. Drug is eliminated primarily as calcium chelate.

Interactions: May lower blood glucose and reduce insulin requirement in diabetic patients (this reaction is thought to be due to chelation of the zinc in the insulin preparation).

Nursing considerations:

- Avoid extravasation. Drug is extremely irritating to tissue; rotate infusion sites.
- Monitor infusion rate closely (rapid infusion can cause hypocalcemic tetany, cardiac dysrhythmias, seizures, or cardiac arrest).
- Keep patient supine for 20 to 30 minutes after infusion to prevent postural hypotension.
- Determine serum calcium level after administering each dose.
- Keep calcium gluconate available for emergency use.
- Monitor patient for early signs of hypocalcemia (paresthesia, mental instability, seizures, carpopedal spasm).
- Ensure that urinalysis and kidney function tests are performed daily during treatment.
- If patient is an insulin-dependent diabetic, determine whether insulin dosage should be reduced.

VOLUME EXPANDER

HUMAN ALBUMIN

Normal Human Serum Albumin (Albuminar 25%) supplies colloid to the blood and expands plasma volume.

Indications: Used to expand plasma volume and maintain cardiac output in the treatment of certain types of shock or impending shock, including that caused by burns, surgery, or hemorrhage. Also used for other conditions involving a circulatory volume deficit.

Usual dosage: Albumin solutions are administered by IV infusion. The concentration of albumin administered depends on the patient's requirements. The usual initial dose for adults is 25 g. If an adequate response is not observed, the same dose may be repeated. Subsequent dosage depends on the patient's condition; up to 125 g a day may be used in some cases. No more than 250 g (5 L of a 5% solution or 1 L of a 25% solution) should be administered within 48 hours. Patients who would need more probably require whole blood transfusion or plasma. *Nephrosis:* usual initial dose of 25-50 g (100-200 ml of a 25% solution), repeated at 1- to 2-day intervals.

Precautions/contraindications: *Cautious use:* restricted sodium intake, low cardiac reserve, pulmonary disease, absence of albumin deficit, hepatic/renal failure, dehydration, hypertension. *Contraindicated:* allergy to albumin, severe anemia, cardiac failure with normal or increased intravascular volume. Safe use during pregnancy has not been established.

Side effects/adverse reactions: Allergic fever, chills, urticaria, circulatory overload, pulmonary edema (with rapid infusion), variable effects on BP, tachycardia.

Nursing considerations:

- Adjust the rate of infusion according to the patient's age and condition. (In adults, initially 500 ml [5% solution] by IV infusion; repeat q 30 min prn.)
- Both the 5% and 25% solutions contain 130-160 mEq of sodium per liter.
- Use solutions within 4 hours or discard (solutions have no preservatives).
- Monitor BP and other vital signs during infusion.
- Monitor output/input ratio.
- Monitor for signs of circulatory overload (dyspnea, restlessness, productive cough).

PLASMA EXPANDERS

DEXTRAN 40

Rheomacrodex

Dextran 40 is a low-molecular-weight polysaccharide with an average molecular weight of 40 kDa. Because it is a hypertonic colloidal solution, it immediately and transiently expands plasma volume by increasing the colloidal osmotic pressure and drawing fluid from the interstitial to the intravascular spaces.

Indications: Used as an adjunct to expand volume and replace fluids in the treatment of shock or impending shock caused by hemorrhage, burns, surgery, or other trauma.

Usual dosage: (IV): First 10 ml/kg of 10% solution may be infused as rapidly as necessary to effect improvement; remainder is given more slowly. *As adjunctive therapy in shock:* Total dose infused during first 24 hours should not exceed 20 ml/kg body weight. First 500 ml may be administered over 15 to 30 minutes with CVP monitoring. Repeated doses (given more slowly for a maximum of 5 additional days) should not exceed 10 ml/kg/day.

Precautions/contraindications: *Cautious use:* restricted sodium intake, active hemorrhage, severe dehydration, chronic liver disease, impaired renal function, susceptibility to pulmonary edema and congestive heart failure (CHF). *Contraindicated:* hypersensitivity to dextran, renal failure, hypervolemic conditions, severe CHF, hemostatic defects. Safe use during pregnancy has not been established.

Side effects/adverse reactions: *Hypersensitivity:* most commonly, allergic reactions (rash, pruritus, nasal congestion, dyspnea, chest tightness, mild hypotension). *Hematologic:* interference with platelet function, prolonging bleeding and coagulation times. *Other:* osmotic nephrosis, oliguria, renal failure.

Pharmacokinetics: Rapidly expands plasma volume, generally one to two times the volume of dextran 40 given, within minutes of infusion; gradually reverses over the next 12 hours. About 75% is excreted in the urine within 24 hours. Dextran molecules with a molecular weight of 50 kDa or higher are degraded to glucose and metabolized to carbon dioxide and water before being excreted.

Nursing considerations:

- Determine patient's hydration status before beginning infusion.
- Obtain a baseline Hct.
- Monitor for signs of fluid overload.
- Monitor vital signs.
- Monitor input/output ratio.
- Remember: 500 ml of dextran 40 in normal saline contains 77 mEq of sodium.

HETASTARCH

Hespan

Hetastarch is a synthetic hydroxyethyl starch closely resembling human glycogen. It has colloidal osmotic properties very similar to those of human serum albumin.

Indications: Used for early fluid replacement and plasma volume expansion when whole blood is not available.

Usual dosage: (IV infusion): *Plasma volume expander:* 500-1,000 ml, not to exceed 1,500 ml a day. Maximum infusion rate for hemorrhagic shock is 20 ml/kg/h. Slower rates are advised with burns and septic shock.

Precautions/contraindications: *Cautious use:* hepatic or renal insufficiency, pulmonary edema, restricted sodium intake. *Contraindicated:* severe bleeding disorders, congestive heart failure, renal failure with oliguria and anuria, treatment of shock without hypovolemia. Safe use in children has not been established. The risk/benefit potential must be considered carefully before this drug is used in pregnant women (FDA pregnancy category C).

Side effects/adverse reactions: *CV:* peripheral overload, edema circulatory overload, heart failure. *Hematologic (with large volumes):* prolonged prothrombin, partial prothrombin, clotting, and bleeding times; decreased Hct. *Hypersensitivity:* ranges from pruritus to anaphylactic reaction. *Other:* vomiting, headaches, mild febrile reaction, chills, pruritus, incontinence.

Pharmacokinetics: Effectively expands plasma volume for about 24 to 36 hours; volume returns to original level after 48 to 72 hours. About 40% of molecules with a molecular weight of 50 kDa or less are easily eliminated by the kidneys within the first 48 hours; the remaining, heavier molecules are metabolized slowly by the mononuclear phagocytic system and blood enzymes to molecules small enough to be excreted over 2 to 3 weeks via urine and bile.

Nursing considerations:

- Monitor input/output ratio.
- Monitor vital signs.
- Observe for easy bruising or bleeding.
- Monitor for signs of circulatory overload (dyspnea, restlessness, productive cough).
- Monitor Hct.
- Remember: 500 ml of hetastarch in normal saline contains 77 mEq of sodium.

PLASMA PROTEIN

Plasmanate

Plasma protein solution is a 5% solution of stabilized human plasma proteins in NaCl containing approximately 88% albumin, 7% alpha-globulin, and 5% beta-globulin. The oncotic action is approximately equivalent to that of human plasma.

Indications: Used in emergency treatment of hypovolemic conditions and shock caused by burns, trauma, surgery, or infection. Can also be used as a temporary measure in the treatment of blood loss when whole blood is not available and to replenish plasma proteins in patients with hypoproteinemia if sodium intake is not restricted. Does not provide labile clotting factors and should not be given to correct coagulation defects.

Usual dosage: (IV): *Hypovolemia or shock:* 250-500 ml, at a rate of up to 10 ml/min. *Hypoproteinemia:* 1-1.5 L (50-75 g of protein) daily, not to exceed 5-8 ml/ min.

Precautions/contraindications: *Cautious use:* restricted sodium intake, low cardiac reserve, no albumin deficiency, hepatic or renal failure. *Contraindicated:* severe anemia, cardiac failure, patient undergoing cardiopulmonary bypass surgery. Safe use during pregnancy has not been established.

Side effects/adverse reactions: A few cases of nausea and vomiting, hypersalivation, and headaches have been reported. *Hypersensitivity:* ranges from tingling sensations, chills, and fever to anaphylaxis. *Other (with rapid IV infusion):* circulatory overload, pulmonary edema. Serious hypotension was reported in surgical patients undergoing extracorporeal circulation following transfusion of earlier plasma protein preparations.

Nursing considerations:

- Infuse at 1-10 ml/h; monitor BP, vital signs, and pulse. Stop infusion if patient becomes hypotensive.
- Monitor for signs of hypervolemia or circulatory overload (dyspnea, restlessness, productive cough).
- Remember: Each liter of plasma protein fraction contains 145 mEq of sodium.

COLONY-STIMULATING MODIFIERS

ERYTHROPOIETIN

Epogen, Procrit

Erythropoietin is a glycoprotein that stimulates the bone marrow to produce RBCs. It is synthesized primarily in the kidneys, although a small amount is also synthesized in the liver.

Indications: Used in the treatment of anemia associated with chronic renal failure to elevate or maintain RBC level and to decrease the need for transfusions. Also used to treat transient anemia related to treatment with zidovudine (azidothymidine, or AZT) in patients with HIV. *Unlabeled use:* to reverse anemia in cancer patients receiving chemotherapy.

Usual dosage: (SC, IV): 300-500 U/kg 3 times a week; recommended initial dosage is 50-100 U/kg 3 times a week (during dose adjustment phase, monitor Hct weekly). If response is not satisfactory, dosage can be increased by 50-100 U/kg 3 times a week. Response should be evaluated q 4-8 wk and the dosage adjusted accordingly in increments of 50-100 U/kg. If condition does not respond to 300 U/kg, higher dosages are unlikely to elicit a response. *Maintenance dose:* After desired response has been achieved, dose should be titrated in response to factors such as variation of AZT dosage or presence of infections; if Hct exceeds 40%, drug should be discontinued until Hct drops to 36%.

Precautions/contraindications: *Cautious use:* pregnancy, nursing mothers. *Contraindicated:* uncontrolled hypertension, known hypersensitivity to mammalian cell-derived products and human albumin.

Side effects/adverse reactions: *CNS:* headaches, seizures. *CV:* hypertension. *GI:* nausea, diarrhea. *Hematologic:* iron deficiency, thrombocytosis, clotting of AV fistula. *Other:* sweating, bone pain.

Pharmacokinetics: When administered intravenously, drug is cleared from plasma with a half-life of approximately 10 hours. After SC injection, peak concentrations in plasma occur within 5 to 24 hours. Drug is metabolized in the plasma.

Nursing considerations:

- Check Hct at least twice a week to ensure initial response.
- If Hct increases more than 4 percentage points over a 2-week period, reduce drug dosage. Once Hct exceeds 30%, reduce weekly dosage and monitor at regular intervals. In some patients initial response may be delayed for 2 to 6 weeks. If Hct does not increase by 5 percentage points after first 2 months of therapy, increase dosage incrementally by 25 U/kg at monthly intervals.

- Remember: response to erythropoietin requires adequate supplies of iron stores; supplemental iron may be needed to support and maintain erythropoiesis.
- Carefully titrate dose to prevent (1) rapid increase in Hct early in treatment and (2) increase in Hct over 36% during maintenance therapy.
- Monitor BP closely throughout treatment. If patient is taking antihypertensive medications, dosage of these drugs may need to be adjusted.

Patients not requiring dialysis:

- Monitor BP and Hct as frequently as with dialysis patients.
- Monitor renal function and fluid and electrolyte balance to determine need to initiate dialysis (need may be obscured by a sense of well-being).
- Follow dose regimen to avoid reaching target Hct too rapidly.
- Check Hct twice a week until target range is reached and maintenance dosage is established; check twice weekly for 2 to 6 weeks if any changes in dosage are made; thereafter, check at regular intervals.
- In patients with CRF, monitor serum chemistry values (creatinine, BUN) at regular intervals.

MYELOID GROWTH FACTORS

The myeloid growth factors, or colony-stimulating factors, are glycoproteins that stimulate the proliferation and differentiation of several types of hematopoietic precursor cells. They also enhance the function of mature leukocytes. The genes for four human colony-simulating factors have been cloned, and recombinant forms of the glycoprotein have been synthesized. These recombinant forms are granulocyte-macrophage colony-stimulating factor (GM-CSF) and granulocyte colony-stimulating factor (G-CSF).

RECOMBINANT HUMAN GRANULOCYTE COLONY-STIMULATING FACTOR
Filgrastim (G-CSF)
Neupogen

Indications: Used to decrease the incidence of infection (as manifested by febrile neutropenia) in patients with nonmyeloid malignancies receiving myelosuppressive anticancer drugs that cause significant neutropenia with fever.

Usual dosage: (SC, IV): initial dosage of 5 μg/kg daily in a single dose; dosage is increased by 5 μg/kg for each chemotherapy cycle.

Precautions/contraindications: *Cautious use:* Pregnancy, nursing mother. *Contraindicated:* hypersensitivity to *Escherichia coli*–derived proteins, simultaneous administration with chemotherapy, myeloid cancers.

Side effects/adverse reactions: *CV:* abnormal depression of ST segment. *Hematologic:* anemia. *GI:* nausea, anorexia. *Other:* bone pain, fever, hyperuricemia.

Pharmacokinetics: Peak blood levels are achieved within 1 hour after SC injection; elimination half-life is 1 to 7 hours. Drug probably is excreted in urine.

Nursing considerations:

- Obtain CBC and platelet count before starting therapy; check these values twice weekly during course of therapy.
- Discontinue drug if patient develops sternal pain.
- Discontinue drug if absolute neutrophil count surpasses 10,000/mm^3 after chemotherapy-induced nadir.

RECOMBINANT HUMAN GRANULOCYTE-MACROPHAGE COLONY-STIMULATING FACTOR
Sargramostim (GM-CSF)
Leukine, Prokine

Indications: Used for myeloid reconstitution after autologous bone marrow transplantation in patients with non-Hodgkin's lymphoma, acute lymphoblastic leukemia, or Hodgkin's disease.

Usual dosage: (IV): 250 μg/m^2 daily infused over 2 hours for 21 days; begin 2 to 4 hours after bone marrow transfusion and not less than 24 hours after last dose of chemotherapy or 12 hours after last radiation therapy.

Precautions/contraindications: *Cautious use:* history of cardiac dysrhythmias, preexisting cardiac disease, hypoxia, congestive heart failure, pulmonary infiltrates, renal and hepatic dysfunction, pregnancy, nursing mother. *Contraindicated:* excessive leukemic myeloid blasts in bone marrow or blood, known hypersensitivity to GM-CSF or yeast products.

Side effects/adverse reactions: *CNS:* lethargy, malaise, headaches, fatigue. *CV:* abnormal depression of ST segment, supraventricular dysrhythmias, edema, hypotension, tachycardia, pericardial effusion, percarditis. *Hematologic:* anemia, thrombocytopenia. *GI:* nausea, vomiting, diarrhea, anorexia. *Other:* bone pain, myalgia, arthralgia, hyperuricemia, fever, pleural effusion, rash, pruritus.

Pharmacokinetics: Onset occurs in 3 to 6 hours; peak effect is achieved 1 to 2 hours after onset. Elimination half-life is 1⅓ to 2½ hours. Drug probably is excreted in urine.

Interactions: *Cautious use:* corticosteroids, lithium; may cause potentiation of myeloproliferative effects.

Nursing considerations:

- Monitor respiration. If patient experiences dyspnea during administration, reduce IV rate 50%; if symptoms worsen, discontinue infusion and notify physician.
- Monitor CBC with differential. If absolute neutrophil count exceeds 20,000/mm³ *or* if platelet count exceeds 500,000/mm³, stop infusion and reduce dose by 50%.
- Assess renal and hepatic function before starting treatment.
- Monitor for edema and cardiac dysrhythmias; also monitor BP.

HEMATINICS

Iron is an essential component of hemoglobin, myoglobin, and a number of enzymes. The total body content is approximately 35 mg/kg in women and 50 mg/kg in men. Approximately two thirds of the body's total iron is found in the hemoglobin molecule of circulating RBCs, the major transporter of oxygen. The remainder is stored in the mononuclear phagocytic cells of the liver, spleen, and bone marrow as hemosiderin or ferritin.

FERROUS SALTS

Indications: Used to correct simple iron deficiency and to treat iron-deficiency anemias. *Unlabeled use:* Iron supplementation may be required by patients undergoing erythropoietin therapy (if ferrous salts are not given, the desired hematologic response may be impaired).

Usual dosage: (PO): *Oral iron replacement:* 750 mg to 1.5 g daily in 3 divided doses. For timed-release formulations, 250-525 mg daily or q 12 h. *Iron supplementation during pregnancy:* 300-600 mg daily in divided doses. *Caution:* Supplemental doses of iron should be considered only for individuals with documented risk factors for iron deficiency.

Precautions/contraindications: *Cautious use:* GI disorders. *Contraindicated:* hemolytic anemia, hemochromatosis, hemosiderosis, patient receiving repeated blood transfusions, pyridoxine-responsive anemia, liver cirrhosis. Safe use during pregnancy has not been established.

Side effects/adverse reactions: Generally minimal. *GI:* primarily GI irritation, anorexia, nausea, vomiting, constipation, diarrhea. Stools may become darker in color. *Other:* temporary staining of teeth, yellow-brown discoloration of eyes, hemosiderosis (rare).

Overdose

Symptoms: A lethal oral dose of iron is about 200-240 mg/kg; however, lesser amounts have also caused fatalities. Symptoms can be observed with doses of 30-60 mg/kg. Acute poisoning produces symptoms in four stages:

Stage 1 Within 1 to 6 hours: lethargy; nausea; vomiting; abdominal pain; tarry stools; weak, rapid pulse; hypotension; dehydration; acidosis; coma.

Stage 2 If dose is not immediately fatal, symptoms may subside for about 24 hours.

Stage 3 Symptoms return 48 hours after ingestion and may include diffuse vascular congestion, pulmonary edema, shock, acidosis, convulsions, anuria, hypothermia and, ultimately, death.

Stage 4 If patient survives, pyloric or atrial stenosis, hepatic cirrhosis, and CNS damage may develop within 2 to 6 weeks of ingestion (see Overdose Treatment under Nursing Considerations).

Pharmacokinetics: In individuals with normal iron stores, only 1 to 2 g are absorbed daily, or 10% of the average daily dietary intake. Absorption is increased 20% to 30% when iron stores are depleted or the rate of erythropoiesis increases. Iron is primarily absorbed from the duodenum and upper jejunum by active transport. The ferrous salt is absorbed three times more readily than the ferric form. The more common iron salt forms (sulfate, gluconate, and fumarate) are absorbed almost milligram for milligram. The amount absorbed varies among the different salt forms because each contains different amounts of elemental iron (Table 12-3). Less iron is absorbed if sustained-release or enteric-coated preparations are used. These formulations are designed to release iron further down the GI tract to prevent gastric irritation; however, the point at which the iron is released is also past the primary absorption sites.

The amount of iron ingested also influences how much will be absorbed; the larger the dose, the more that is absorbed. Food can decrease iron absorption by 40% to 66%. This may not be avoidable with gastric intolerance, which necessitates that iron be administered with food.

Iron is transported via the blood bound to transferrin. Daily loss of iron from urine, sweat, and sloughing of intestinal mucosal cells amounts to approximately 0.5 to 1 mg in healthy men and in women who are not menstruating. In menstruating women, the average daily loss is 1 to 2 mg.

Interactions: 12 to See Table 12-4.

Table 12-3

APPROXIMATE ELEMENTAL IRON CONTENT OF VARIOUS IRON SALT PREPARATIONS

Generic name	Trade name	Iron content (per 100 mg)
Ferrous fumarate	Femiron, Feostat	33 mg
Ferrous gluconate	Fergon, Ferralet	12 mg
Dried ferrous sulfate (exsiccated iron sulfate)	Fer-In-Sol (capsule), Feosol (tablet)	30 mg
Ferrous sulfate	Feratab, Feosol (liquid), Fer-In-Sol (liquid)	20 mg

Table 12-4

DRUG INTERACTIONS WITH VARIOUS IRON SALTS (ORAL)

Drugs	Effect of interaction with iron salts
Antacids	May decrease GI absorption of iron
Ascorbic acid	May enhance absorption of iron
Chloramphenicol	May increase serum iron
Cimetidine	May decrease GI absorption of cimetidine
Levodopa	Decreased absorption of levodopa
Methyldopa	Decreased absorption of methyldopa
Penicillamine	Decreased absorption of penicillamine
Quinolones	Decreased absorption of quinolones
Tetracyclines	Decreased absorption of tetracyclines and iron salts

Nursing considerations:

- Confirm that anemia is caused by iron deficiency.
- Monitor Hb and reticulocyte values during therapy.
- Stools may appear darker in color.
- Because iron-containing liquids may cause temporary staining of teeth, dilute liquid preparations with water and have patient drink with a straw.

Overdose treatment:

1. Induce vomiting within the first hour of ingestion using ipecac or, preferably, lavage. Lavage solution should be tepid water or 1% to 5% sodium bicarbonate solution or 5% phosphate solution. Iron-chelating agents (e.g., deferoxamine mesylate) should also be administered.
2. Be ready to use supportive measures for dealing with shock, dehydration, blood loss, or respiratory failure.
3. Do not perform gastric lavage after first hour of ingestion because of the danger of perforation from gastric necrosis.

Patient teaching:

- Take medicine on empty stomach to enhance absorption if possible, but if upset stomach occurs, take after meals or with food.
- Avoid taking antacids, tetracyclines, or fluoroquinolones with iron preparation.
- Do not chew or crush sustained-release preparations.
- Store iron preparations out of reach of children.

IRON DEXTRAN
Imferon

Iron dextran is a dark brown liquid containing ferric hydroxide with dextran.

Indications: Used to treat iron deficiency in patients with documented iron deficiency for whom oral administration of iron is unsatisfactory or impossible.

Usual dosage: (IM, IV): Solution contains the equivalent of 50 mg of elemental iron per milliliter. *Maximum adult daily dose:* 2 ml (100 mg) IM or IV. Dosage is determined from a table that correlates the patient's weight and Hb and the number of milliliters required for iron replacement. IM: Daily doses usually do not exceed 0.5 ml (25 mg of iron). IV (intermittent): 2 ml (100 mg) or less per day.

Precautions/contraindications: *Cautious use:* rheumatoid arthritis, ankylosing spondylitis, impaired hepatic function, history of allergies and/or asthma. *Contraindicated:* hypersensitivity to the drug; all anemias except iron-deficiency anemia. Safe use during pregnancy has not been established.

Side effects/adverse reactions: *CNS:* headaches, shivering, paresthesia, dizziness, coma, seizures. *CV:* peripheral vascular flushing (with rapid IV infusion), hypotension, precordial pain or feeling of pressure, tachycardia, fatal cardiac dysrhythmia, circulatory collapse. *GI:* nausea, vomiting, transient loss of sense of taste, abdominal pain. *Hypersensitivity:* urticaria, skin rash, pruritus. *Other:* sterile abscess and brown discoloration of skin at IM injection site, local phlebitis at IV infusion site, hemosiderosis, hepatic damage.

Pharmacokinetics: After IM administration, most of the drug is absorbed from the injection site through the lymphatic system. The remainder (10% to 50%) becomes fixed locally and is gradually absorbed over several months or longer. Iron dextran is slowly cleared from plasma by the mononuclear phagocytic system. Small amounts cross the placenta. Traces are excreted in urine, bile, and feces and distributed into breast milk.

Interactions: Clinical response may be delayed if patient is also receiving chloramphenicol.

Nursing considerations:

- Confirm diagnosis of iron-deficiency anemia with appropriate laboratory test.
- Give test dose of 0.5 ml over 5 minutes regardless of route of administration. Because fatal anaphylactic reactions have occurred, epinephrine (0.5 ml of 1:1,000 solution) should be available.
- Give IM injections only into muscle mass in upper outer quadrant of buttock; Z-tract technique is recommended to prevent drug leakage along needle track and brown staining of subcutaneous tissue.
- After IV administration, keep patient supine for 30 minutes to prevent orthostatic hypotension. Monitor BP and pulse.
- Periodically check Hb, Hct, and reticulocyte count to guide therapeutic planning.

REFERENCES

1. American Cancer Society: *Cancer facts and figures—1992*, Atlanta, Ga, 1992, The Society.

2. American Pain Society: *Principles of analgesic use in the treatment of acute and chronic cancer pain*, Washington, DC, 1989, The Society.

3. Appelbaum R: Bone marrow transplantation. In Wittes R, editor: *Manual of oncologic therapeutic*, Philadelphia, 1989, JB Lippincott.

4. Baird SB, McCorkle R, Grant M: *Cancer nursing: A comprehensive textbook*, Philadelphia, 1991, SB Saunders.

4a. Beare PG, Myers JL: *Principles and practice of adult health nursing*, St. Louis, 1990, Mosby.

5. Belcher AE: *Cancer nursing*, St. Louis, 1992, Mosby.

6. Blume K, Faiman S, O'Donnell M, et al: Total body irradiation and high-dose etoposide: A new preparatory regimen with bone marrow transplantation in patients with advanced hematologic malignancies, *Blood* 69(4):1015-1020, 1987.

7. Brookoff D, Polomano R: Treating sickle cell pain like cancer pain, *Ann Intern Med* 116:364-368, 1992.

8. Brundage DJ: *Renal disorders*, St. Louis, 1992, Mosby.

9. Cain J, Hood-Barnes J, Spangler: Myelodysplastic syndromes, *Oncol Nurs Forum* 18(1):113-117, 1991.

10. Canobbio MM: *Cardiovascular disorders*, St. Louis, 1990, Mosby.

11. Capizzi R, et al: Methotrexate therapy of head and neck cancer: Improvement in therapeutic index by the use of leucovorin "rescue," *Cancer Res* 30:1782.

12. Chipps E, Clanin NJ, Campbell VG: *Neurologic disorders*, St. Louis, 1992, Mosby.

13. Corcoran-Buchsel P: Long term complications of allogeneic bone marrow transplantation: Nursing implications, *Onc Nurs Forum* 13(6): 61-70, 1986.

14. Duigon A: Anticipatory nausea and vomiting associated with cancer chemotherapy, *Onc Nurs Forum* 13(1):35-40, 1986.

15. Eilers J, Beger AM, Petersen MC: Development, testing, and application of the oral assessment guide, *Onc Nurs Forum* 15(3): 325-330, 1988.

16. Ellerhost-Ryan J: Complications of the myeloproliferative system: infection and sepsis, *Semin Onc Nurs* 1(4):244-250, 1985.

17. Ford R, Ballard B: Acute complications after bone marrow transplantation, *Semin Onc Nurs* 4(1): 15-24, 1988.

18. Fraser MC, Tucker MA: Late effects of cancer therapy: chemotherapy-related malignancies, *Onc Nurs Forum* 15(1):67-77, 1988.

19. Freedman S, Shivnan J, Tilles J, Klemm P: Bone marrow transplantation: overview and nursing implications, *Crit Care Q* 13(2): 51-62, 1990.

20. Froberg J: The anemias: Causes and courses of action, *RN* 52:24-29, 1989.

21. Froberg J: The anemias: Causes and courses of action. Part II, *RN* 52:52-57, 1989.

22. Gale R: Management of acute leukemias part I: Bone marrow transplants, *Clin Advan Onc Nurs* 1(2): 1-6, 1989.

23. Gilyon K, Kuzel T: Cutaneous T-cell lymphoma, *Oncol Nurs Forum* 18(5): 901-908, 1991.

24. Grimes DE: *Infectious diseases*, St. Louis, 1991, Mosby.

25. Groenwald SL, Frogge MJ, Goodman M, Yarbro CH: *Cancer nursing: Principles and practice*, Boston, 1990, Jones & Bartlett.

26. Gullatte M, Graves T: Advances in antineoplastic therapy, *Onc Nurs Forum* 17(6):867-876, 1990.

27. Gullo SM: Safe handling of antineoplastic drugs: translating the recommendations into practice, *Onc Nurs Forum* 15(5): 595-601, 1991.

28. Haeuber D: Future strategies in the control of myelosuppression: the use of colony-stimulating factors, *Onc Nurs Forum* 18(2):16-21, 1991.

29. Hagie ME: Implantable devices for chemotherapy: access and delivery, *Semin Onc Nurs* 3(2):96-105, 1987.

29a. Halma C, Daha MR, Van Es LA: In vivo clearance by the mononuclear phagocyte systems in humans: an overview of methods and their interpretation, *Clin Exper Immunol* 89(1):1-7, 1992.

30. Herman C, et al: Effects of coping style and relaxation on cancer chemotherapy side effects and emotional responses, *Onc Nurs Forum* 13(5): 308-315, 1990.

31. Holleb AI, Fink DJ, Murphy GP: *American Cancer Society textbook of clinical oncology*, Atlanta, Ga, 1991, The Society.

32. Kane N, Lehman M, Dugger R, Hansen L, Jackson D: Use of patient-controlled analgesia in surgical oncology patients, *Onc Nurs Forum* 15(1): 29-32, 1988.

33. Kaplan H: Historic milestones in radiobiology and radiation therapy, *Semin Onc* 4:479-490, 1979.

34. Kim MJ, McFarland GK, McLane AM: *Pocket guide to nursing diagnoses*, ed. 5, St. Louis, 1993, Mosby.

35. Konradi D, Stockert P: A close-up look at leukemia, *Nursing* 89:34-42, 1989.

36. Krakoff IH: Cancer chemotherapeutic agents, *CA Canc J Clin* 37:97-105, 1987.

37. Kramer S, Hanks G, Diamond J, et al: The study of patterns of clinical care in radiation therapy in the United States, *CA Cancer J Clin* 34:75-85, 1984.

38. Lotze MT, Rosenberg BA: The immunologic treatment of cancer, *CA Canc J Clin* 38(2):68-89.

39. McCaffery M, Beebe A: *Pain: a clinical manual for nursing practice*, St. Louis, 1989, Mosby.

40. McCance KL, Huether SE: *Pathophysiology: the biologic basis for disease in adults and children*, St. Louis, 1990, Mosby.

41. McGuire D, Yarbro C: *Cancer pain management*, Orlando, Fla, 1987, Grune & Stratton.

42. Mourad LA: *Orthopedic disorders*, St. Louis, 1991, Mosby.

42a. Mudge-Grout C: *Immunologic disorders*, St. Louis, 1992, Mosby.

43. National Institutes of Health: *The integrated approach to the management of pain*, Bethesda, Md, 1986, NIH.

44. Nims J and Strom S: Late complications of bone marrow transplant recipients: Nursing care issues, *Semin Onc Nurs* 4(1): 47-54, 1988.

45. Otto SE: *Oncology nursing*, St. Louis, 1991, Mosby.

46. Powers LW: *Diagnostic hematology*, St. Louis, 1989, Mosby.

46a. Robbins S, Cotran RS, Kumar V: *Pathologic basis of disease*, ed 4, Philadelphia, 1989, WB Saunders.

47. Schneiderman E: Thrombocytopenia in the critically ill patient, *Crit Care Nurs Q*, 13(2):1-6, 1990.

48. Schryber S, Lacasse C, Barton-Burke M: Autologous bone marrow transplantation, *Onc Nurs Forum* 14(4): 74-80, 1987.

49. Seeley RR, Stephens TK, Tate P: *Anatomy and physiology*, ed 2, St. Louis, 1992, Mosby.

50. Seidel HM et al: *Mosby's guide to physical examination*, ed. 3, St. Louis, 1993, Mosby.

51. Spross JA, McGuire DB, Schmitt RM: ONS position paper on cancer pain (part I), *Onc Nurs Forum* 17(4):595-614, 1990.

52. Spross JA, McGuire DB, Schmitt RM: ONS position paper on cancer pain (part II), *Onc Nurs Forum* 17(5):751-760, 1990.

53. Spross JA, McGuire DB, Schmitt RM: ONS position paper on cancer pain (part III), *Onc Nurs Forum* 17(6):943-955, 1990.

54. Strohl RA: The nursing role in radiation oncology: symptom management of acute and chronic reactions, *Onc Nurs Forum* 15(4):429-434, 1988.

55. Tenenbaum L: *Cancer chemotherapy: a reference guide*, Philadelphia, 1989, WB Saunders.

56. Thompson JM et al: *Mosby's clinical nursing*, ed. 3, St. Louis, 1993, Mosby.

57. Tilkian S, Conover M, Tilkian A: *Clinical implications of laboratory tests*, St. Louis, 1987, Mosby.

58. Vander AS, Sherman JH, Luciano DS: *Human physiology: The mechanisms of body function*, ed 4, New York, 1990, McGraw-Hill.

59. Wickham R: Managing chemotherapy-related nausea and vomiting: the state of the art, *Onc Nurs Forum* 16(4): 563-574, 1989.

60. Wilson SF, Thompson JM: *Respiratory disorders*, St. Louis, 1990, Mosby.

61. Yasko J: *Care of the client receiving radiation therapy*, Reston, Va, 1982, Reston.

Index

RESOURCES, ORGANIZATIONS, AND AGENCIES

American Cancer Society (ACS), National Headquarters
1599 Clifton Road NE
Atlanta, GA 30329
(404) 320-3333
Phone numbers for local units and divisions are listed in the white pages of the telephone book.
Programs include the following service and rehabilitation programs for persons with cancer and their family/significant others: Can Surmount; I Can Cope; Reach to Recovery; Resources, Information, and Guidance Services; Road to Recovery; Laryngectomy Rehabilitation; Ostomy Rehabilitation; Look Good. . .Feel Better (see related listings)

Association of Community Cancer Centers
11600 Nebel Street, Suite 201
Rockville, MD 20852
(301) 984-9496

Cancer Fax
NCI International Cancer Information Center
9030 Old Georgetown Road
Building 82, Room 219
Bethesda, MD 20892
(301) 402-5874 on fax machine handset
(301) 496-8880 for technical assistance
FAX # (301) 402-0212

Cancer Information Service
1-800-4-CANCER
1-800-638-6070—Alaska
524-1234—Hawaii; in Oahu, dial direct; call collect from neighboring islands

Leukemia Society of America, Inc.
600 Third Avenue
New York, NY 10016
(212) 573-8484

National Hemophilia Foundation
110 Greene Street, Suite 303
New York, NY 10012
(212) 219-8180
1-800-42-HANDI

National Marrow Donor Program
3433 Broadway Street, NE, Suite 400
Minneapolis, MN 55413
(414) 257-8325
Hotline # 1-800-654-1247
Office # 1-800-526-7809

National Maternal and Child Health Clearinghouse
8201 Greensboro Drive, Suite 600
McLean, VA 22102
(703) 821-8955 ext 254 or 265

Oncology Nursing Society (ONS)
501 Holiday Drive
Pittsburgh, PA 15220-2749
(412) 921-7373

Physician Data Query (PDQ): National Cancer Institute (NCI) Computerized Data Base for Physicians
NCI Building 82, Room 123
9030 Old Georgetown Road
Bethesda, MD 20892
(301) 496-4907

Sickle Cell Disease Branch
Division of Blood Diseases and Resources
Federal Building, Room 508
7550 Wisconsin Avenue
Bethesda, MD 20892
(301) 496-6931